Classic Papers in Breast Disease

Classic Papers in Breast Disease

Edited by

Michael Baum MD ChM FRCS
Emeritus Professor of Surgery and
Visiting Professor of Medical Humanities
University College London
The Portland Hospital
London, UK

and

Craig Henderson MD
Adjunct Professor
Hematology/Oncology UCSF
Program Member
UCSF Comprehensive Cancer Center
San Francisco, CA, USA

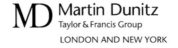
Martin Dunitz
Taylor & Francis Group
LONDON AND NEW YORK

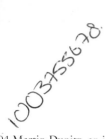

© 2004 Martin Dunitz, an imprint of the Taylor & Francis Group plc

First published in the United Kingdom in 2004
by Martin Dunitz, an imprint of the Taylor and Francis Group plc,
11 New Fetter Lane, London EC4P 4EE

Tel.: +44 (0) 20 7583 9855
Fax.: +44 (0) 20 7842 2298
E-mail: info@dunitz.co.uk
Website: http://www.dunitz.co.uk

Although every effort has been made to ensure that drug doses and other information are presented
accurately in this publication, the ultimate responsibility rests with the prescribing physician.
Neither the publishers nor the authors can be held responsible for errors or for any
consequences arising from the use of information contained herein. For detailed
prescribing information or instructions on the use of any product or procedure
discussed herein, please consult the prescribing information or
instructional material issued by the manufacturer.

A CIP record for this book is available from the British Library.

ISBN 1 90186 583 5

Distributed in the USA by
Fulfilment Center, Taylor & Francis,
10650 Toebben Drive, Independence, KY 41051, USA
Toll Free Tel.: +1 800 634 7064
E-mail: taylorandfrancis@thomsonlearning.com

Distributed in Canada by
Taylor & Francis, 74 Rolark Drive, Scarborough,
Ontario M1R 4G2, Canada
Toll Free Tel.: +1 877 226 2237
E-mail: tal_fran@istar.ca

Distributed in the rest of the world by
Thomson Publishing Services, Cheriton House,
North Way, Andover, Hampshire SP10 5BE, UK
Tel.: +44 (0) 1264 332424
E-mail: salesorder.tandf@thomsonpublishingservices.co.uk

Typeset by
J&L Composition, Filey, North Yorkshire, UK

Printed and bound
in Spain by Grafos SA

Contents

Contributors

Michael Baum MD ChM FRCS
Emeritus Professor of Surgery and
Visiting Professor of Medical Humanities
University College London
The Portland Hospital
London, UK

Jack Cuzick PhD
Department of Surgery
The Institute of Surgical Studies
University College London Medical School
London, UK

J Michael Dixon BSc MBChB MD FRCS FRCSEd
Consultant Surgeon and Senior Lecturer
Edinburgh Breast Unit
Western General Hospital
Edinburgh, Scotland

Mitchell Dowsett BSc PhD
Head of Department
Academic Department of Biochemistry
The Royal Marsden Hospital NHS Trust
London, UK

Lesley Fallowfield DPhil
Professor of Psycho-Oncology
Director of the Cancer Research UK Psychosocial Oncology Group
Brighton and Sussex Medical School
University of Sussex
Falmer, Brighton, UK

A Patrick Forrest MD ChM FRCS FRCPE FRSE
Emeritus Professor of Surgery
Edinburgh University
Edinburgh, Scotland, UK

Jay R Harris MD
Department of Radiation Oncology
Brigham and Women's Hospital and
Dana-Farber Cancer Institute
Harvard Medical School
Boston, MA, USA

Craig Henderson MD
Adjunct Professor
Hematology/Oncology UCSF
Program Member
UCSF Comprehensive Cancer Center
San Francisco, CA, USA

Daniel B Kopans MD
Professor of Radiology
Harvard Medical School
Boston, MA, USA

Marc E Lippman MD
John G. Searle Professor and Chairman
Department of Internal Medicine
University of Michigan School of Medicine
Ann Arbor, MI, USA

Caroline Lohrisch MD
Medical Oncologist
British Columbia Cancer Agency
Vancouver, British Columbia, Canada

Robert Mansel MB BS MRCS LRCP FRCS MS
Professor of Surgery
Chairman, Division of Surgery
University of Wales College of Medicine,
Cardiff

Anne-Marie Martin
University of Pennsylvania Cancer Center
Philadelphia, PA, USA

Klim McPherson PhD FFPH FMedSci
Professor of Public Health Epidemiology
Department of Social Medicine
University of Bristol
Bristol, UK

William Miller BSc PhD DSc
Edinburgh Breast Unit Research Group
University of Edinburgh
Western General Hospital
Edinburgh, Scotland, UK

David L Page MD
Department of Pathology
Vanderbilt University Medical Center
Nashville, TN, USA

Martine J Piccart MD PhD
Head of Chemotherapy Unit
Jules Bordet Institute
Brussels, Belgium

Kathleen I Pritchard MD FRCPC
Head, Clinical Trials & Epidemiology
Toronto Sunnybrook Regional Cancer Centre
Professor, Department of Medicine
Faculty of Medicine
University of Toronto
Ontario, Canada

Barbara L Weber MD
Professor of Medicine and Genetics
Director, Breast Cancer Program, Abramson Cancer Center; Director, Cancer Genomics
Program, Abramson Family Cancer Research Institute
University of Pennsylvania
Philadelphia, PA, USA

Preface

All cultivated men and women, including most medical practitioners, pride themselves on their love of the 'classics'. By this we usually mean works of music, literature, and the plastic arts that have stood the test of time. The 'test of time' is rigorous and has little patience for transient 'pop culture' or fashion. The test of time determines which works of art inform us of the human condition with knowledge that transcends the current era and geographic boundaries. The same test will ultimately determine those beauties and verities that are so sublime as to inform and enhance the lives of men and women from the 18th to the 21st century from Europe to Asia and from artisans to the professional classes. These values alone are relevant to medicine, as witnessed by the current movement of 'Medical Humanities' as a reaction to the brutalism of molecular reductionism; but before we get carried away waxing lyrical, the same principles of 'classicism' can apply to medical science and its literature.

There is a 'pop culture' in medicine and there are fashionable subjects in medical research. In fact, the recognition of this phenomenon has often lead to bitter attacks on the peer review system. Yet there is an ever present danger here of a logical syllogism, namely 'William Harvey was a genius who wasn't recognized in his lifetime, I am not being recognized in my lifetime therefore I am a genius!' Fortunately, once more we have the test of time to guide us. What papers have stood this test? Here we are not looking for the recondite values of the Arts but the accumulated wisdom of the scientific process. This process consists of two steps: the elaboration of a testable hypothesis and its formal testing. Hypothesis generation is a complex process consisting of making observations coupled with leaps of imagination. Therefore some classic papers might be the original observations that lead to the flight of fancy. Other classic papers might be those that fully elaborated a testable and fruitful hypothesis. Yet others might be the experimental testing of the hypothesis either in the laboratory or in the clinic. Finally, others might describe the development of instrumentation that allowed the observations in the first place or the description of the statistical and epidemiological tools that gave the testing scientific credibility. All of these classic papers must also share in common their place as building blocks, as judged by the refraction of history, in the current knowledge base or current research program of the subject.

As far as medicine is concerned – and in particular breast cancer – the final outcome measures are the length and quality of life of our patients. Putting it another way, therefore: What are the papers, as judged by the test of time, that have either directly or indirectly contributed to improvements in the length or quality of life of patients with breast cancer?

All of this is fine in principle, but surely making such choices has to be subjective and to an extent reflect the prejudices of the reviewer? That we concede. Certainly, if it was just left to the two of us, notorious for our prejudices, that would be the case. We can therefore offer up the first genuine defence for a multi-author textbook. To help us with the 16 chapters in this book are authors whom we have selected as recognized experts in their fields and balanced in their viewpoints. We have only rarely had to exercise our editorial perogative in the selection or annotation process.

So what use can be made of this compilation? All subjects have their canon of literature that should be studied before a serious student can advance in his or her chosen field. We would like to lay claim to this and suggest that what is provided between the covers of this book is an instant access to the bedrock of the knowledge about breast cancer painfully accumulated over the last hundred or so years. We fervently hope that specialists of the future will start here, learn from the mistakes of the past, learn of the scientific process, learn a few 'facts', and then be prepared to make contributions of their own. Who knows but in the fullness of time some of our readers will add to this canon, proving yet again that the scientific process is a neverending quest.

MICHAEL BAUM

CRAIG HENDERSON

CHAPTER 1

Historical perspectives

CRAIG HENDERSON AND MICHAEL BAUM

Progress far from consisting of change, depends on retentiveness ... Those who cannot remember the past are condemned to fulfil it

George Santayana, *Life of Reason* (1905–06)

Introduction

The history of this subject can be viewed in two ways. First, there is the conventional viewpoint, as a slow progression from ignorance to enlightenment as a result of the accumulation of scientific facts. Alternatively, the history of our knowledge about breast cancer can be looked upon like any other scientific endeavor as a sequence of conceptual models of the disease, with revolution rather than evolution shifting the paradigms along the way. The trouble with conceptual models of any disease process is that the belief in the model might be more powerful than the evidence that supports it. Furthermore, each conceptual model has a therapeutic consequence, and this explains the many tragedies that litter the history of our subject over the last two millennia. As will be seen from our selection of classic papers, this is much closer to the truth and also much more helpful in looking to the future. A deterministic linear approach in our thinking will only get us so far. We must encourage revolutionary thoughts yet not fall into the trap of believing that every revolutionary is a prophet in his own time.

Starting with the ancients, we may recall the wisdom of the Egyptian physician writing in the Edwin Smith papyrus, who distinguished bulging tumors of the breast that were hot from bulging tumors of the breast that were cold (Paper 1). The former (abscesses) were considered treatable by the knife whereas the latter (cancers) were deemed inoperable. This advice would have stood the test of time until the last two decades of the19th century, but sadly was ignored by generations of meddlesome doctors.

The ancient Greeks, to their credit, distinguished disease processes from spiritual afflictions. Aristotle was the first to describe a system of pathology that led to the humoral theory of cancer. These teachings were ultimately codified by Galen in the Graeco-Roman period of the 2nd century AD. Breast cancer was considered a systemic disorder resulting from the accumulation of black bile (melancholia) within the breast tissue. This is described by De Moulin (Paper 2), who provides translations of some of the most influential of these documents. The therapeutic consequence of this belief was 1500 years of cupping, leaching, venesection, purgation, and crank diets. These treatments did nothing to improve the length or quality of life – quite the opposite – and yet their persistence demonstrated the danger of a fundamentalist belief in an unproven biological model. These concepts and the treatments that evolved from them persisted well into the 19th century (some neo-Galenic doctrine can be witnessed today in the practice of alternative medicine), as documented by Velpeau in his treatise on surgical treatments for breast cancer (Paper 3).

The development of a new concept or therapy is frequently the result of new techniques or new instrumentation. A prime example is the development of the microscope by Anthony van Leeuwenhoek in mid 17th century Holland. This ultimately led to the description of the cellular nature of biological matter and Müller's first description of the cellular nature of breast cancer at the beginning of the 19th century, although it took close on another 50 years before the humoral theory of breast cancer was replaced by the cellular model of the disease.

In the mid 19th century, Virchow's elegant anatomical dissections of women dying with advanced breast cancer described the lymphatic spread of the disease to the regional lymph nodes. These observations suggested a mechanistic model of breast cancer, with the regional lymph nodes acting as filters to inhibit the onward spread of the disease. The therapeutic consequences of these teachings did not have to wait long, as the discoveries of the germ theory of infection by Pasteur, of antisepsis by Lister, and of anesthesia by Simpson allowed the development of the classic radical mastectomy towards the end of the 19th century. Although William Halsted at the Johns Hopkins Hospital in Baltimore takes credit for this procedure that has become eponymous, Meyer in Berlin and Handley in London described similar procedures at around the same time, and both the 'unified concept of the operation' and the techniques used in the radical mastectomy had evolved from the work of Petit and Velpeau in Paris a century earlier. With the wisdom of hindsight, the classic radical mastectomy is considered an unnecessary mutilation, yet it was certainly the best that could be offered in its time. The majority of cancers were locally advanced at presentation, and without radiotherapy or chemotherapy the radical mastectomy was probably the best way of achieving local control, allowing the woman to die of distant metastases, free of the ravages of uncontrolled breast cancer on her chest wall.

The Halsted radical mastectomy was rapidly established as the 'treatment of choice', and held sway with various modifications and extensions well into the 1970s. This again reflected the durability of the therapeutic consequence of an untested biological hypothesis. Even Sir Jeffrey Keynes' advocacy of lumpectomy and radium needle insertion in the years prior to World War II was radical in intent although conservative in outcome (Paper 5). Although the radical mastectomy is rarely performed today, the underlying Halstedian concept still dominants our thinking. Control of the primary is the first goal of most treatment plans. Therapies that follow are referred to as 'adjuvant', even though they may have a much greater impact on the patient's survival.

Frustration and dissatisfaction with the radical approach gradually accumulated in the middle years of the 20th century. Although Halsted had described his procedure as a 'cure' for breast cancer, his observations were limited almost entirely to the local behavior of the disease. Local control served as a sort of surrogate for improved survival. If local disease-free survival were improved by the surgery, then surely overall survival benefits would follow. (This mistake has been repeated more recently in the use of chemotherapy, especially high-dose chemotherapy and autologous bone marrow transplantation – see Chapter 16.) Two of the surgeons on the faculty of Johns Hopkins who had been trained by Halsted, Dean Lewis and William Francis Rienhoff, demonstrated the poor correlation between improved local control and survival in 1932 when they provided long-term follow-up of the patients treated by Halsted and his immediate successors (Paper 6). The survival of these patients was no better and the percentage who died of causes other than breast cancer was no better than that of an untreated population from the 19th and early 20th centuries described by Bloom *et al.* (Paper 8). This important paper by Lewis and Rienhoff apparently had little impact at the time.

Another tool, as important as the microscope in its impact on the modern management of breast cancer, was introduced late in the 19th century. This was statistical analysis, which was based on the recognition that chance events easily obscure real effects (or the lack of effect) from therapy. Over a period of nearly two centuries, clinical research slowly evolved from studies and descriptions of one patient at a time, to observations on a series or group of patients, to randomized trials that enrolled thousands of patients, and to meta-analyses that included tens of thousands of patients. As important as the number of patients in these studies was, were the emphasis on comparing like with like and the recognition that, even with careful staging, patients from one era or one hospital were more likely to differ from those in another era or another hospital merely by chance than because of a therapeutic intervention. The first randomized trials comparing therapeutic interventions were begun shortly after World War II, and among the first of these were two breast cancer trials performed at the Christie Hospital in Manchester, England and reported by Ralston Paterson (Paper 9). One of these demonstrated that the use of radiotherapy to the chest wall immediately following mastectomy improved local control but had little impact on patient survival. The other tested the concept that breast cancer is a systemic disease and that survival can be affected by the early use of systemic therapies. This study used oophorectomy, which had first been shown by Beatson a half-century earlier to induce regression of metastatic lesions. Although described at about the same time as classic radical mastectomy, ovarian ablation was little used until disillusion with radical surgery had set in. In the Christie trial, patients randomized to ovarian ablation had a better survival than those in the control group, but the evidence from this and other similar trials that followed had little impact on practice until meta-analyses of these studies 30 years later overcame the lack of statistical power of the individual trials.

Paradigmatic shifts do not occur easily. First they require recognition that outcomes cannot be adequately explained by existing paradigms. Second, there must be a new, compelling concept that emerges, and by the end of the 20th century new concepts had to be supported by laboratory data. Finally, there must be an available technology (or treatment) to test the new concept. Observations by Lewis and others on the lack of survival benefit from radical mastectomy started the first of these processes, but it took another three to four decades before surgeons seriously questioned the Halstedian dogma. On the European side of the Atlantic, it may have been the seminal paper by Brinkley and Haybittle (Paper 11) that impelled surgeons to question this approach. Brinkley and Haybittle studied the long-term outcomes of 704 cases treated by radical mastectomy in the late 1940s and early 1950s at Addenbrooke's Hospital, Cambridge. Over a 35-year period of follow-up, they demonstrated a continuous excess mortality for the treated patients over an age-matched population. This raised important questions about the curability of the disease by local therapy alone. In the USA, Fox (Paper 12) raised similar doubts by demonstrating that many of the patients diagnosed with breast cancer in the 1950s and 1960s were probably not represented in historical series of untreated patients and that this new group of patients had a disease with very limited malignant potential. At the same time, a smaller subset of patients with a more aggressive form of the disease appeared to have the same mortality as the untreated patients in the historical series, in spite of the fact that they had all undergone a mastectomy. It seems plausible that the subset of patients whose tumors had low malignant potential resulted from a redefinition of breast cancer as a histological rather than clinical entity during the course of the 20th century. This created the illusion of greater progress in control of the disease than had actually occurred. However, Fox also explored another recurring theme in the history of breast cancer concepts by suggesting that this is not one disease and that one paradigm will never encompass all those who carry this diagnosis.

A revision of the biological model had to wait a long time, however – until the development of syngeneic strains of mice allowed experimentation to challenge the mechanistic view of the spread of breast cancer. These early experiments in the 1960s carried out by George Crile at the Cleveland Clinic and of Bernard Fisher at the Presbyterian Hospital in Pittsburgh paved the way for the next revolution (Paper 10). Their studies suggested that – at least in experimental models of the disease – the lymphatic system was not the only mode of dissemination. Nor were the lymph nodes effective barriers to progression. It was likely, therefore, that the major route for dissemination that led to the establishment of potentially fatal metastases was via the bloodstream. Furthermore, this dissemination probably occurred very early and perhaps in the preclinical setting, before the cancer was diagnosable. If that was the case, then radical surgery was shutting the stable door after the horse had bolted, with biological factors becoming more important than chronological factors in determining prognosis. In other words, according to Devitt, 'lymph node metastases are an expression, not the determinant of prognosis'. This new belief system is now described for convenience as 'biological predeterminism', a term first defined by Ian MacDonald (Paper 7) to distinguish it from the mechanistic anatomical model of its antecedents. The therapeutic consequences of this belief were profound. They opened the gates to trials of adjuvant systemic therapy and also encouraged surgeons to explore alternatives to radical mastectomy that allowed breast conservation (see Chapter 10). The new therapies that permitted randomized trials to test the new belief system included ovarian ablation, a variety of endocrine therapies starting with stilbestrol right after World War II, tamoxifen in the 1970s, and now aromatase inhibitors, and finally the cytotoxic agents that were introduced to treat many different cancers starting in the late 1940s.

This then brings us nearly up to the present day, where we know with extreme statistical confidence that breast-conserving techniques are equal in outcome as far as survival is concerned compared with the radical techniques of the past, and that adjuvant systemic therapy prolongs survival and for all we know improves the cure rate. This latter assertion is suggested by recent statistics showing a sudden and significant fall in breast cancer age-specific mortality in both the USA and the UK. The drop in mortality in the UK from a higher baseline than the USA is of the order of 30% and started abruptly round about 1985, which coincidentally was the date of the first meta-analysis of the trials of systemic therapy (see Chapters 12–14). As we enter the new millennium, we must not lose sight of our historical perspective. It is likely that the contemporary biological model that has served us so well is incomplete and has yet to explain some of the enigmatic behavior of the disease. Some exciting new developments in molecular biology and genetics (see Chapters 4 and 5) are paving the way for the next conceptual revolution.

Paper 1

The Edwin Smith Papyrus

Author

Anonymous

Translator

Breasted JH

Reference

The Edwin Smith Papyrus. Chicago: University of Chicago Press, 1930: 403–406

Summary

If thou examinest a man (person) having bulging tumours of his breast and thou findest that swellings have spread over his breast; if thou puttest thy hand upon his breast upon these tumours, and thou findest them very cool, there being no fever at all herein when thy hand touches him; they have no granulations, they form no fluid, they do not generate secretions of fluid and they are bulging to thy hand. Thou shouldst say concerning him. There is no treatment.

This translation of the Edwin Smith surgical papyrus was published in 1930. Many scholars have suggested that this is evidence that the ancient Egyptians distinguished inflammatory mastitis from carcinoma of the breast. We would go further and suggest that this passage describes locally advanced breast cancer perhaps with satellite nodules and demonstrates the wisdom of the ancient and anonymous author in recognizing the futility of any intervention. This therapeutic nihilism must have resulted from the accumulated experience in vainly trying to influence the natural history of the advanced disease. The advice with 'there is no treatment' was perhaps the soundest advice that could have been provided to the medical profession up until, say, the last decade of the 19th century.

Related reference **(1)** Robbins GF (ed). *Silvergirl's Surgery – The Breast.* Austin, TX: Silvergirl, Inc., 1984: 9–16.

Key message

In medicine, there is an old maxim 'there are many conditions you cannot help but there are none you cannot make worse'. This perhaps is the first recorded example of this principle.

Why it's important

One should always understand the natural history of a disease before starting to treat it. This ancient document demonstrates the importance of observation of clinical signs of disease.

Relevance

This remains a fundamental principle to this day. Or, as Aristotle might have said, 'Primum non nocere'.

Paper 2

A Short History of Breast Cancer

Author

De Moulin D

Reference

A Short History of Breast Cancer. Boston: Martinus Nijhoff, 1983

Summary

This monograph provides a brief summary of important concepts regarding the natural history of breast cancer that begot various treatments used from ancient times to 1982. The text is organized by historical periods including antiquity, the Middle Ages, the Renaissance, and each of the last four centuries. Hippocrates' somewhat nihilistic attitudes about the treatment of breast cancer, Celsius' treatise from the 1st century AD – the oldest extant clinical description of the disease – and the dominance of Galen's ideas for nearly 1500 years are described. De Moulin explores the basis for popular ideas that arose in later centuries, and often provides the social context for the application of treatments. He demonstrates how increased knowledge of anatomy led eventually to an understanding of how the disease spread from a single focus in the breast to many areas of the body and how the introduction of the microscope led to cellular concepts of disease spread. He illustrates the point that in the 20th century the application of statistics led to more reliable evaluation of treatment effects.

   The idea that breast cancer is, at least in part, a systemic disease is not a revolutionary idea unique to the latter half of the 20th century. The ancients often ascribed the disease to various humors and used systemic therapies along with surgical extirpation. Breast cancer was considered to be a contagion four centuries ago because pockets of high incidence were noted. Similar observations still provide the basis for many epidemiological studies. And whether spread of the tumor is contiguous through lymphatics or widely disseminated through the bloodstream has been a recurring theme.

Related references (1)   Mansfield CM. *Early Breast Cancer: Its History and Results of Treatment.* Basel: Karger, 1976.
             (2)   Robbins GF (ed). *Silvergirl's Surgery – The Breast.* Austin, TX: Silvergirl, Inc., 1984.

Key message

Ideas that we think are revolutionary have frequently been explored in previous generations.

Why it's important

Viewing ideas that are intuitively attractive in a different setting – in this case a historical setting – provides perspective. This, in turn, forces the clinician or investigator to consider the possibility that very compelling ideas may look equally ridiculous when more knowledge becomes available at a future date.

Strengths

The book is short and well written, with enough detail to make it interesting. It is scholarly and well referenced. The author does not impose a bias or attempt to develop a simplistic theme.

Weakness

Each chapter could easily become a separate book if one wishes to explore all of the details.

Relevance

There is still not a simple paradigm that explains the many clinical manifestations of this disease.

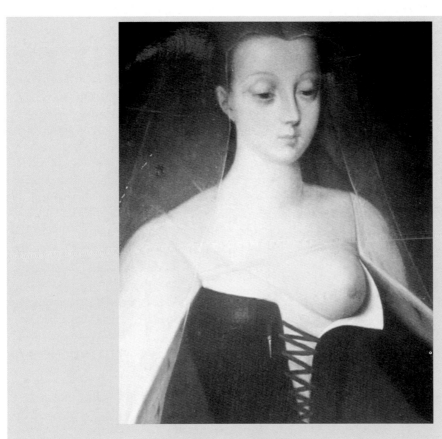

Agnes Sorrell, Mistress of the King of France
(C15th Unknown English artist).

Paper 3

A Treatise on the Disease of the Breast and Mammary Region

Author

Velpeau AALM

Reference

A Treatise on the Disease of the Breast and Mammory Region. London: Sydenham Society, 1856 (Translation by M Henry of *Traite des Maladies du Sein et de la Region Mammaire.* Paris: Masson, 1854). In: *Silvergirl's Surgery – The Breast* (Robbins GF, ed). Austin, TX: Silvergirl, Inc., 1984: 37–44

Summary

Alfredo-Armand-Louis-Marie Velpeau (1795–1867), one of the most highly regarded surgeons of his era, wrote extensively, and persuasively argued the case for surgical management of the disease. This is a very detailed description of 'radical' surgical techniques pre-microscope, pre-anesthesia, and pre-Halsted. Velpeau recommends removal of the tumor *en bloc* with wide margins along with skin and lymph nodes when the tumor appears to extend to these areas. He classified breast tumors on the basis of their physical characteristics and recognized the importance of lymph node involvement. However, he also recognized that lymphadenopathy could represent either involvement by tumor or an inflammatory reaction. This article includes a description of many non-surgical approaches such as bloodletting, purgatives, hemlock, arsenic, iodine, gold, and quinine that were popular at that time. Velpeau wrote long before objective evidence was required to bolster arguments for or against a particular treatment. He argues that results from surgery are superior on the basis of either his experience with or his 'natural disinclination' toward various non-surgical approaches.

Then, as now, the clinician struggled with the true nature of the disease in each patient he treated. Velpeau was certain that many breast tumors should not be treated – either because they were benign or because the tumor had already spread. 'People can only believe in the cure of cancer, when they have either been unable or unwilling to distinguish malignant from innocent tumors.'

Related reference   **(1)**   De Moulin D. *A Short History of Breast Cancer.*
                                    Boston: Martinus Nijhoff, 1983 (Paper 2 in this chapter).

Key message

Long before pathologists had agreed that breast cancer could be defined histologically or that tumor grades were a reflection of underlying aggressiveness, before anyone understood the differences between hormone-responsive and non-responsive tumors or the differences between tumors that did and did not overexpress HER2/*neu*, clinicians understood that this diagnosis subsumed a variety of conditions with different natural histories.

Why it's important

The recognition of this heterogeneity and using this knowledge to select appropriate treatment for individual patients is a persistent theme in the study of breast cancer extending back for many centuries. The importance of heterogeneity is appreciated today even though we have still not perfected the definitions of patient subsets to minimize toxicity for patients who will do well without a treatment or who will do poorly in spite of it.

Strength

This article gives a detailed description of treatments used in the 18th and 19th centuries, especially surgical approaches.

Weakness

Radical surgery was abandoned for a variety of other radical treatments nearly a half century ago, making this less relevant than it once was.

Relevance

The development of new paradigms and new treatments that we often attribute to a single individual (e.g. Halsted) usually evolve from the observations of many scientists over long periods of time.

Paper 4

The results of operations for the cure of cancer of the breast performed at the Johns Hopkins Hospital from June, 1889 to January, 1894

Author

Halsted WS

Reference

Johns Hopkins Hospital Bulletin 1894–95; No.4:297

Summary

In this paper, Halsted describes 50 cases operated upon by his method of radical mastectomy, which includes in some cases dissection of the supraclavicular fossa. He claims only 6% local recurrence, which he compares favorably with other selected series that describe up to 80% local recurrence after differing extents of the operation in other hands. In addition, he describes 8 cases as suffering from 'regionary recurrence'. He claimed that the surgeon could not be responsible for this class of recurrence, which was outside of the scope of the operation and originated from invisible foci of the disease within the skin flaps.

Related references

(1) Meyer W. An improved method of the radical operation for carcinoma of the breast. *Medical Record* 1894; **46**:746.

(2) Sampson Handley W. Parasternal invasion of the thorax in breast cancer and its suppression by the use of radium tubes as an operative precaution. *Surgery, Gynecology and Obstetrics* 1927; **45**:721.

Key message

In the days when the disease most often presented in the advanced stages, radical surgery was associated with acceptable levels of local recurrence.

Why it's important

This paper is probably the first attempt to maintain a careful audit of the outcome of a surgical procedure for breast cancer. It was a remarkable achievement to complete this kind of surgery in the very early days of antisepsis and anesthesia with such low surgical morbidity and mortality. Given that the disease was advanced at presentation, a generous interpretation of these data shows acceptable levels of local control. In the days before the availability of radiotherapy and chemotherapy, this was the best that could be expected.

Strength

This is a careful description of a surgical technique with an audit of short-term outcomes.

Weaknesses

The follow-up was extremely short, with a maximum amongst survivors of 3 years and 7 months. The definition of local recurrence was self-serving and uncritical. Furthermore, comparisons with other series would be subject to case selection bias, since only the fittest of patients would have been selected for such major surgery (and also those with the lowest tumor burden).

Relevance

The relevance of this study today is as an excellent illustration of the danger of selection bias and historical controls in exaggerating the benefit of a new innovation. With this shaky foundation based on an obsolete model of the disease, the classical radical mastectomy remained the 'treatment of choice' for the following 70 years. The danger remains to this day that unproven treatments based on a plausible hypothesis will be translated into therapeutic dogma unless there is eternal vigilance (namely high-dose chemotherapy and stem cell rescue).

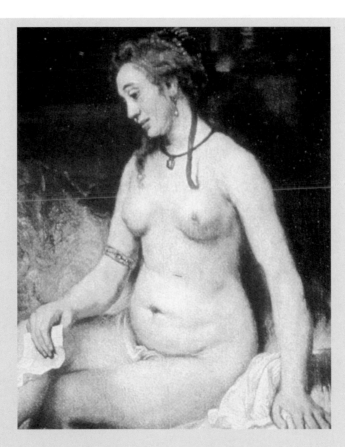

Bathsheba at her toilet (Rembrandt, 1655).

Paper 5

The radium treatment of carcinoma of the breast

Author

Keynes J

Reference

British Journal of Surgery 1931–32; **19**:425

Summary

This paper describes 171 cases treated by excision of the primary tumor, with radium needles being inserted into the breast, the axilla, and supraclavicular fossa. The cases were 'staged' as class one (no glands palpable), class two (glands palpable), and class three (inoperable). Of those treated 3 or more years earlier, 77.7% of class one were alive, 36.3% of class two, and 46.1% of class three. This was compared favorably with a similar group of patients treated at University College Hospital, London by classic radical mastectomy.

Related reference   (1)   Keynes G. *The Gates of Wisdom.* Oxford: Clarendon Press, pp. 211–18.

Key message

Breast-conserving surgery by local excision and radical radiotherapy produced results equivalent to those of the classical radical mastectomy in vogue at the time. This paper also described a simple approach to the staging of breast cancer and the calculation of results with percentage outcomes rather than absolute numbers.

Why it's important

This was one of the earliest attempts at treating breast cancer whilst conserving the breast. Keynes recognized the significance of the psychological and physical morbidity of radical surgery, yet his pioneering attempts were ignored for nearly 50 years and he was vilified by the surgical establishment for his efforts. (See his autobiography, related reference 1)

Strength

This was a bold attempt to challenge surgical dogma with a careful audit of results.

Weaknesses

Although the outcome of treatment was conservative, the field of treatment was still radical. The follow-up time was short, failing to recognize the long natural history of the disease.

Relevance

In the days before radomized controlled trials, this was certainly *a priori* evidence that conservative surgery could produce the same order of outcomes as radical mastectomy. One could argue that the onus was on the proponents of radical surgery to demonstrate more favorable results to justify the costs of an increase in physical and psychological morbidity. This is a good illustration of a prophet before his time and a sad reflection of the conservative nature of the surgical profession.

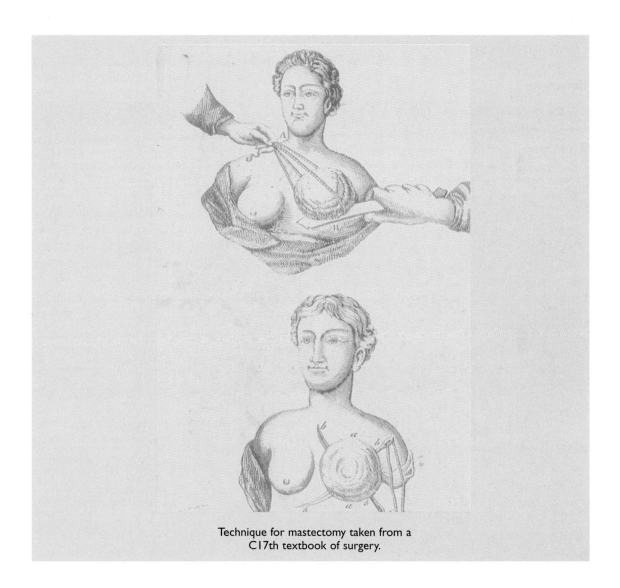

Technique for mastectomy taken from a
C17th textbook of surgery.

Paper 6

A study of the results of operations for the cure of cancer of the breast performed at the Johns Hopkins Hospital from 1889 to 1931

Authors

Lewis D, Rienhoff WF Jr

Reference

Annals of Surgery 1932; **95**:336–400

Summary

Lewis and Rienhoff were surgeons at The Johns Hopkins Hospital in Halsted's unit. In this report, they provide follow-up on 950 consecutive patients operated on by Halsted and the surgeons he trained. Of these patients, 420 (44%) were known to have died and accurate data on the postoperative course and cause of death were available. An additional 209 patients had been lost to follow-up, and 97 were know to be alive and well, 65 of these for more than 5 years. Among those who had died, the median survival was less than 3 years. The survival rates at 3, 5, 10, 15, and 20 years were 43%, 22%, 7%, 4%, and 3%, respectively (excluding perioperative deaths, these numbers were 46%, 24%, 8%, 4%, and 3%). The last 2 deaths occurred in year 32. Breast cancer was the cause of death in 96% of the patients for which this could be accurately determined. This study provides interesting insights into the relationship between delay in diagnosis and outcome and between the surgical procedure and local recurrences.

The survival of the patients treated by Halsted and his associates over a 42-year period is analyzed and reported with extensive details about the nature of the cancers treated, the frequency of various kinds of recurrence, the time of death, and the cause of death.

Related references **(1)** Bloom HJG, Richardson WW, Harries EJ. Natural history of untreated breast cancer (1805–1933). *British Medical Journal* 1962; **ii**:213–220 (Paper 8 in this chapter).

(2) Henderson IC, Canellos GP. Cancer of the breast: the past decade. *New England Journal of Medicine* 1980; **302**:17–30.

Key message

Halsted's original report describing the radical mastectomy was entitled 'The results of operations for the cure of cancer of the breast …'. This report changed the way in which breast cancer was treated in Europe and the USA, and radical mastectomy became standard treatment until well into the 1950s in Britain and the early 1970s in the USA. However, Halsted's original report focused primarily on local recurrence rate rather than survival. In this follow-up study by Lewis and Rienhoff, it is clear that the survival of these patients was not much different from that of untreated patients during the same era. (See Bloom *et al.* (related reference 1), where the median survival was 2.7 years and the survival rates at 3, 5, 10, and 15 years were 44%, 18%, 4%, and 1%, respectively.) There is little evidence that any of Halsted's patients were truly cured.

Why it's important

In Halsted's paper, local recurrence is used as a surrogate for cure. Because the natural history of breast cancer is so long, it is always tempting to find early evidence of treatment effects that will reliably predict long-term outcomes. The dangers of doing this are well illustrated here. Clearly, this operation did not cure many (if any) patients, but the perception of superiority generated by results using the surrogate endpoint led to excessive and toxic treatment of millions of women.

Strength

It is uncommon for the first report of an innovative therapy to be followed by an analysis of outcomes based on follow-up in excess of 20 years. This paper provides this information with unusual detail for one of the seminal reports in the breast cancer literature: Halsted's description and early results from using radical mastectomy.

Weakness

The patients treated by these surgeons are like the untreated patients described by Bloom, but are very different from those commonly seen in practice today.

Relevance

Since prolongation of survival is an important goal of treatment for many (if not most) patients, the relationship between survival and surrogate endpoints, such as freedom from local recurrence, disease-free survival, or the disappearance of tumor markers, must be demonstrated empirically.

Paper 7

Biological predeterminism in human cancer

Author

MacDonald I

Reference

Surgery, Gynecology and Obstetrics 1951; **92**:443–458

Summary

MacDonald analyzed data derived from studies of a number of tumor types to determine whether there was a correlation between early diagnosis, defined as a short duration of symptoms, and tumor characteristics associated with good outcomes, such as a limited number of positive lymph nodes or small tumor size. While there was generally a correlation, he observed that within each category there was still a wide range of values. For example, 19% of breast cancer patients with symptoms for less than 1 month had tumors measuring less than 1 cm, but 5% of patients with tumors that had been observed for more than 1 year prior to presentation were also in this size group. The converse was also true. Of the patients with short duration of symptoms, 12% had tumors larger than 5 cm, but even after a delay of more than 1 year, only 22% of the tumors had reached this size.

There was, at best, only a weak correlation between tumor characteristics that suggested a limited duration of growth and the observed duration of symptoms prior to diagnosis. MacDonald concluded that for many (possibly all) tumors there was no time when the tumor was both detectable and sufficiently localized that it could be entirely removed by mastectomy. As a result, he felt that a patient's survival was determined more by the intrinsic biology of the tumor than by the therapeutic intervention.

Related references (1) Devitt JE. The enigmatic behavior of breast cancer. *Cancer* 1971; **27**:12–27.

(2) Baum M. The curability of breast cancer. *British Medical Journal* 1976; **1**:439–442.

Key message

Many, most, or all breast cancers are 'incurable' (i.e. unaffected by mastectomy) either because they have spread to distant organs before they can be detected or because they have little metastatic potential and limited, if any, lethality.

Why it's important

This was the first of a number of thoughtful papers that challenged the paradigms that had become dogma over the previous century. By questioning the validity of these paradigms, these authors opened up the possibility that more limited surgery (or no surgery) might result in survival at least equal to that achieved with mastectomy and that the early use of systemic treatments, such as ovarian ablation and chemotherapy, would have a greater impact on survival than surgery. The importance of these reports is evidenced by the intensely emotional response they evoked from leading surgeons on both sides of the Atlantic.

Strength

Extensive data from carefully observing patient signs and symptoms were educed to support the arguments.

Weakness

A much more powerful study design to test these hypotheses is the randomized clinical trial.

Relevance

Exploration of new paradigms is not possible until the old ones have been at least challenged and possibly discredited.

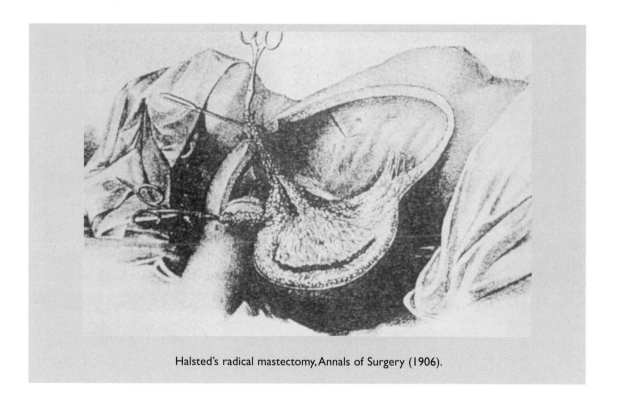

Halsted's radical mastectomy, Annals of Surgery (1906).

Paper 8

Natural history of untreated breast cancer (1805–1933)

Authors

Bloom HJG, Richardson WW, Harries EJ

Reference

British Medical Journal 1962; **ii**:213–220

Summary

The cancer ward at the Middlesex Hospital in London was among the first established anywhere in the world primarily for the treatment of cancer. In this retrospective study, Bloom *et al.* reviewed all records of breast cancer patients treated at Middlesex and identified 356 who had received no treatment, the first of these having presented in 1805. There was adequate information on 250 women to include them in the study, and histological material was available on 86 cases seen between 1902 and 1933. The median time between the initial symptoms, as reported by the patient, and death was 2.7 years. The longest interval was 18 years and 3 months. The survival rates at 3, 5, 10, and 15 years were 44%, 18%, 4%, and 1%, respectively. Five percent of the patients died of causes other than breast cancer. Retrospective grading of the tumors for which histological material was available demonstrate a correlation with grade and survival.

This is a retrospective study of untreated patients. In the 19th century, there were limited treatments, especially for patients who presented late in the course of their disease. In the early 20th century, radiotherapy, more extensive surgical procedures, and ovarian ablation were being used, so a higher percentage of the 20th century patients were self-selected.

Related references (1)   Bloom HJG, Field JR. Impact of tumor grade and host resistance on survival of women with breast cancer. *Cancer* 1971; **28**:1580–1589.

(2)   Fox MS. On the diagnosis and treatment of breast cancer. *Journal of the American Medical Association* 1979; **241**:489–494 (Paper 12 in this chapter).

(3)   Henderson IC, Canellos GP. Cancer of the breast: the past decade. *New England Journal of Medicine* 1980; **302**:17–30.

Key message

This study demonstrated that the natural history of breast cancer is very long even without treatment.

Why it's important

Very few (if any) patients would agree to participate in a randomized trial in which the control arm was 'no treatment of any kind at any time' for the remainder of their life. Thus, our comparison of current treatments with no treatment at all must depend on historical controls. When patients have a long life after diagnosis, we usually attribute this to our treatment. This study demonstrates that this is often an incorrect assumption. If the 5% of patients in this study who died of causes other than breast cancer had been in a modern study, we would almost certainly have counted them as 'cures' resulting from our interventions.

Strengths

There are at least a half dozen other observational studies of untreated patients. This is one of the largest, the follow-up is very long, and necropsy material is available on a substantial number of the patients. The population of patients from which this cohort was drawn is well defined and was carefully combed to identify those included in the study.

Weaknesses

As in all historical series of this type, the patients were self-selected. Although treatments used in the 19th century probably had little impact on the survival of breast cancer patients, this is a disease that has been treated for more than three millennia, as described in several of the other classic papers discussed in this chapter. It cannot be assumed that these patients are necessarily like all others presenting in the years covered by this study. Many presented for the first time very late in the course of their disease and presumably had a variant that was more tolerable and/or less aggressive than the average may have been. (However, see related reference (2).)

Relevance

This paper is a good starting point for every student of breast cancer. It is important to understand the disease without treatment if one is to objectively evaluate the effects of therapy.

Paper 9

Breast cancer: A report of two clinical trials

Author

Paterson R

Reference

Journal of the Royal College of Surgeons of Edinburgh 1962; 7:243–254

Summary

The first of these two trials enrolled 720 women between 1948 and 1952. Eligible patients under age 70 with newly diagnosed breast cancer were treated with a Halsted radical mastectomy and then randomized to receive kilovoltage radiotherapy to the anterior chest wall and the apex of the axilla ('quadrate technique'). Another 741 patients were randomized between 1953 and 1955 using a 'peripheral technique' that aimed at irradiating the internal mammary, axillary, and supraclavicular lymph nodes as well as the chest wall. Those randomized to the control or 'watched group' received radiotherapy if and when a local recurrence was found. The incidence of local recurrences were reduced by nearly two-thirds among those treated with radiotherapy immediately following mastectomy, but the percentage of patients with uncontrolled disease at the time of death was nearly the same in the two groups of patients. There was no significant difference in survival. In the second trial, 598 pre- and perimenopausal women were randomized after primary treatment to ovarian irradiation (450 r) or no ovarian ablation. The survival of the irradiated patients was superior to that of the control group at 10 and 15 years, but this did not reach conventional levels of statistical significance ($p=0.07$ at 10 years). One hundred and forty-nine women with inoperable breast cancer were also randomized in the same fashion, and ovarian ablation did not result in a survival advantage for this group.

These two studies are the first results of randomized trials evaluating treatments of patients with early breast cancer. The first demonstrated that radiotherapy after mastectomy would reduce local recurrences but not increase long-term local control of the disease or improve survival. The second showed that the survival of premenopausal women might be prolonged by the use of adjuvant ovarian ablation. The trial design and rationale for the studies is provided in this report, but related references (1)–(3) must also be read to obtain the mature results of the studies that are summarized above.

Related references **(1)** Easson EC. Post-operative radiotherapy in breast cancer. In: *Prognostic Factors in Breast Cancer* (Forrest APM, Kunkler PB, eds). Edinburgh: E & S Livingstone, 1968: 119–127.

(2) Cole MP. A clinical trial of an artificial menopause in carcinoma of the breast. *Inserm* 1975; **55**:143–150.

(3) Cole MP. Prophylactic compared with therapeutic X-ray artificial menopause. In: *The Clinical Management of Advanced Breast Cancer, 2nd Tenovus Workshop* (Joslin CAF, Gleave EN, eds). Cardiff: Alpha Omega Alpha Publishing, 1970: 2–11.

(4) Early Breast Cancer Trialists' Collaborative Group. Effects of radiotherapy and surgery in early breast cancer. An overview of the randomized trials. Early Breast Cancer Trialists' Collaborative Group. *New England Journal of Medicine* 1995; **333**:1444–1455 [Erratum 1996; **334**:1003].

(5) Early Breast Cancer Trialists' Collaborative Group. Ovarian ablation in early breast cancer: overview of the randomised trials. *Lancet* 1996; **348**:1189–1196.

Key message

It is possible to randomly allocate patients to one of two treatment plans and obtain reliable results on the benefits (or lack of benefit) from these treatments – an approach that was radical and extremely controversial when these studies were performed. The results of these two trials have been largely confirmed by later studies (related references 4 and 5). Although evidence from recent overviews demonstrates that better local control of the disease will improve survival, the effects are much smaller than anticipated prior to these first, pivotal studies. Ovarian ablation was not considered an important treatment for decades because of this and subsequent small trials in which a treatment effect was seen but not taken seriously because the *p*-value exceeded 0.05. It is now clear that it is one of the most effective treatments available.

Why it's important

These studies changed the way that breast cancer treatments (and treatments of almost all medical conditions) are evaluated. It is remarkable that these very large studies at the Christie Hospital in Manchester, England were begun at almost the same time as a much smaller study of tuberculosis treatment that is often cited as the first randomized trial performed in the clinic. In the half-century following these studies, more than 150 000–200 000 women with breast cancer have been randomized in clinical trials. Very few diseases have been studied as systematically as breast cancer using this technique, now considered to be the gold standard for evaluating treatments of all types.

Strengths

This was a randomized clinical trial in which the patient populations were well defined and were followed for decades to fully assess the outcomes. At the time of relapse, patients on the control arms were offered the treatment initially withheld so that it was possible to evaluate early versus late interventions. Almost no other trial of local treatment followed patients for the remainder of their life to assess long-term local control.

Weaknesses

Today the techniques for radiotherapy and ovarian ablation used in these studies would be considered substandard. Although there is no evidence of bias in the randomization, it was technically possible for the physician to know in advance which treatment his/her patient might receive. This would be unacceptable in a randomized trial performed now. Both studies were seriously underpowered to detect the relatively small benefits that we now know exist when these therapies are used.

Relevance

Uncontrolled trials or those using historical comparisons are likely to seriously over- or underestimate the benefits of treatment. Randomized trials that are underpowered may result in the same error.

Paper 10

The Surgical Dilemma in the Primary Therapy of Invasive Breast Cancer: A Critical Appraisal

Author

Fisher B

Reference

The Surgical Dilemma in the Primary Therapy of Invasive Breast Cancer: A Critical Appraisal. Chicago: Year Book Publishers (Current Problems in Surgery), 1970

Summary

This monograph summarizes 5 years of animal experimentation using syngeneic groups of mice, exploring the relationship between transplanted murine breast cancers and 'the host'. Ingenious experimental models were set up to study the putative role of the regional lymph nodes (RLN) in filtering out cancer cells from the afferent lymph and the role of the RLN in inducing an immune response to a subsequent challenge with the same tumor. These experiments demonstrated that the RLN do not have a filtration capacity and that cancer cells could bypass the nodes by lympho-venous channels or by direct invasion of the venous system. Furthermore, the surgical removal of the RLN inhibited the induction and maintenance of an immune response capable of the recognition and rejection of a subsequent challenge with the same tumor.

Fisher then went on to elaborate his hypothetical model of 'biological predeterminism', which stated that the outcome of treatment for early breast cancer was determined by the burden of micrometastases present at the time of diagnosis. The involvement of the lymph nodes was an expression of a poor prognosis, and their removal in an attempt at cure was equivalent to 'shutting the stable door after the horse had bolted', while the removal of uninvolved nodes was on the one hand unnecessary and on the other hand potentially harmful in abrogating acquired cellular immunity to the primary cancer.

Related references (1) Macdonald I. Biological predeterminism in human cancer. *Surgery, Gynecology and Obstetrics* 1951; **92**:443–458 (Paper 7 in this chapter).

(2) Devitt JE. The significance of regional lymph node metastases in breast carcinoma. *Canadian Medical Association Journal* 1965; **93**:289–294.

Key message

If the outcome of surgery is predetermined by the extent of micrometastases present at the time of diagnosis, then the notion of 'early' breast cancer needs to be reconsidered and the role of surgery redefined. If the disease is thus a systemic disorder by the time it is diagnosable, then improvements in cure may only be achieved by systemic modalities such as cytotoxic, endocrine, and immune therapies. The role of surgery then becomes relegated to that required for diagnostic purposes, local control, and staging. If all of these can be achieved equally well by breast-conserving techniques, then so much the better.

Why it's important

It cannot be overestimated how much Bernard Fisher's work influenced surgical thinking in the 1970s. It led to a true paradigm shift in the way we considered the fundamental nature of the disease. Furthermore, this biological framework paved the way for the clinical trials of breast-conserving surgery and adjuvant systemic therapy.

Strengths

This was a powerful attempt to bring modern biological sciences to the service of an enigmatic disease where progress was illusionary. A long programme of animal research was planned to challenge the prevailing dogmas of the period.

Weaknesses

The syngeneic strain of mice with transplantable tumors was a poor model of human breast cancer. In particular, the artificiality of the experiments involving hind limb amputations with or without RLN dissection led to a decade of futile research into immunotherapy as treatment for both early and advanced stages of the disease. The deterministic model also fails to explain many recent observations of the disease, in particular the biphasic pattern of relapse with twin peaks at 3 and 7–10 years and the impact of postoperative radiotherapy on long-term cause-specific mortality.

Relevance

Fisher's work remains relevant to this day in planning trials of both adjuvant and local therapy, but in the opinion of this reviewer the biological model is 'past its sell-by date' and it is time for *another* paradigm shift!

Paper 11

The curability of breast cancer

Authors

Brinkley D, Haybittle JL

Reference

Lancet 1975; **ii**:95–99

Summary

A total of 704 patients treated at Addenbrooke's Hospital, Cambridge by radical mastectomy between 1947 and 1952 were followed up for 25 years. They were divided into two groups: stage I and II (Manchester classification) and stage III. There survival was then compared with that of an age-matched cohort and the results were plotted on a semilogarithmic graph. Parallelism in survival between the breast cancer group and the normal cohort was not reached until over 20 years, at which point a population of patients 'cured' by surgery could be defined. This was less than 30% for the most favorable group.

Related reference **(1)** Brinkley D, Haybittle JL. A 15 year follow up of patients treated for carcinoma of the breast. *British Journal of Radiology* 1968; **41**:215–219.

Key message

Haybittle's mathematical help to define the curability of the disease, applied to this large prospective collected series, critically damaged the complacency of the surgical establishment. To add insult to injury, the more mature data published in the *Lancet* 10 years later demonstrated that up to 35 years of follow-up there was still a significant excess breast cancer mortality in the treated group compared with the controls. Furthermore, if there was a group 'cured' by surgery alone, it could only be on the order of 10%!

Strengths

A large cohort of patients were treated by a radical mastectomy in a single institution with complete and extremely long-term follow-up. Added to the revolutionary teaching of Bernard Fisher, this paper probably put the nail in the coffin of classical radical mastectomy as the unchallenged treatment for early breast cancer.

Weaknesses

This work did not allow for the fact that the very long-term survivors might still have survived even if untreated, albeit with progressive disease on the chest wall.

Relevance

There are still no convincing data that breast cancer, once invasive and clinically detectable, is curable by local therapy alone. Furthermore, with the risk of cause-specific mortality ever present, therapeutic strategies for young women must include trials that allow, say, a 25-year follow-up. Research-funding organizations are still reluctant to accept this reality.

Paper 12

On the diagnosis and treatment of breast cancer

Author

Fox MS

Reference

Journal of the American Medical Association 1979; **241**:489–494

Summary

This study is an analysis of the relative survival of patients diagnosed with breast cancer in the state of Connecticut between 1950 and 1973. The data were collected by the End Results Section, Biometry Branch, US National Cancer Institute during a time when the incidence of breast cancer was increasing (an 18% increase from 1936 to 1965 and 50% from 1965 to 1975) but mortality remained constant. The relative annual mortality of all patients included in the study dropped from about 12% in the first year following diagnosis to 2.5% at 10 years. It remained constant at about 2.5% per year thereafter. Because of the relatively sharp break in the curve at 10 years, the author hypothesized that there are two distinct patient populations. One died at a rate of 25% per year. These patients were all dead by year 10. The second group died at a rate of 2.5% per year. Half of these patients would have survived 30 years in the absence of other causes, and they constituted about 60% of the population of breast cancer patients in the registry. The relative mortality of this second group was calculated to be nearly equal to that of cigarette smokers. Among those patients with localized or stage I disease, 85% fell in the group with an annual mortality rate of 2.5%, compared with only 40% of those with regional or stage II breast cancer. Fox applied the same analysis to untreated patients in the Middlesex Hospital series (related reference 1), and found that those patients died at an annual rate of 25%!

Related references (1)   Bloom HJG, Richardson WW, Harries EJ. Natural history of untreated breast cancer (1805–1933). *British Medical Journal* 1962; **ii**:213–220 (Paper 8 in this chapter).

(2)   Bross IDJ, Blumenson E, Slack NH, Priore RL. A two-disease model for breast cancer. In: *Prognostic Factors in Breast Cancer* (Forrest APM, Kunkler PB, eds). Edinburgh: E & S Livingstone, 1968: 289–299.

(3)   Haagensen CD, Cooley E, Miller E, *et al.* Treatment of early mammary carcinoma: a cooperative international study. *Annals of Surgery* 1969; **170**:875–899.

Key message

Heterogeneity of behavior is a fundamental characteristic of breast cancer. There are some patients with breast cancer whose risk of dying from the disease is so low that the benefits from treatment, especially radical and toxic therapies, are questionable. The results of this study suggest that the majority of breast cancer patients diagnosed in more recent years have a less lethal form of the disease than those with no treatment at all who were included in a number of retrospective analyses, such as those in the series by Bloom *et al.* (related reference 1). This might be explained by the difference in the way breast cancer was diagnosed in these two eras. By 1950, the diagnosis of breast cancer was based entirely on histology. Histology was available on only one-third of the untreated patients, and in most cases this was necropsy material.

Why it's important

The heterogeneity of the disease is one important reason why the relative benefit of various treatments for breast cancer can only be properly addressed with a randomized trial. Inappropriate comparisons between patients treated in different eras and different locations resulted in the widespread use of radical mastectomy (see related reference 3). The idea that there are distinctly different subsets of breast cancer patients with a different natural history is a recurring theme (see related reference 2).

Strength

The study used a large population-based registry with long-term follow-up.

Weakness

The observations were sufficient to provide support for the idea that distinct subsets of breast cancer patients might exist. This study does not prove this point, however, and provides no practical guidance to prospectively place a particular patient in one or the other of the two groups of patients defined by the study.

Relevance

Beware of all conclusions based on studies comparing groups that are defined by any criteria other than randomization.

CHAPTER 2

Biostatistics

JACK CUZICK

Introduction

A choice of papers that highlights pivotal biostatistical contributions to breast cancer is particularly difficult, not only because of the scope of 'biostatistics' but also its intrinsic interaction with the subject under study. At one extreme, relevant major advances in theoretical statistics have a much wider applicability than breast cancer alone, whereas at the other extreme important applied statistical work generally makes a major contribution to the subject matter, so that a particular paper is also appropriate to another chapter in this book. In this case the distinction between a classic 'biostatistical' contribution or a classic paper about treatment improvements or risk factors becomes largely semantic.

The choice of historically important versus more modern classics is also difficult. Probably, the first statistical analysis related to breast cancer was that of Rigoni-Stern [1] who noticed that unmarried women had a strikingly higher ratio of breast cancer to uterine cancer deaths (including uterine cervix) than married women. However, the absence of controls made it unclear which of these cancers was affected. Farr's work, as the first statistician in the UK General Registrar's Office, of annually publishing mortality rates for a range of diseases [2], beginning in 1837, was also notable, as was Greenwood's work [3] on actuarial methods for survival. In these cases one might argue that the major contributions were more epidemiological than biostatistical, although Greenwood's calculation of variances for actuarial survival curves foreshadowed the classic work of Kaplan and Meier (Paper 4).

However, to start with I have chosen Fisher's classic work (Paper 1) on the design of experiments in which the importance of randomization was clearly enunciated. This early work was not concerned with breast cancer, or even medicine, but with the assignment of treatments to crops in field experiments. However, the power of this concept was so great, and its influence on breast cancer trials so universal, that it seemed imperative to include it. Other major contributions to statistical theory, such as significance testing, confidence intervals, likelihood ratios, normal, chi-squared, and binomial distributions are also fundamental, but their role is so basic to all of statistics that I have chosen not to highlight them here.

Another major biostatistical development of great importance for breast cancer was the development of methodology for observational studies. Again, the motivation and utility of these ideas extends far beyond their use in studies of breast cancer. A now classic development is the case–control study, and among the many contributors to its development I have selected Cornfield's early work (Paper 3) on odds ratios and McNemar's observation (Paper 2) about the need to use different methods of analysis for matched and unmatched studies. Many others have made important contributions to the design and analysis of case–control studies including Breslow, Day, Prentice, Pike, and Gart. Other novel approaches to observational studies including case–cohort studies [4] and approaches to genetic determinants of risk, such as sib-pairs, cases and parents, and case-only studies [5] but their impact has been greater in other areas. However, I have included the famous 1966 paper of Mantel (Paper 5) which applies the use of (stratified) odds ratios to life tables to derive the fundamental Mantel–Haenszel or logrank test. This paper provided a bridge between methods for trials and observational studies. This paper was followed by several important works on clinical trials, but the unification achieved by Cox (Paper 6), using the concepts of partial likelihood and proportional hazards model stands out among the rest. A later pair of papers under the names of a host of pre-eminent statisticians (Paper 7) was highly influential in spelling out the details of good trial design and analysis.

The need for large numbers of patients to detect moderate treatment differences led to the development of the overview of all trials addressing the same question. The importance of collecting and updating follow-up on an individual patient basis was first demonstrated by Cuzick *et al.* (Paper 9) and led to important changes in the use of radiotherapy. Larger efforts, looking at all aspects of breast cancer treatment, were subsequently undertaken by the Early Breast Cancer Trialists Collaborative Group and an important exposition of overview methodology was published in one of their early reports (Paper 12). The analysis of overviews continues to be a fruitful area, and the use of random effect models to deal with treatment heterogeneity is an important new development.

Quality of life has been another new direction for breast cancer trials, and fundamental new concepts have been developed by Gelber *et al.* (Paper 10) to balance length of life against quality. Screening has also led to new developments, again built-up over time through a range of papers, but the paper of Walter and Day (Paper 8) has probably been the most influential.

Genetics is the new frontier for many diseases, including breast cancer, and has generated a host of statistical problems. The linkage analysis study for BRCA1 (Paper 13) stands out as pivotal, but many investigators have made important contributions, and undoubtedly there is more to come. The identification of risk is vital for chemoprevention trials and other interventions in high-risk groups, and the paper by Gail *et al.* (Paper 11) is an important first step in developing a risk assessment based on risk multiple factors.

Any selection from such a rich field is unavoidably subjective, both in the choice of specific topics and the selection of the key paper for each specific topic. Many other areas have produced important statistical developments, including repeated measurements, frailty models, generalized estimating equations, and others. No doubt other 'classics' will emerge as the field continues to develop and expand.

References

[1] Rigoni-Stern D. Fatti statistici relativi alle mallattie cancrose che servirono de base alle poche cose dette dal dott. *G Servire Progr Pathol Terap Ser* 2. 2:07–517, 1842. Translated by B de Stavola. *Statistics in Medicine* 1987; **8**:881–884.

[2] Registrar General's Statistical Review for England and Wales (1837–1838). London: HMSO.

[3] Greenwood M. The natural duration of cancer. *Reports on Public Health and Medical Subjects* 1926; **33**:1–26. London: HMSO.

[4] Prentice RL. A case–cohort design for epidemiologic cohort studies and disease prevention trials. *Biometrika* 1986; **73**:1–11.

[5] Khoury MJ, Flanders WD. Nontraditional epidemiologic approaches in the analysis of gene–environment interaction: case–control studies with no controls! *American Journal of Epidemiology* 1996; **144**:207–213.

Paper 1

The design of experiments

Author

Fisher RA

Reference

The Design of Experiments, 1st edn. Edinburgh: Oliver & Boyd, 1935; 8th edn. New York: Hafner Publishing Co, 1966

Summary

This was a comprehensive treatise on a range of aspects of the design of experiments. The general goal was to provide designs which eliminated bias and reduced random error. There are extensive sections on complex combinatorial designs such as Latin squares and partially replicated factorial designs, but there are also crucial basic sections on the importance of randomization and a discussion of the ability of replication to minimize random errors. Sections 9–11 on randomization and replication are fundamental and chapter IV (sections 22–30) which describes the randomized block design are particularly relevant. Although written with agricultural applications in mind, this treatise is a landmark for all investigations of interventions in complex systems, where modelling of all the relevant effects is not reliable, and the key safeguard against bias is randomization.

Related references **(1)** Bradford Hill A. *Principles of Medical Statistics*, 3rd edn. London: The Lancet, 1942; 12th edn (with ID Hill). London: Edward Arnold, 1991.

(2) Paterson R. Breast cancer: a report of two clinical trials. *Journal of the Royal College of Surgeons of Edinburgh* 1962; 7:243–254.

Key message

Randomization is the only sure way to eliminate bias in clinical trials.

Why it's important

Randomization is the keystone of modern evaluations of new treatments. In human subjects the potential for selection bias is so great that unless a treatment is overwhelmingly effective, the only way to reliably assess its value is via a randomized trial. The dangers of not randomizing treatment allocation have now been repeatedly observed in clinical studies where subsequent randomized trials have clearly shown that major inaccuracies were reported in the non-randomized precursor trials.

Strengths

1. Universality of the concept.
2. There is a clear exposition of the need for randomization.

Weaknesses

1. There is no application to human subjects.
2. No advice is given as to how to deal with ethical issues of informed consent.

Relevance

This remains a fundamental requirement for valid treatment evaluation.

Paper 2

Note on the sampling error of the difference between correlated proportions or percentages

Author

McNemar Q

Reference

Psychometrika 1947; **12**:153–157

Summary

This was an early paper pointing out the dangers of using convention tests for 2×2 tables when the observations were obtained from matched case–control studies. The appropriate test using only the discordant pairs was developed and the sampling distribution was given.

Related references

(1) Pike MC, Hill AP, Smith PG. Bias and efficiency in logistic analyses of stratified case-control studies. *International Journal of Epidemiology* 1980; **9**:89–95.

(2) Breslow NE, Day NE (eds). *Statistical Methods in Cancer Research*, Vol. 1 – *The Analysis of Case–Control Studies* (Chapters V and VII). Lyon: IARC, 1980.

Key message

When paired or matched samples are collected, it is imperative to use a matched analysis in which information is only contributed for samples that are discordant.

Why it's important

This was a very early paper and formed the basis for the conditional analysis of matched data. The paper itself was limited to developing a test, but the ideas led to subsequent appreciation of the difference between matched and unmatched odds ratios. Subsequent work expanded this concept into the conditional logistic regression model where estimates could be obtained for risk factors, and precisely described the biases inherent in not using a matched analysis for a matched design.

Strengths

It is observed that a matched study requires a matched analysis, and that much power can be lost if this is not done. Also use of an unmatched analysis for a matched design leads to a bias towards the null hypothesis.

Weakness

This paper focused only on the testing questions. Later papers developed the appropriate estimators.

Relevance

The importance of looking only at discordant pairs for a matched case–control study formed the basis for conditional logistic regression which is widely used today. The simple discordant pairs test also remains a standard for matched pair studies when there are no covariates.

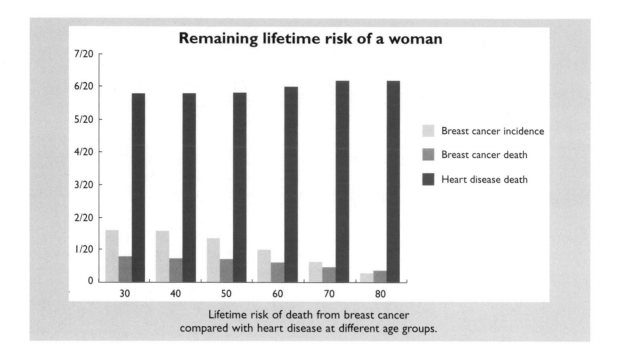

Lifetime risk of death from breast cancer
compared with heart disease at different age groups.

Paper 3

A method of estimating comparative rates from clinical data

Author

Cornfield J

Reference

Journal of the National Cancer Institute 1951; **11**:1269–1275

Summary

This paper provides the statistical justification for case–control studies. The key observation is that by focusing on odds ratios (rather than relative risks or other parameters) valid estimates could be derived as easily from case–control studies as from prospective cohort studies.

Related references (1) Cornfield J. A statistical problem arising from retrospective studies. In: Neyman J (ed.) *Proceedings of the Third Berkeley Symposium on Mathematical Statistics and Probability*, Vol. 4. Berkeley: University of California Press, 1956: 135–148.

(2) Breslow NE, Day NE (eds). *Statistical Methods in Cancer Research – The Analysis of Case-Control Studies*, Vol. 1. Lyon: IARC, 1980.

(3) MacMahon B, Cole P, Lin TM, *et al.* Age at first birth and cancer of the breast. A summary of an international study. *Bulletin of the WHO* 1970; **43**:209–221.

(4) Feinstein AR. Methodologic problems and standards in case-control research. *Journal of Chronic Disease* 1979; 32:35–41.

Key message

By using odds ratios as the effect measure, the exposure variable and disease categories are interchangeable and retrospective case-control studies can estimate odds ratios just as well as prospective cohort studies.

Why it's important

A theoretical basis was provided which laid the foundation for the now ubiquitous case–control study. The key outcome variable was identified and retrospective studies could now be undertaken at a fraction of the cost and time required by prospective cohort studies.

Strengths

1. A solid theoretical base was provided for the conduct of case–control studies.
2. This paper identified the odds ratio as the key parameter measuring effect.
3. The method of analysis was simple.

Weaknesses

1. There are difficulties in the unbiased selection of controls.
2. There are difficulties in recall of exposures that occurred years ago or are affected by disease status (e.g. diet).

Relevance

Case–control studies remain the workhorse of the epidemiologist, and their cost-effectiveness makes it possible to do studies that could not be justified using prospective methods.

Paper 4

Non-parametric estimations from incomplete observations

Authors

Kaplan EL, Meier P

Reference

Journal of the American Statistical Association 1958; **53**:457–481

Summary

This paper developed the so-called 'product limit' estimator for a survival function when the data are subject to non-informative censoring. In this way all the data could be used in estimating survival curves, e.g. individuals followed for only 2 years still make a contribution to the estimated 5-year survival rates. The product-limit estimate takes the form of a product of terms of the form $(1 - d_i/n_i)$, where there is one term for each failure time $t_1 < t_2 \dots < t_k$, indexed in increasing order, d_i is the number of failures at time t_i and n_i is the 'number at risk' just before time t_i.

Related references (1) Greenwood M. The natural duration of cancer. *Reports on Public Health and Medical Subjects* 1926; **33**:1–26. London: HMSO.

(2) Nelson W. Theory and applications of hazard plotting for censored failure data. *Technometrics* 1972; **14**:945–965.

(3) Cutler SJ, Ederer F. Maximum utilization of the life table method in analyzing survival. *Journal of Chronic Diseases* 1958; **8**:699–712.

Key message

Efficient unbiased estimates of survival probabilities can be computed for a study at a time when follow-up is still ongoing.

Why it's important

The paper established the method by which survival curves are now computed in clinical studies with incomplete follow-up. It was a major advance over the procedure of only using patients with potentially complete follow-up to the time point in question (e.g. 5 years), and minimized both the potential for biased ascertainment and the random error of the estimate. The approach refined actuarial methods originally used by Major Greenwood as early as 1926, and also by Cutler and Ederer, and eliminated the need for stratification of the time intervals used in their earlier works. Subsequent work by Nelson, Aalen and others developed an analogous estimator based on the more general theory of counting processes.

Strengths

1. This work uses all of the data to obtain a survival estimator.
2. It is able to deal with both left truncation (late entry) and incomplete follow-up (right censoring).

Weaknesses

1. This approach is limited to single-sample situations, so cannot deal with covariates.
2. The estimate becomes unstable at long follow-up times, where there are few patients in the risk set.

Relevance

This is still the standard method for computing survival curves.

Paper 5

Evaluation of survival data and two new rank order statistics arising in its consideration

Author

Mantel N

Reference

Cancer Chemotherapy Reports 1966; **50**:163–170

Summary

The life-table approach developed in 1958 by Kaplan and Meier (Paper 4) was extended to allow comparison of two or more life-tables via the so-called logrank test. Comparison of survival curves was reduced to estimating the common odds ratio in a series of 2 × 2 tables. The proportional hazards concept was introduced and a simple estimate of the odds ratio was developed as a weighted average of the odds ratios from the individual tables. Sampling properties of the test and estimator were deduced. Extensions to more than two survival curves were also indicated.

Related references
  (1) Mantel N and Haenszel W. Statistical aspects of the analysis of data from retrospective studies of disease. *Journal of the National Cancer Institute* 1959; **22**:719–748.
  (2) Mantel N. Chi-square tests with one degree of freedom: Extensions of the Mantel–Haenszel procedure. *Journal of the American Statistical Association* 1963; **58**:690–700.
  (3) Peto R and Peto J. Asymptotically efficient rank in variant procedures (with discussion). *Journal of the Royal Statistical Society, Series B* 1972; **135**:185–206.
  (4) Prentice RL. Linear rank tests with right censored data. *Biometrika* 1978; **65**:167–179.

Key message

An efficient test and estimator for comparing two survival curves was provided that could handle censored data.

Why it's important

This paper provided an efficient and unbiased method for comparing two survival curves that were generated by incomplete data. This test (variably referred to as the Mantel–Haenszel test or the logrank test) has become the standard method for comparing two treatments in a clinical trial. Previous approaches of comparing proportions at a fixed follow-up time or overall crude failure rates, were inefficient and subject to bias in ascertainment or length of follow-up.

Strength

This is an efficient, robust, stable and intuitive method for comparing two survival curves. In addition to providing a test for the equality of two survival curves, a robust estimator for the relative failure rate of the two arms was given.

Weakness

It is not able to handle patient-specific covariates. The estimator of the relative failure rate is inefficient when the differences are large.

Relevance

This remains the standard method for comparing two survival curves when there are no covariates.

Paper 6

Regression models and life-tables

Author

Cox DR

Reference

Journal of the Royal Statistical Society Series B 1972; **34**:187–200

Summary

This paper presented a sweeping unification and extension of the previous work on survival data which allowed for the study of individual covariates and multivariate analysis. The finely stratified conditional analysis for individual failure times developed previously by Kaplan and Meier for a single survival curve and by Mantel and Haenszel for two or more curves (in terms of 2 × 2 contingency tables) was generalized to the conditional logistic model. The fundamental role of the proportional hazards model was emphasized and a comprehensive calculus was developed using the novel idea of partial likelihood. Highly flexible models allowing individual time-varying exposures, multiple events, and stratification of different sorts could be constructed and analysed in a coherent framework.

Related references	(1)	Cox DR. Partial likelihood. *Biometrika* 1975; **62**:269–276.
	(2)	Anderson PK, Gill RD. Cox's regression model for counting processes. A large sample study. *Annals of Statistics.* 1982; **10**:1100–1120.
	(3)	Kalbfleisch JD, Prentice RL. *The Statistical Analysis of Failure Time Data.* New York: Wiley, 1980.

Key message

Life-table methods could be extended to deal with individual covariates.

Why it's important

This paper has been absolutely fundamental to our thinking about models for survival problems. It provided a unifying concept for building models and a wealth of fertile new ideas for developing a whole range of models for life events. It continues to be the mainstay for detailed analyses of problems involving survival analysis and the framework developed in this paper has formed a foundation for much subsequent development. Subsequent work developed far reaching models using counting process models and Martingale methods.

Strengths

1. This paper provided a rich structural model that unified previous work and gave a foundation for future developments.
2. It provided a flexible, robust method for comparing treatments when individual covariates need to be accommodated, and censoring is present.

Weakness

It relies on the proportional hazards assumption, which is not always appropriate.

Relevance

This continues to be the standard method of analysis of survival data with covariates. It provides flexible framework for modelling failure processes.

Paper 7

Design and analysis of randomized clinical trials requiring prolonged observation of each patient

Authors

Peto R, Pike MC, Armitage P, *et al.*

References

British Journal of Cancer 1976; **34**:585–612 (Part I. Introduction and design); *British Journal of Cancer* 1977; **35**:1–39 (Part II. Analysis and examples)

Summary

This was a very influential paper which provided much practical advice about the design, conduct and analysis of clinical trials. It had a major impact on the introduction of life-table methods into clinical trials and the use of the logrank (Mantel–Haenszel) test statistic.

Related reference   (1)   Bradford Hill A. *Principles of Medical Statistics*, 3rd edn. London: The Lancet, 1942; 12th edn (with ID Hill). London: Edward Arnold, 1991.

Key message

For studies of survival or recurrence, conduct large randomized trials and analyse them by life-table methods without any exclusions.

Why it's important

This was a key translational paper that explained the importance of using modern methods in clinical trial analysis. The paper was accessible to non-specialists, and the detailed description and worked examples helped clinicians to feel comfortable with the new techniques. A range of practical issues and pragmatic questions were dealt with, and statistical issues in both design and analysis were discussed. The importance of large trials that could detect moderate differences, as opposed to the then current trials that only had adequate power for unrealistic large treatment effects, was made clear. Also the now well established requirement to include all randomized patients in the main analysis without exclusions, and the dangers of early stopping for marginally significant apparent treatment differences, were very clearly explained.

Strengths

1. This was a widely accessible paper promoting good practice in clinical trials.
2. It provided an enormous stimulus to conduct large simple trials.

Weakness

It was somewhat dogmatic and occasionally hindered acceptance of other appropriate methods of analysis.

Relevance

This was a key paper in promoting and explaining modern clinical trial methods to clinicians.

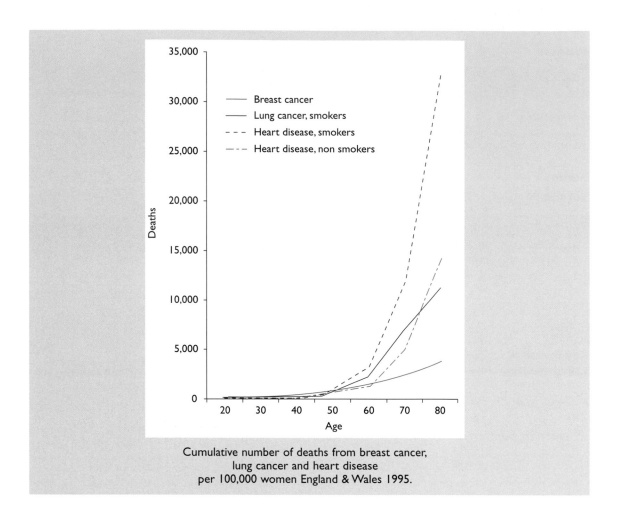

Cumulative number of deaths from breast cancer,
lung cancer and heart disease
per 100,000 women England & Wales 1995.

Paper 8

Estimation of the duration of a pre-clinical disease state using screening data

Authors

Walter SD, Day NE

Reference

American Journal of Epidemiology 1983; **118**:865–886

Summary

This paper developed a robust model based on the length of the pre-clinical state and the sensitivity of the screening test. The model used data on the detection rate of cancer at each screen, and the rate of interval cancers. The key model parameters were the screening sensitivity and the incidence rate of (symptomic) disease in the absence of screening. A distinction was made between the prevalent (first) screening test and subsequent (incident) tests. This leads to estimates of lead-time bias and length bias. The data from the first breast cancer screening trial (HIP, New York) were used to illustrate the method. When an exponential model was used, the sensitivity was estimated to be 82% and the mean lead time was 1.71 years in this trial.

Related references (1) Tabar L, Fagerberg CG, Gad A, *et al.* Reduction in mortality from breast cancer after mass screening with mammography: randomised trial from the Breast Cancer Screening Working Group of the Swedish National Board of Health and Welfare. *Lancet* 1985; **i**:829–832.

(2) Nystrom L, Rutqvist LE, Walls S, *et al.* Breast cancer screening with mammography: overview of Swedish randomised trials. *Lancet* 1993; **341**:973–978.

(3) Zelen M, Feinleib M. On the theory of screening for chronic diseases. *Biometrika* 1969; **56**:601–613.

Key message

Useful models for breast screening must include allowance for test sensitivity and must separately analyse cancers found on the prevalence screen, incidence screen, and those interval cancers found between screens.

Why it's important

Several previous papers on screening had been published based on renewal theory ideas. This paper provided a more realistic model by also including screening sensitivity into the model. Subsequent papers have refined and developed this approach, but the same basic model is used. A robust model for the results of an intervention on breast cancer natural history allowed one to use the results of screening trials not only to estimate mortality reduction, but also to study the effect of changes to the screening parameter such as interval between screens, age at starting and stopping, sensitivity, etc. on the programme effectiveness.

Strengths

1. A unified framework was provided for dealing with test sensitivity and lead-time bias.
2. It was simple enough to estimate screening parameters from readily available data.

Weakness

It did not deal with age-dependent screening sensitivity or other factors affecting sensitivity, such as radiographically dense breasts.

Paper 9

Overview of randomized trials of postoperative adjuvant radiotherapy in breast cancer

Authors

Cuzick J, Stewart H, Peto R, *et al.*

Reference

Cancer Treatment Reports 1987; **71**:15–29

Summary

This was the first overview of randomized trials in which individual patient information was collected and updated. Previously, reviews relied on published data, but here the trialists all collaborated in updating their databases so that a unified central analysis of all the data could be undertaken. The results proved surprising, and highlighted the existence of a late non-cancer mortality effect associated with radiation. Subsequent reports have identified this to be cardiovascular disease associated with the radiation field, but they also have suggested a balancing benefit in terms of reduced breast cancer mortality, especially for node positive tumours.

Related references **(1)** Cuzick J, Stewart H, Rutqvist L, Houghton J, Edwards R, *et al.* Cause-specific mortality in long term survivors of breast cancer who participated in trials of radiotherapy. *Journal of Clinical Oncology* 1994; **12**:447–453.

(2) EBCTCG. Favourable and unfavourable effects on long-term survival of radiotherapy for early breast cancer: an overview of the randomised trials. *Lancet* 2000; **355**:1757–1770.

Key message

There are late mortality effects of radiotherapy and associated with the irradiation of cardiac tissue and the major vessels.

Why it's important

This paper was important both for methodologic and subject-related reasons. Methodologically, it established the feasibility and importance of overviews using individual patient data. The importance of analysing results from all randomized patients in all relevant trials without exclusion was emphasized, and the use of the stratified logrank test to combine trials was established. The importance of large numbers and long-term follow-up was illustrated by the clear demonstration of unexpected late mortality in these trials.

Strengths

1. This was the first cancer overview using individual patient data.
2. The importance of large numbers and long-term follow-up was established.
3. The late side-effects of radiotherapy were established.

Weaknesses

1. Detailed causes of late mortality were not given. (This was done in a subsequent publication.)
2. Long-term effects always relate to treatments used many years ago, and may not be relevant to new treatments. This is especially important for breast cancer, where radiotherapy, surgery and adjuvant therapy have all changed markedly.

Relevance

Overviews have become the standard for evaluating new treatments subject to trial by several groups. With the advent of breast conserving surgery, radiotherapy is now being used more for good prognosis patients, where late mortality from cardiovascular disease is a particularly serious side effect. It is still unclear as to whether newer techniques can minimize this outcome.

Paper 10

A quality-of-life oriented endpoint for comparing therapies

Authors

Gelber RD, Gelman RS, Goldhirsch A

Reference

Biometrics 1989; **45**:781–795

Summary

A new endpoint for clinical trials, the time without symptoms of disease (TWiST), was defined and heralded the integration of quality-of-life into primary endpoints for clinical trials. This is particularly important for evaluating therapies which lead to only small survival differences, but have markedly different toxicities. The method consisted of subtracting time with toxicity from time to relapse in making comparisons. Subsequent work looked at survival (Goldhirsch *et al.* 1989) and gave non-zero coefficients (in fact 0.5 in this paper) to the toxicity time and also the time after relapse when making comparisons. This led to the so-called Q-TWiST analysis. Actuarial methods were extended to analyse this type of data.

Related references **(1)** Goldhirsch A, Gelber RD, Simes RJ, Glasziou P, and Coates AS. Costs and benefits of adjuvant therapy in breast cancer: a quality-adjusted survival analysis. *Journal of Clinical Oncology* 1989; 7:36–44.

(2) Gelber RD, Cole BF, Goldhirsch A, *et al.* Adjuvant chemotherapy plus tamoxifen compared with tamoxifen alone for postmenopausal breast cancer: meta-analysis of quality-adjusted survival. *Lancet* 1996; **347**:1066–1071.

(3) Gelber RD, Goldhirsch A. A new endpoint for the assessment of adjuvant therapy in post-menopausal women with operable breast cancer. *Journal of Clinical Oncology* 1986; **4**:1772–1779.

Key message

Time with toxicity or symptoms should be discounted when comparing treatments.

Why it's important

This paper provided a method for integrating quality of life measures into the overall evaluation of a treatment. Weight factors are unavoidably subjective, but for any given set of weights a trade-off analysis could be done to determine under what conditions one treatment is superior to another. If one treatment is superior for all weights, then it is clearly better; whereas if not, subjective decisions about trade-offs between time with symptoms and increased overall survival need to be made.

Strengths

1. This paper created a way of putting quality-of-life data on the same footing as recurrence and survival data.
2. 'Equivalence trials' with small expected differences in survival can be further analysed using Q-TWiST.

Weakness

The weighing of the 'quality of life' for different disease states is subjective and universal weights cannot be agreed.

Relevance

Many toxic treatments provide only small gain in life expectancy. Evaluating both length and quality-of-life remains an important issue.

Paper 12

Treatment of early breast cancer: worldwide evidence 1985–1990

Authors

Early Breast Cancer Trialists Collaborative Group

Reference

Treatment of Early Breast Cancer, Vol 1: *Worldwide Evidence 1985–1990*. Oxford: Oxford University Press, 1990

Summary

This was a major worldwide effort involving 61 trials and almost 30,000 randomized women. It demonstrated the power and importance of collecting individual patient information on all the randomized trials worldwide related to a specific question. A detailed methodologic section provided a widely accessible description of and justification for overviews and dealt with issues about combining similar but not identical trials, and the need for large numbers to reliably detect moderate but important differences. Use of the 'forest plot' to graphically summarize the results of similar trials was introduced. The paper was particularly important in increasing the use of tamoxifen in early breast cancer which has led to worldwide improvements in survival.

Related references

(1) Systemic treatment of early breast cancer by hormonal, cytotoxic, or immune therapy – Part I. *The Lancet* 1992; **339**:1–15. Part II. *The Lancet* 1992; **339**:71–85.

(2) EBCTCG. Tamoxifen for early breast cancer: an overview of the randomised trials. *The Lancet* 1998; **351**:1451–1467.

Key message

Overviews are needed to properly review all of the evidence on treatment question. Clear benefits of both tamoxifen and chemotherapy were established.

Why it's important

This paper established a clear statistical foundation for conducting overviews in terms of the stratified logrank statistic. A detailed justification for combining similar but non-identical trials was given in a widely accessible manner. The associated data collection activity also created a framework in which collaborators were prepared to contribute their data on an ongoing basis to a central group, who synthesized it and produced a combined analysis which was extensively discussed. This activity has now become almost routine and has resulted in a much more rapid appreciation of the value of the different treatments used in breast cancer. The widespread collaboration in the projects has also led to more rapid implementation of the findings.

Strengths

1. Large numbers give reliable results on important clinical questions.
2. There was collaborative activity to review *all* randomized evidence on a particular question.

Weakness

The process was limited to data that was already available for most trials, so only major endpoints and factors could be studied.

Relevance

This approach has become a standard activity in breast cancer and forms a quinquennial focus for discussing the value of available treatments.

Paper 13

Linkage of early-onset familial breast cancer to chromosome 17q21

Authors

Hall JM, Lee MK, Newman B, *et al.*

Reference

Science 1990; **250**:1684–1689

Summary

Linkage analysis was used to pinpoint the first breast cancer gene (*BRCA1*) on chromosome 17q21. A total of 146 cases of breast cancer from 23 extended families were studied by linkage analysis of 183 polymorphic markers. LOD scores (logarithms of odds ratios) were calculated using a multi-locus autosomal-dominant model, and strong linkage (10^6:1) for a highly polymorphic marker (D17S74) on chromosome 17q was found for early-onset families. In contrast, no increased risk was associated with this marker in late-onset families, indicating heterogeneity of risk and the likely existence of other breast cancer genes. Subsequent work led to the discovery of the first breast cancer gene (*BRCA1*).

Related references (1)   Easton DF, Bishop DT, Ford D, Crockford GP, and the Breast Cancer Linkage Consortium. Genetic linkage analysis in familial breast and ovarian cancer: results from 214 families. *American Journal of Human Genetics* 1993; **52**:678–701.
(2)   Ford D, Easton DF, Peto J. Estimates of the gene frequency of *BRCA1* and its contribution to breast and ovarian cancer incidence. *American Journal of Human Genetics* 1995; **57**:1457–1462.
(3)   Miki Y, Swensen J, Shattuck-Eidens D *et al.* Isolation of *BRCA1*, the 17q-linked breast and ovarian cancer susceptibility gene. *Science* 1994; **266**:66–71.

Key message

Statistical analysis of genetic data from breast cancer families pinpointed the location of the first breast cancer gene.

Why it's important

This was the first paper to clearly pinpoint the location of a gene associated with breast cancer. The gene was found a few years afterwards. Similar methods were used to locate a second breast cancer gene.

Strengths

1. Linkage analysis can be used even when the gene in question is unknown.
2. The method makes maximum use of complex family data from multiple loci.
3. This is an important first-line screening method for gene discovery.

Weaknesses

1. It is only really useful for highly penetrant genes.
2. It is typically only possible to localize genes to within about 10^6 base pairs, so considerable additional work is needed to find the gene.

Relevance

The multipoint linkage analysis method continues to be an important standard method in localizing highly penetrant genes that segregate with disease. The availability of markers that span the full genome makes this a standard gene hunting method.

CHAPTER 3

Epidemiology

KLIM McPHERSON

Introduction

The epidemiology of breast cancer is largely hormonal – although the precise meaning that this may have is uncertain! Since the relationship is highly complex and important and since hormonal contraception quickly became, in the 1960s, a vital component of the further emancipation of women the relationship of oral contraception with breast cancer risk is important for women, for public health and of course for understanding how to prevent the disease. In terms of the epidemiology of breast cancer this question had dominated research into its aetiology. It is a reflection of the complexity – both social and scientific – that we still know relatively little about preventing breast cancer although, of course, the selective estrogen receptor modulators (SERMs) seem to offer some considerable hope. The complexity of the relationships is profound and the determinants of epidemiological effort somewhat obscure. In the end epidemiology must take a perspective that invokes the whole life course of different exposures and different host characteristics. To imagine, as is the prevailing tendency, that exposures do or don't cause disease through life – is pathologically naïve.

Breast cancer remains enigmatic and the role of oral contraceptives relatively uncertain. However, it is simply too early to know the real relationship from the vast natural experiments of widespread effective contraception. The problem is that learning from them is possibly too confounded with the varied implications of the outcome. It is clear that while mortality is falling quite dramatically in many countries, including the UK, incidence among those women not old enough to be part of the screening programme is rising.

References

[1] Cummings SR, Eckert S, Krueger K, *et al.* The effect of raloxifene on the risk of breast cancer in post menopausal women: results from the MORE randomised trial. *Journal of the American Medical Association* 1999; **281**:2189–2197.

[2] Peto R, Borham J, Clarke, *et al.* UK and USA breast cancer deaths down 35% in year 2000 at ages 20–69 years. *Lancet* 2000, **355**:1822.

Paper 1

Evaluation of rare adverse effects of systemic contraceptives

Authors

Doll R, Vessey M

Reference

British Medical Bulletin, 1970; **26**:33–38

Summary

The introduction of oral contraception presented the medical profession with a new problem, in that it involves the prescription of highly potent drugs for healthy young people over prolonged periods. In some ways, the problem is comparable to that created by the use of alcohol, tobacco and marihuana, save that these substances are taken without medical prescription and the responsibility of the profession in relation to them is limited to defining their effects and suggesting how they can be controlled. The oral contraceptives, by contrast, are generally available only on prescription, and alternative methods of contraception exist, some of which are without risk, though they are less certainly effective in preventing pregnancy. When the hazards of pregnancy are slight, methods of contraception need to be extremely safe, and serious reactions give rise to concerns, even when they are very uncommon.

Jones and Malden (related reference 1) estimated that in mid-1967 about 13 million women around the world were using oral contraceptives, and the number has increased rapidly since then. Every type of disease that occurs normally among adult women must, therefore, be expected to occur among women who are taking oral contraceptives and it is not surprising that many reports of illnesses that are presumed to be adverse reactions to oral contraceptives have been published in the medical literature.

This paper alludes to the possibility that causes of important disease like (breast) cancer can act at a very early stage in their progression and that this can take as long as 30 years. Therefore, they mention the fact that while an exposure like oral contraception may not seem to affect cancer risk immediately after use is completed, that does not mean that the risk will not be altered some time (they say 10–15 years) later. For some reason, those responsible for evaluating the safety of drugs like oral contraceptives seem to be oblivious of this point. Yet it is absolutely crucial when there are good reasons to suspect initiation or speeding up the initiation processes. Clearly, the uncertainties that come from its recognition and understanding are most unsettling – particularly for those engaged in reducing unwanted pregnancies.

Related references (1) Jones GW, Malden WP. *Studies in Family Planning* 1967; **24**:1.
(2) Skegg D. Pitfalls of pharmacoepidemiology. *British Medical Journal* 2000; **321**:1171–1172.

Key message

The particular problems associated with studying the consequences of, particularly hormonal, contraception, are complex in some respects and straightforward in others. Since the confounding with risk factors will generally be difficult to disentangle and patterns of use are likely to change with age and time, the pertinent exposure will be changing but at least the dosages will be commonly recorded and the compliance with stated doses will also be reliable. But pharmacovigilance, in this case, will not be straightforward.

Why it's important

This paper presents a perceptive analysis of the contemporary epidemiological problems associated with assessing the safety of oral contraceptives, commonly ignored in practice.

Strength

This was a profound study, written by leading epidemiologists who were concerned with the major health issues of the time – oral contraceptives and jaundice, venous and pulmonary thromboembolism, and ischaemic heart disease. It is essential to understand the particular and specific problems associated with designating a particular exposure as a putative risk factor. All interpretations of epidemiology depend on this understanding, particularly of negative studies.

Weakness

There was a tendency to understate what is now known about the possible length of the process between initiation and diagnosis of cancer. Indeed breast cancer is not mentioned at all, which was odd, because ever since oral contraceptives were introduced the possibility of any relationship was universally held to be serious.

Relevance

In terms of interpreting the epidemiology of the association of 'systemic' contraception and disease this is clearly a comprehensive and profound study but oddly limited by its time.

Paper 2

Age at first birth and breast cancer risk

Authors

MacMahon B, Cole P, Lin TM, *et al.*

Reference

Bulletin of the WHO 1970; **43**:209–221

Summary

An international collaborative study of breast cancer and reproductive experience was carried out in seven areas of the world. In all areas studied, a striking relation between age at first birth and breast cancer risk was observed. It was estimated that women having their first child when aged under 18 years have only above one-third the breast cancer risk of those whose first birth is delayed until the age of 35 years or more. Births after the first, even if they occur at an early age, have no, or very little, protective effect. The reduced risk of breast cancer in women having their first child at an early age explains the previously observed inverse relationship between total parity and breast cancer risk, since women having their first birth early tend to become ultimately of high parity. The association with age at first birth requires different kinds of aetiological hypotheses from those that have been invoked in the past to explain the association between breast cancer risk and reproductive experience. Almost all subsequent work on breast cancer aetiology cites this or derivative publications.

Related reference   (1)   Pike MC, Spicer DV, Dahmoush L, Press MF. Estrogens, progestogens, normal breast cell proliferation and breast cancer risk. *Epidemiological Reviews* 1993; **15**:17–35.

This summarises more recent evidence about the complexity of the relationship with age at first birth pointing out that the protective effect of early birth is not apparent until age 40, but few authors point to the possibility of effect modification of first pregnancy.

Key message

This was a seminal paper in the understanding of the epidemiology of breast cancer. Many studies had investigated the role of early reproductive factors in the risk of disease and had come to conflicting conclusions. In particular, lactation was thought to be protective on the basis of considerable evidence. This paper, by assiduous collection of data from many sources, was able to identify with some reliability the role of the first term pregnancy in altering the risk of breast cancer. Thus the now familiar three-fold increase in risk associated with a late first pregnancy was established. The total duration or lactation as a protective factor was seen to be a consequence of confounding with early pregnancy. Clearly any other putative risk factor needs not to be associated with age at first pregnancy for confounding not to be a plausible cause of any association.

Why it's important

This work consolidated an important role for reproductive factors in breast cancer aetiology.

Strength

There was an intelligent use of many sources of data to extract a clear relationship.

Weakness

This may be possibly seen by modern standards to be a rather cavalier use of meta-analytic methods.

Relevance

This study provided clarity to a confused situation for the aetiology of breast cancer. The determination of a risk factor is important – but more important may be that by thus understanding a mechanism a strong clue about effect modification is obtained.

Paper 3

Cancer risk as related to use of oral contraceptives during fertile years

Authors

Paffenbarger R, Fasal E, Simmons M, *et al.*

Reference

Cancer 1977; **39**:1887–1891

Summary

A case–control study of 452 breast cancer patients, aged less than 50 years, and 872 age-, race-, and religion-matched control patients generated relative risk estimates of breast cancer associated with oral contraceptive practices. The relative risk of breast cancer from ever-use of oral contraceptives was 1.1, not significant. Relative risks did not differ by age, interval since first use, interval since last use, or time periods in which steroid compounds differed in composition and potency. However, the relative risks of breast cancer from current use, from 2 to 4 years of ever-use, from 6 or more years of use by women with prior benign breast disease, and from use before first childbirth were increased significantly. The findings suggested that the malignant process may be quickened if transformed cells are present during oral contraceptive use. Yet, the findings did not indicate that oral contraception induces breast cancer nor did they exonerate female steroid hormones. They did encourage continued surveillance of steroid contraception for cancer induction or promotion. The authors argued that, in addition to duration of oral contraceptive use and other measures of dose response, future observations should pay especial attention to use by women before first childbirth and by women with already established benign breast disease.

Related references

(1)   Bone, M. *The Family Planning Services: Changes and Effects*. London: HMSO, 1979.

(2)   McPherson K, Vessey MP, Neil A, Doll R, Jones L, Roberts M. Early oral contraceptive use and breast cancer: results of another case–control study. *British Journal of Cancer* 1987; **56**:653–660.

Key message

This study generated the hypothesis that oral contraceptive use could have an effect on breast cancer when used before first pregnancy at a time when such use was relatively uncommon. The authors reported an apparent increased risk, for ever-use of oral contraceptives, of around three-fold. They postulated sensible mechanisms and alerted the public to the possibility that early oral contraceptive use may uniquely increase breast cancer risk. By the late 1970s prolonged oral contraceptive use by young, unmarried and nulliparous women was rapidly becoming the norm.

Why it's important

A possible epidemiological association is found for which a plausible mechanism exists.

Strength

This is the first paper to suggest a clear link between the use of oral contraceptives and breast cancer risk

Weakness

This was clearly largely a data-derived hypothesis, based on a small study.

Relevance

A key hypothesis arose from basic understanding of the possible biological processes. 'The data presented here shed little new light on whether or how oral contraceptives may be carcinogenic, but neither do they clear these drugs of complicity.' The authors go on to say: 'And on the basis of very limited observation, we must ask whether it is wise for young women to use oral contraceptives to defer their first childbirth.' A commendably modest, but possibly germane, conclusion.

Paper 4

Malignant breast tumours among atomic bomb survivors: Hiroshima and Nagasaki

Authors

Tokunaga M, Norman JE, Agano M

Reference

Journal of the National Cancer Institute 1979; **62**:1347–1359

Summary

For 1950–74, 360 cases of malignant breast tumors were identified among the 63 000 females of the Radiation Effects Research Foundation's (Hiroshima and Nagasaki) Extended Life-Span Study sample of survivors of the 1945 atomic bombings of Hiroshima and Nagasaki; 288 of these females were residing in one of these two cities at the time of bombing. Two-thirds of all cases were classified as breast cancers on the basis of microscopic review of slides, and 108 cases received an estimated breast tissue dose of at least 10 rad. The number of cases of radiogenic breast cancer could be well estimated by a linear function of radiation dose for tissue doses below 200 rad. Excess risk estimates, based on this function, from women 10–19, 20–29, 30–39, and 50 years old or older at the time of bombing were 7.3, 4.2, 2.6, and 4.7 cases per million women per year per rad, respectively. Women irradiated in their forties showed no dose effect. Among all women who received at least 10 rad, those irradiated before age 20 years will have experienced the highest rates of breast cancer throughout their lifetimes. Separated excess risk estimates for Hiroshima and Nagasaki did not differ significantly, which indicates that for radiogenic breast cancer the effects of neutrons were about equal. Radiation did not reduce the latency period from the development of breast cancer, which was at least 10 years. The distribution of histologic types of cancers did not vary significantly with radiation dose.

This study shows that irradiation before menarche confers a greater risk of breast cancer subsequently than after menarche and the effect is, as far as can be measured, dose related. Clearly, any effect of a breast carcinogen that is potent before menarche must work via some systemic route and must have a delayed effect on breast tissue yet to develop. In this case the effect is apparent 20 or 30 years after exposure among young women.

Related reference (1)

McGregor D, Land C, Choi K, *et al.* Breast cancer incidence among atomic bomb survivors, Hiroshima and Nagasaki, 1955–69. *Journal of the National Cancer Institute* 1997; **59**:799–811.

Key message

This study shows that breast cancer initiation is possible before breasts are formed, and certainly among developing breasts, and that the effects may not be apparent in terms of increased incidence for as long as 30 years later.

Why it's important

This paper illustrates and demonstrates that exposure to a known carcinogen, ionizing radiation, increases the risk of breast cancer. However, the major finding is that it does so in a manner in which exposure at a young age has a dose-related increased risk of breast cancer which is more potent than later exposure. Interestingly, the greatest potency manifest among girls age 10–19 at the time of the atomic bomb and among women aged 50+. Moreover, the increased risk among the young at time of exposure was delayed for 20 years, before which no increase was apparent.

Strength

This was an assiduous and careful analysis of a horrendous 'natural' experiment on two devastated communities which led to fairly unambiguous conclusions.

Weakness

Reliable dosage determination was clearly problematic.

Relevance

We understand much better the effect of ionizing radiation on breast cancer induction and that early exposure, even before puberty, are important in the aetiology.

Paper 5

Breast cancer, pregnancy and the pill

Author

Drife JO

Reference

British Medical Journal 1981; **283**:778–779

Summary

The authors claim that there is no satisfactory explanation for the effect of pregnancy on the risk of breast cancer. Breast cancer is commoner among women who have never borne children than among parous women and the longer a woman delays her first pregnancy the more she increases her risk of developing the disease. It has been suggested that prolonged use of oral contraceptives before first full-term pregnancy may increase the risk of breast cancer, although after this pregnancy the risk is probably unaffected by taking the pill.

Clearly the first full-term pregnancy does something to alter a woman's risk of developing breast cancer. Before this pregnancy the breast is at greater risk of precancerous change: afterwards the risk diminishes. Whether or not a woman breast-feeds is probably irrelevant: so far as the breast is concerned the important thing is that a full-term pregnancy has occurred. There are three possible explanations for this. One is that a woman's hormonal state is permanently altered by her first pregnancy. This has been investigated but no consistent answer has emerged. A second possibility is that during the first pregnancy cells that have undergone precancerous change are destroyed, immunologically or otherwise. There is no evidence that this occurs, and indeed since pregnancy is period of increased immunological tolerance such a phenomenon seems unlikely. The third explanation is that the breast epithelium itself is permanently changed by pregnancy. There is good evidence that such a change occurs.

Related references	(1)	Drife JO, Mclelland DBL, Pryde A, Roberts M, Smith II. Immunoglobulin synthesis in the resting breast epithelium. *British Medical Journal* 1976; **2**:503–506.
	(2)	Pike MC, Henderson BE, Casagrande JT, Rosario I, Gray GE. Oral contraceptive use and early abortion as risk factors for breast cancer in young women. *British Journal of Cancer* 1981; **43**:72–76.

Key message

Drife's evidence came from studies of *in vitro* DNA synthesis in which he claimed to see no cyclical pattern among nulliparous women compared with a pronounced pattern among parous women, increasing in the luteal phase. Thus he postulated that the breast epithelium is rendered more capable of responding to circulating progesterone after the first birth. Before then, the epithelium cannot respond to the low concentrations present during the menstrual cycle, and hence Drife speculated on the possible connection between the use of oral contraceptives and the epidemiology.

Why it's important

Drife's postulate was that the breast epithelium was permanently changed by a term pregnancy. Drife goes on to speculate that oral contraception before first pregnancy might thus be effectively unopposed and hence that the effect of oral contraceptives before first pregnancy on breast cancer might therefore differ from a similar exposure after first pregnancy.

Strength

From a clinician who is a strong proponent of hormonal contraception, and from work in the laboratory, this speculative paper attempted to make biological sense of a recent paper from Pike and colleagues that purported to show a strong effect of the pill and other influences on hormonal milieu among young users on breast cancer risk.

Weakness

This paper attempted to tie too many loose ends with too little solid theory, but admittedly was speculative.

Relevance

It recognized, and described well, plausible mechanisms supported by laboratory work, clearly invoking a life-course mode of thinking.

Paper 6

Breast cancer in mothers given diethylstilbestrol in pregnancy

Authors

Greenberg ER, Barnes AB, Resseguie L, *et al.*

Reference

New England Journal of Medicine 1984; **311**:1393–1398

Summary

This reports a massive piece of work in the USA in which the incontinent use of the non-hormonal steroid diethylstilbestrol to prevent miscarriage in the 1950s was studied with respect to the long-term breast cancer risks on the mothers. (The daughters had been studied after a consequential and massive increase in the risk of adenocarcinoma of the vagina had become apparent quite quickly.) This study followed mothers, both given the drug and not given the drug during a pregnancy between 1940 and 1960, for 40 years. Such was the use of this drug in the practice styles of the time that it can be safely assumed that providers believed in its (ultimately shown to be ineffectual) effect on preventing miscarriage or they did not. Selection by intrinsic breast cancer risk seemed to be unimportant. But the risk of breast cancer was doubled among those exposed but not until 40 years after exposure. The period between exposure and 20 some years later is completely devoid of any excess risk among the exposed group. The possibility that such a profound, and unique, effect could be attributable to bias or confounding must be quite fanciful.

Related references	(1)	Herbst AL, Ulfender H, Poskanzer DC. Adenocarcinoma of the vagina: association of maternal stilbestrol therapy with tumor appearances in young women. *New England Journal of Medicine* 1971; **284**:878–881.
	(2)	Dieckmann WJ, Davies ME, Rynkiewicz LM *et al.* Does the administration of diethylstilbestrol during pregnancy have therapeutic value? *American Journal of Obstetrics and Gynecology* 1953; **66**:62–81.

Key message

Exposure to diethylstilbestrol while pregnant causes an increase in breast cancer, but the increase is not seen until 20 years after exposure.

Why it's important

Ionizing radiation is known to have a delayed effect on cancer incidence but is clearly carcinogenic or responsible for cancer initiation. Diethylstilbestrol on the other hand probably is not and therefore is more likely to have a promoting effect and hence not a long latent period associated with any effect on cancer. This work seems therefore to show that promoters might act during the initiation period by otherwise enhancing the possibility of initiation or very soon afterwards, and may thus also themselves be associated with a long latency.

Strength

Clearly this is the key study of the long-term effect of diethylstilbestrol on breast cancer.

Weakness

Confounding will always remain an implausible explanation for the finding.

Relevance

Large careful studies are capable of discerning complicated relationships between relatively unexpected exposures and breast cancer.

Paper 7

Oral contraception use influences resting breast proliferation

Authors

Anderson TJ, Battersby S, King RJ, *et al.*

Reference

Human Pathology 1989; **20**:1139–1140

Summary

The controversy surrounding oral contraceptive use and breast cancer risk arose from epidemiologic studies, yet the direct effect of such use on breast tissue remained undefined. Breast epithelial proliferation was assessed by [^{3}H]thymidine labelling of normal lobular units dissected from benign biopsies of 347 females aged 14–48 years. Factors shown to influence this response included cycle phase, time since menarche (breast age), and parity status. Multivariate analysis allowing for these influences was used to compare activity of natural cycles and those artificially regulated by oral contraceptives. The increased activity in nulliparous oral contraceptive users was highly significant ($p < 0.005$). Comparing the effect of differences in oral contraceptive type, whether combined, triphasic, progestin only, or according to oestrogen or progestin content, showed a heterogeneity in response that was significant ($p < 0.01$). Examined specifically, the formulation of oral contraceptive according to progestin content did not have a significant influence although progestin-only oral contraceptives were most active, while the influence of increasing oestrogen content was significant ($p < 0.05$). However, emphasis was placed on acknowledging the multiple factors and interactive processes responsible for breast epithelial stimulation when considering strategies or intervention.

Observational data on the mitotic activity of these samples from the resting breast thus demonstrated, when adjusting for breast age and phase of the menstrual cycle, that current oral contraceptive use is associated with a significant increase. This increase is, however, confined to nulliparous women, there being no effect among parous women. This effect appears to be related to the oestrogen dose of the pills.

Related references **(1)** Ferguson DJP, Anderson TJ. Morphological evaluation of cell turnover in relation to the menstrual cycle in the 'resting' human breast. *British Journal of Cancer* 1981; **44**:177–181.

(2) Thijssen JH. Oestrogen, progestins and breast proliferation. *Zentralblatt-Gynakologie* 1997; **119**(Suppl 2):43–47.

(3) Jerstrom HCB. Effects of oral contraception on endogenous hormones, body constitution, and breast epithelium in healthy young women. Thesis: the Jubileum Institute, Dept Oncology, Lund University, Sweden, 1989.

Key messages

This work demonstrates that mitotic activity in the breast epithelium is clearly cyclical, with higher rates in the luteal phase both for natural cycles and oral contraceptive cycles – in direct contrast to the endometrium. But also that oral contraceptive cycles have an important effect on the breast epithelium of nulliparous women.

Why it's important

Tom Anderson's work on the proliferation of resting breast tissue tells us more about Drife's hypothesis. Interestingly, the higher mitotic activity, adjusting for the menstrual phase of the sampling, associated with oral contraceptive use was confined to nulliparous women. This oral contraceptive effect was demonstrably higher for higher doses of oestrogen in the pills, although the progesterone dose was not significant. The interaction of nulliparity was highly significant. Increased mitotic activity gives rise to plausible co-initiation properties of oral contraceptives, which are themselves unlikely to be initiators *per se*.

Strength

This was the largest systematic analysis of a sample of normal breast tissue in which detailed assessment of exogenous exposure to hormones on breast tissue can be related to cycle, breast age and obstetric events.

Weakness

Sample size was quite small and the number of relevant exposure variables large. It is possible that the breast sample tissues were taken from a non-representative group of women.

Relevance

If breast carcinogenesis is related to the mitotic activity, due to the greater opportunity for carcinogenesis, of the resting breast then these observations may prove to be of profound significance.

Paper 8

Is the CASH study really negative?

Author

Peto J

Reference

Lancet 1989; **i**:552

Summary

The results of the very large Cancer and Steroid Hormone Group (CASH) case–control study of breast cancer were widely regarded as providing strong evidence against the conclusions of several other studies that had produced evidence of a significant increase in breast cancer among young women who had used oral contraceptives. For example, the CASH researchers had stated that their results 'suggest that use of oral contraceptives by young women in the United States has no effect on the aggregate risk of breast cancer before 45 years of age'.

By amalgamating existing published tabulations from the massive CASH study, Peto demonstrated that the data seemed to indicate a strong association for oral contraceptive use before first pregnancy and breast cancer risk – which was not the interpretation of the study authors.

Related references   (1)   Stadel BV, Lai S, Schlesslman JJ, Murray P. Oral contraception and pre-menopausal breast cancer in nulliparous women. *Contraception* 1988; **38**:287–299.

(2)   Stadel BV. Oral contraception and breast cancer. *Lancet* 1989; **i**:1267–1268.

(3)   Wingo PA, Lee NC, Ory HW *et al.* Oral contraceptives and the risk of breast cancer [discussion]. In: Mann RD (ed.) Oral Contraceptives and breast cancer, Chapter 4 Carnforth UK: Parthenon Publishing; 1990. pp. 79–84.

Key message

The conclusions drawn by investigators or large epidemiological studies may be other than what their data suggest. The astonishing aspect of this is that the then Chair of the Committee on Safety of Medicine stated that Stadel was unable to confirm Peto's re-analysis (related reference 2). The estimated relative risks were actually identical (with a significant trend) in every exposure cell except the longest (12 years use), for which Peto estimated 1.8 and Stadel, on his own data, estimated 2.7. Such is the relationship of epidemiology with policy.

Why it's important

The classical USA case–control study by the CASH group was easily the largest ever conducted investigating the effect of oral contraceptives on breast cancer. Repeated publications sought to demonstrate no important association of oral contraceptive use with breast cancer in these data. In particular the possibility of a delayed effect of early oral contraceptive use was rarely properly investigated, in part because use of oral contraceptives will nulliparous was rare at the time the cases and controls were themselves nulliparous.

Strength

This was a clever, daring and cheeky analysis of the published data from other people's study. The qualitative interpretation of this paper was subsequently completely confirmed in an apparent denial by the CASH team. This interpretation has never been refuted from a study cited many times as entirely negative.

Weakness

This was clearly a derivative publication based only on published tabulations.

Relevance

The social importance of this observation was clearly profound because by now effective contraception among the young relied on long-term prescription of oral contraceptives. None the less, this letter is rarely cited.

Paper 9

Oral contraceptive and breast cancer. A meta-analysis

Authors

Delgado-Rodriguez M, Sillero Arenas M, Rodriguez-Contreras R, *et al.*

Reference

Revue Epidemiologique Sante Publique 1991; **39**:165–181

Summary

Since the relationship between oral contraceptive use and breast cancer had not been consistent, the authors undertook a meta-analysis of studies published to date. Papers were located by searching the MEDLINE database, supplemented by a hand search of all the references in the articles recovered. Studies were graded as to quality. Those judged as probably unbiased were included in the analysis. The method of Woolf was used to combine relative risks. Forty-seven studies were collected: 40 case–control and 7 cohort studies. Thirty-nine of these were considered unbiased. The main results observed were that the relative risk was 1.06 (1.02–1.10) for all studies and 1.14 for premenopausal cancer. For premenopausal cancer, higher relative risks were observed in women who early used oral contraceptive with a significant linear dose–response effect: 1/25 (1.10–1.44) in oral contraceptive users before age 25, and 1.17 (1.06–1.30) in users before the first full-term pregnancy. The authors concluded that oral contraceptive use may be a risk factor for premenopausal breast cancer.

This fearless first meta-analysis found that premenopausal breast cancer was not affected by ever use of oral contraceptives but use before age 25 appeared to be associated with an increase in risk according to duration of use. Subsequent analysis of the same data set confirmed a similar (correlated) effect of oral contraceptive use before first-term pregnancy.

Key message

Oral contraceptive use may have a particular detrimental effect on breast cancer risk, depending on when used as well as for how long.

Why it's important

This was one of the first attempts to perform a meta-analysis of the entire epidemiology of the relationship between oral contraceptives and breast cancer.

Strength

It was perceptive and bold.

Weakness

This analysis was not based on individual data from all the studies but on summary statistics.

Relevance

Notwithstanding the prevailing view that oral contraceptives had no relationship with breast cancer risk, these analyses based on almost all of the research suggested otherwise.

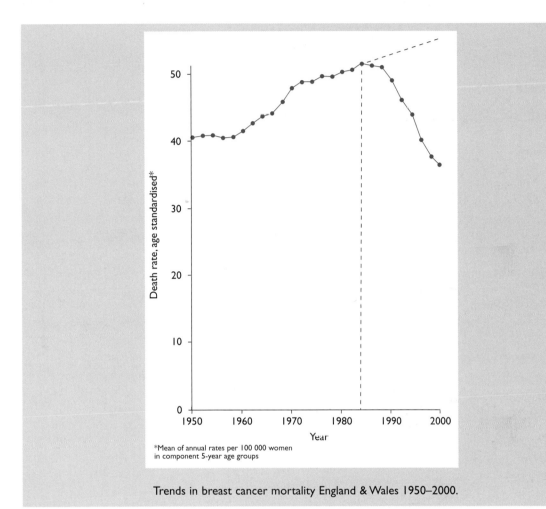

*Mean of annual rates per 100 000 women
in component 5-year age groups

Trends in breast cancer mortality England & Wales 1950–2000.

Paper 10

Latent effects in the interpretation of any association between oral contraceptives and breast cancer

Author

McPherson K

Reference

In: *Benign Breast Disease* (Mansel RE, ed). Carnforth, UK: Parthenon, 1994

Summary

This paper tried to link the epidemiology with the biology of contemporary oral contraceptive use patterns. Basically, it pointed out, on the basis of computer simulations, that plausible mechanisms might give rise to epidemiological results that underestimate the true effect until well into the twenty-first century.

Related references (1)   McPherson K, Coope PA, Vessey MP. Early oral contraceptive use and breast cancer: theoretical effects of latency. *Journal of Epidemiology and Community Health* 1986; **40**:289–294.
(2)   Rothman KJ. Induction and latent periods. *American Journal of Epidemiology* 1981; **114**:235–239.

Key message

Since, until sufficient time has elapsed, the main problem will be the paucity of relevant data, it is as well to understand the power against these hypotheses, and the precision of current studies.

Strength

This paper was speculative and wide ranging.

Weakness

The paper is purely theoretical; it does not advance the substantive knowledge base, only consolidates the uncertainty.

Relevance

This paper reports the results of computer simulations in which the effect on the epidemiology is quantified with respect to calendar time, should there be a delayed effect of early use consequent upon a possible co-initiating effect. Data on the prevalence of prolonged use before first pregnancy was shown to be strongly related to calendar time and plausible delays in any attributable effect implied that current epidemiological estimates of effect, which do not take latency into account might thus be seriously attenuated. The implications therefore on the interpretation of, for example, the above meta-analysis, and certainly the CASH study, would be that the estimated relative risks may be conservative, once follow-up can be as long as (say) 40 years after exposure.

Paper 11

Breast cancer and hormonal contraception: Further results

Authors

Collaborative Group on Hormonal Factors in Breast Cancer

Reference

Contraception 1996: **54**(Suppl 3):1S–106S

Summary

The Collaborative Group on Hormonal Factors in Breast Cancer brought together and reanalysed the world-wide epidemiological evidence on breast cancer risk and use of hormonal contraceptives. Original data from 54 studies, representing about 90% of the information available on the topic, were collected, checked and analysed centrally. The 54 studies were performed in 26 countries and included a total of 53 297 women with breast cancer and 100 239 women without breast cancer. The studies were varied in their design, setting and timing. Most information came from case–control studies with controls chosen from the general population; most women resided in Europe or North America and most cancers were diagnosed during the 1980s. Overall 41% of the women with breast cancer and 40% of the women without breast cancer had used oral contraceptives at some time; the median age at first use was 26 years, the median duration of use was 3 years, the median year of first use was 1968, the median time since first use was 16 years, and the median time since last use was 9 years.

The main findings, summarized elsewhere (related reference 1), were that there is a small increase in the risk of having breast cancer diagnosed in current users of combined oral contraceptives and in women who had stopped use in the past 10 years but that there was no evidence of an increase in the risk more than 10 years after stopping use. In addition, the cancers diagnosed in women who had used oral contraceptives tended to be less advanced clinically than the cancers diagnosed in women who had not used them.

Despite the large number of possibilities investigated, few factors appeared to modify the main findings either in recent or in past users. For recent users who began use before age 10 the relative risks were higher than for recent users who began at older ages. For women whose use of oral contraceptives ceased more than 10 years before, there was some suggestion of a reduction in breast cancer risk in certain subgroups, with a deficit of tumours that had spread beyond the breast, especially among women who had used preparations containing the highest doses of oestrogen and progestogen. These findings were unexpected.

Although these data represented most of the epidemiological evidence then available on the topic, there was still insufficient information to comment reliably about the effects of specific types of oestrogen or of progestogen. What evidence there was suggested, however, no major difference in the effects for specific types of oestrogen or of progestogen and that the pattern of risk associated with use of hormonal contraceptives containing progestogens alone might be similar to that observed for preparations containing both oestrogens and progestogens.

On the basis of these results, there appeared to be little difference between women who had and had not used combined oral contraceptives in terms of the estimated cumulative number of breast cancers diagnosed during the period from starting use up to 20 years after stopping. The cancers diagnosed in women who had used oral contraceptives were, however, less advanced clinically than the cancers diagnosed in never users.

Related references **(1)** Collaborative Group on Hormonal factors on breast cancer. Breast cancer and hormonal contraceptive. *The Lancet* 1996; **347**:1713–1727.

(2) McPherson K. Type 3 Errors, pill scares, and the epidemiology of oral contraception and health. *Journal of Epidemiology and Community Health* 1999; **53**:258–260.

(3) Collaborative Group on Hormonal Factors in Breast Cancer. Familial breast cancer: collaborative reanalysis of individual data from 52 epidemiological studies including 58,209 women with breast cancer and 101,986 women without the disease. *Lancet* 2001; **358**:1389–1399.

(4) Collaborative Group on Hormonal Factors in Breast Cancer. Breast Cancer and breastfeeding: collaborative reanalysis of individual data from 47 epidemiological studies in 30 countries including 50,302 women with breast cancer and 96,973 without the disease. *Lancet* 2002; **360**;187–195.

Key message

This overview, easily the most comprehensive of its kind, finds small and short-term effects of oral contraceptive use on breast cancer risk. Whether the use of oral contraceptives among young women may have an important effect more than 20 years after stopping use is left open.

Why it's important

Any comprehensive overview of virtually all the data in the world – analysed on an individual basis in the way this was – must be of unrivalled relevance to the question examined.

Strength

This study was massive and involved the active collaboration of essentially everyone involved in investigating this question. The analyses were comprehensive and illuminating.

Weaknesses

Overviews of observational epidemiology may be subject to unknown biases which overviews of randomized controlled trials will escape. The data in this study are nonetheless very sparse for long-term use more than 20 years before diagnosis (76 cases and 85 controls). For these the estimated relative risk is around unity.

Relevance

The role of oral contraceptive use and the short-term risk of breast cancer are now as well understood as is possible. The conclusions are stated in very reassuring manner – illegitimately so in my view.

Paper 12

Risks and benefits of estrogen plus progestins in healthy postmenopausal women: Principal results from the Women's Health Initiative randomized controlled trial

Authors

Rossou JE *et al.*: Writing Group of the WHI investigators

Reference

Journal of the American Medical Association 2002; **288**:321–333

Summary

Despite decades of accumulated observational evidence, the role of exogenous hormones on breast cancer has remained unclear. This prospective double-blind randomized trial of 16 608 post-menopausal women with an intact uterus, recruited in 40 US centres between 1993 and 1998, tested experimentally the attributable role of combined equine oestrogen and medroxyprogesterone acetate when compared with placebo. The plan was to follow these women for 8.5 years, but after an average of 5.2 years the trial was stopped when a predetermined index of risks and benefits was exceeded, with the balance indicating that risks exceed benefits. This was a large measure due to the excess cases of invasive breast cancer, which had accumulated 290 new cases. After 4 years of follow-up data, the accumulation of breast cancer cases separated between active hormone replacement therapy (HRT) and placebo, until after 7 years with 166 cases in the active arm compared with 124 in the placebo arm. The balance between the two groups indicates a hazard ratio of 1.26 (1.00–1.59) against exogenous hormones.

This formidable study was the first randomized controlled trial to demonstrate a specific effect of specific hormones on breast cancer risk. Clearly, it could turn out to be wrong, but is so consistent with the observational evidence, in spite of unknown biases, that this seems unlikely. The residual issue has to do with which of the two exogenous hormones is responsible and also on what this effect might have on death from breast cancer. Neither question is addressable on the basis of these data, but the current trial of oestrogen alone among women who have had a hysterectomy will provide useful information on the former.

Related reference   (1)   Collaborative Group on Hormonal Factors in Breast Cancer. Breast cancer and hormone replacement therapy: collaborative reanalysis of data from 51 epidemiological studies of 52,705 women with breast cancer and 180,411 women without breast cancer. *Lancet* 1997; **350**:1047–1059.

Key message

If the observational evidence on the safety with respect to breast cancer of prophylactic hormones (and other widely used preparations) is not clear, or uncomfortable, then it pays to go to (apparently) extreme lengths to randomize as early as possible. In the case of HRT, it was too easy to believe the (false) protective effect on coronary heart disease, derived from biased studies, and hence systematically to play down the evidence suggesting an increased risk of breast cancer. These are important questions, which deserve to be addressed rigorously.

Why it's important

This study demonstrated that the role of hormones on breast cancer risk could be investigated properly and the size of the effect reliably measured. Clearly, the reliability was in the end compromised by the necessity to terminate the trial early – since pursuing the randomized blind schedules could not be justified knowing what was 7 or so years after the study began.

Strengths

Randomization and double-blind assessment simply have enormous strengths for understanding the effects of interventions. This work probably implicates these two hormones in late-stage disease, and the questions will now concentrate on how and why, and on what circulating endogenous hormones through life could moderate that effect. Not least will be the question of and effect of past exposure to oral contraceptives, and of childbearing early in life, on risk with and without exogenous hormones at the menopause. Detailed analyses taking account of actual use of HRT may be indicated, since the proportion of women in this study who changed medication consisted of about 35% who gave up HRT and 10% on placebo who took up HRT during the study.

Weakness

This study possibly happened too late, given what a dispassionate observer could have known in the late 1980s.

Relevance

This work is absolutely core to the aetiology of breast cancer and to the prevention of disease among women.

CHAPTER 4

Genetics

ANNE–MARIE MARTIN

BARBARA L WEBER

Introduction

Enormous strides have been made in recent years in the understanding of genetic factors that contribute to the development of breast cancer. The first description of hereditary breast cancer was by the French surgeon Paul Broca in 1866 (Broca P. *Traité des Tumeurs*. Paris: Asselin, 1866) documenting the occurrence of breast cancer in four generations of his wife's family. Such families have now been well studied and, at least in some cases, molecularly defined. In particular, the past 30 years have seen great advances in understanding the basis of familial clustering of breast and ovarian cancers.

Although non-genetic factors clearly play a role in the familial clustering of breast cancer, 5–10% of all breast cancers can be explained by the inheritance of mutations in one of two major breast cancer susceptibility genes, *BRCA1* and *BRCA2*. The identification of these two genes has paved the way to studies designed to determine the function of these genes and their gene products. But most importantly from a clinical standpoint, the identification of *BRCA1* and *BRCA2* has allowed for the screening of at-risk individuals and the identification of founder mutations in specific ethnic groups. Based on this information, individuals who carry germline mutations in *BRCA1* and/or *BRCA2* can be assigned a risk assessment and appropriate management strategies can be implemented.

Finally, prophylactic surgical methods have been developed and now studies, that clearly reduce the lifetime risk for developing breast and/or ovarian cancers in high-risk individuals. One study (Hartmann *et al.*, Paper 10) provided evidence that surgical prophylaxis is effective in reducing both risk for developing breast cancer and related mortality. Another study by Rebbeck *et al.* (related reference 1 for Paper 10) indicates that prophylactic oopherectomy not only reduces risk for developing ovarian cancer, but also reduces the risk for developing breast cancer in high-risk women. The studies described in this chapter detail the seminal accomplishments in this area and lay the groundwork for ongoing efforts to ultimately prevent this disease.

Paper 1

Familial association of breast/ovarian carcinoma

Authors

Lynch HT, Mulcahy GM, Harris RE, Guirgis HA, Lynch JF

Reference

Cancer 1978; **41**:1543–1549

Summary

Twelve pedigrees showing a clustering of breast and ovarian cancers among female relatives were analyzed. Ninety-one female relatives of the 12 subject probands were found to have breast cancer ($n = 60$), ovarian cancer ($n = 28$) or both ($n = 3$). The age of cancer diagnosis was typically earlier (50 years for breast cancer and 52.4 years for ovarian cancer) among affected individuals than in the general population. Mother to daughter and father to daughter transmission of elevated breast and ovarian cancer risk was observed in the 12 pedigrees studied. Excluding the proband or index case, the estimated cumulative risk of breast and ovarian cancer to daughters of affected mothers was 46% for the age interval 20–80 years, suggesting that affected mothers in these pedigrees transmit a cancer susceptibility gene to half of their daughters. In addition there was evidence for male transmission of breast and ovarian susceptibility in eight sibships.

This paper is a concise documentation of the inheritance of both breast and ovarian cancer susceptibility in families. It suggests the presence of at least one cancer-susceptibility gene and describes the mode of disease transmission as likely to be autosomal dominant.

Related reference (1)   Lynch HT, Krush AJ. Carcinoma of the breast and ovary in three families. *Surgery, Gynecology and Obstetrics*, 1971; **133**:644–648.

Key message

There is likely to be at least one autosomal dominant susceptibility allele for breast and ovarian cancer.

Why it's important

This paper was the first clear documentation that at least one dominant susceptibility gene for hereditary breast and ovarian cancer was likely to exist and that these susceptibility alleles could be transmitted both maternally and paternally, suggesting the gene(s) was located on an autosome. Previous papers documented familial clustering of breast and ovarian cancer but did not provide a genetic analysis of affected families.

Strengths

1. There was an aggregation of 12 informative pedigrees for analysis.
2. This was a comprehensive genetic and statistical report of 12 families with clustering of breast and ovarian cancers.
3. It was recognized that both the mother and the father can transmit breast and ovarian cancer susceptibility, suggesting an autosomal dominant susceptibility allele.

Weakness

The collection of families was small and not subjected to a formal segregation analysis.

Relevance

This paper led to subsequent work with segregation analyses, linkage studies and positional cloning, ultimately leading to the identification of *BRCA1* and *BRCA2*.

Paper 2

Genetic epidemiology of breast cancer: segregation of 200 Danish pedigrees

Authors

Williams WR, Anderson DE

Reference

Genetic Epidemiology 1984; **1**:7–20

Summary

This study was an investigation into the genetic epidemiology of breast cancer using segregation analysis of a cohort of 200 Danish families. The study suggested that the observed distribution of breast cancer in these families was consistent with autosomal-dominant transmission of disease susceptibility, conferred solely by one major gene. The gene frequency of the mutant allele was estimated to be much less than 1% in the general population but accounting for a significant proportion of breast cancer among women with an early age of diagnosis. The authors concluded that among older women with breast cancer, the majority are phenocopies.

This was the largest sample set subjected for segregation analysis at that time. The paper described the most likely model of inheritance for each family tested and rejected all models except autosomal dominant susceptibility transmission caused by one major gene.

Related references (1)	Dublin N, Pasternack BS, Strax P. Epidemiology of breast cancer in a screened population. *Cancer Detection and Prevention* 1984; 7:87–102.
(2)	King MC, Elston RC. Genetic epidemiology of breast cancer: a comment on heterogeneity. *Genetic Epidemiology* 1985; **2**:167–169.
(3)	Williams WR, Anderson DE. Genetic epidemiology of breast cancer: further clarification and a response to King and Elston. *Genetic Epidemiology* 1985; **2**:170–176.

Key message

The only model of inheritance of breast cancer risk in these kindreds supported by this study was a single autosomal-dominant susceptibility allele.

Why it's important

This was the first statistical analysis to document that an autosomal-dominant susceptibility allele for breast cancer existed, setting the stage for family ascertainment and subsequent linkage analyses.

Strengths

1. A large sample set was analyzed.
2. All models of genetic transmission of breast cancer susceptibility were convincingly rejected except an autosomal-dominant model.

Weaknesses

None

Relevance

This segregation analysis defined the phenotype of families necessary for subsequent studies.

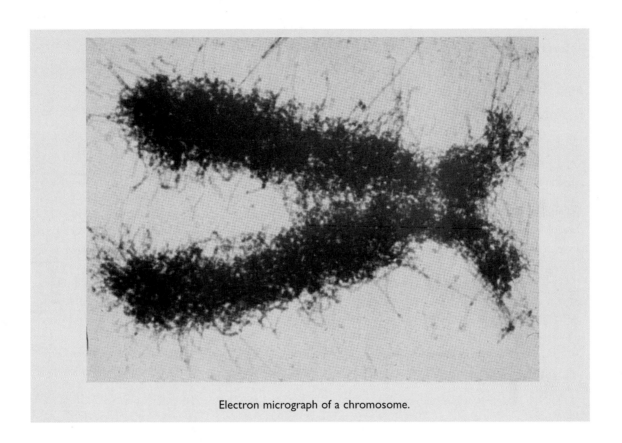

Electron micrograph of a chromosome.

Paper 3

Linkage of early-onset familial breast cancer to chromosome 17q21

Authors

Hall JM, Lee MK, Newman B, *et al.*

Reference

Science 1990; **250**:1684–1689

Summary

Using linkage analysis of 23 extended breast cancer families with 146 affected individuals, inherited susceptibility to breast cancer among families with an early age of diagnosis (<45 years) was mapped to chromosome 17q21 in a region close to the VNTR (variable number tandem repeat) genetic marker D17S74. Genetic analysis yielded a LOD (logarithm of the likelihood of ratio for linkage) score of 5.98 for linkage of breast cancer susceptibility among families with an early age of breast cancer diagnosis. A negative LOD score was calculated when families with a late age of breast cancer diagnosis.

Early-onset breast cancer susceptibility is linked to the D17S74 locus on chromosome 17q21. This finding was confirmed and further investigated to show that ovarian cancer susceptibility is also linked to this locus (see related reference 1). In this subsequent study, five large families with a hereditary predisposition to breast and ovarian cancer were investigated with three families showing evidence of linkage, the largest family having an individual LOD score of 2.72. These findings confirmed that a gene at 17q12–q23, shown by King and colleagues in this paper to contain a gene for early-onset breast cancer, is also associated with a proportion of hereditary ovarian cancers.

Related references

(1) Narod SA, Feunteun J, Lynch HT, *et al.* Familial breast–ovarian cancer locus on chromosome 17q12-q23. *Lancet* 1991; **338**:82–83.

(2) Easton DF, Bishop DT, Ford D, *et al.* Genetic linkage analysis in familial breast and ovarian cancer: results from 214 families. The Breast Cancer Linkage Consortium. *American Journal of Human Genetics* 1993; **52**:678–701.

Key message

A breast cancer susceptibility gene resides on human chromosome 17q21.

Why it's important

This was the first documentation of the location of a gene responsible for hereditary susceptibility to breast cancer. In addition, there is evidence of disease heterogeneity in the families tested noted by different ages of diagnosis of disease.

Strengths

1. This was a large and conclusive study of 23 extended breast cancer families with 329 participating relatives.
2. To avoid statistical error, all pathology records were reviewed on all affected family members.
3. To verify results, four statistical methods of evaluating linkage were applied.
4. Analyses defined families with an early age of breast cancer diagnosis as the key phenotype predicting linkage to this locus.

Weakness

The interval in which the gene could be found was not well defined by the use of a single genetic marker; however, relatively few markers were available at that time.

Relevance

This was the first definitive proof that a gene exists that is responsible for hereditary breast and ovarian cancer susceptibility. This paved the way to identifying the gene itself, which has subsequently allowed the identification of at-risk individuals and the initiation of appropriate management strategies.

Paper 4

A strong candidate for the breast and ovarian cancer susceptibility gene BRCA1

Authors

Miki Y, Swensen J, Shattuck-Eidens D, *et al.*

Reference

Science 1994; **266**:66–71

Summary

BRCA1 was isolated in 1994. The cDNA encodes a protein of 1863 amino acids and the gene encompasses 100 kb of genomic sequence. Sequences encoding a zinc finger (RING) functional motif were identified at the 5′-end of the gene. The gene was found to be expressed in a number of tissues including breast and ovarian tissues, with highest transcript levels present in the testes and thymus.

Sequence analysis of *BRCA1* in kindreds with linkage between early-onset breast and ovarian cancer and markers flanking *BRCA1* identified a number of disease-associated mutations.

Related references (1)   Castilla LH, Couch FJ, Erdos MR, *et al.* Mutations in the *BRCA1* gene in families with early-onset breast and ovarian cancer. *Nature Genetics* 1994; **8**:387–391.

(2)   Futreal PA, Liu Q, Shattuck-Eidens D, *et al. BRCA1* mutations in primary breast and ovarian carcinomas. *Science* 1994; **266**:120–122.

(3)   Friedman LS, Ostermeyer EA, Szabo CI, *et al.* Confirmation of *BRCA1* by analysis of germline mutations linked to breast and ovarian cancer in ten families. *Nature Genetics* 1994; **8**:399–404.

Key message

The 17q-linked breast cancer susceptibility gene, *BRCA1*, was identified by positional cloning. The gene is expressed in numerous tissues including breast and ovary. Disease-associated germline mutations were identified in a number of kindreds.

Why it's important

This paper was a huge breakthrough in the field of breast cancer genetics. Not only was it the first documentation of a gene mutation known to cause familial breast cancer, but also it was the first to describe specific disease-causing mutations in *BRCA1*.

Strengths

1. This was the first discovery of a major gene conferring susceptibility to a common adult cancer.
2. Sequence motifs suggesting that *BRCA1* may play a role in transcription were identified.

Weaknesses

1. There was a cloning artifact in the original cDNA that was thought to be exon 4 which has subsequently been removed from the sequence.
2. Germline mutations were not identified in all linked families.

Relevance

With the discovery of the *BRCA1* gene, germline mutations responsible for breast cancer etiology have been determined and large-scale commercial testing for at-risk individuals is now in place. Studies aimed at determining the function of BRCA1 and the development of breast cancer in the absence of BRCA1 protein are underway.

Paper 5

Identification of the breast cancer susceptibility gene BRCA2

Authors

Wooster R, Bignell G, Lancaster J, *et al.*

Reference

Nature 1995; **378**:789–792

Summary

Shortly after the discovery of *BRCA1*, Stratton and colleagues localized and then isolated the second autosomal-dominant breast cancer susceptibility gene, *BRCA2*. *BRCA2* was initially positioned in a 6 cM region on chromosome 13q12–q13 between the genetic markers D13S289 and D13S267. Using a set of Icelandic families, many of which included cases of male breast cancer, the interval in which *BRCA2* lies was refined by microsatellite mapping to a 600 kb interval. Finally, using yeast artificial chromosomes and P1 artificial chromosomes, 14 overlapping clones were organized into a contig. To identify putative coding sequences, DNA from at least one affected member of 46 breast cancer families, which had shown linkage to *BRCA2*, was examined for sequence variants in candidate genes within the contig. Six different disease-associated mutations in *BRCA2* were identified in these breast cancer families. As with the isolation of *BRCA1*, germline disease-associated mutations in *BRCA2* were identified in a number of the breast cancer families tested. An association between *BRCA2* germline mutations and male breast cancer was documented.

Related references (1) Wooster R, Neuhausen SL, Mangion J, *et al.* Localization of a breast cancer susceptibility gene, *BRCA2*, to chromosome 13q12-13. *Science* 1994; **265**:2088–2090.

(2) Tavtigian SV, Simard J, Rommens J, *et al.* The complete *BRCA2* gene and mutations in chromosome 13q-linked kindreds. *Nature Genetics* 1996; **12**:333–337.

(3) Couch FJ, Farid LM, DeShano ML, *et al. BRCA2* gemline mutations in male breast cancer cases and breast cancer families. *Nature Genetics* 1996; **13**:123–125.

Key message

The 13q-linked breast cancer susceptibility gene, *BRCA2*, was identified and is associated with susceptibility to both female and male breast cancer. Disease-associated germline mutations were identified.

Why it's important

This paper provided the first documentation of a second gene associated with familial breast cancer. Disease-causing mutations were identified, and for the first time mutations in *BRCA2* were associated with an increased incidence of male breast cancer.

Strengths

1. This is a definitive and elegant example of positional cloning.
2. This was the discovery of an important breast cancer susceptibility gene.

Weakness

The coding sequence and N-terminus of the gene are incomplete. Complete sequencing of the gene was subsequently provided by another group (see related reference 2).

Relevance

The identification of a second breast cancer susceptibility gene allows a more complete understanding of breast cancer etiology and pathogenesis, as well as a more comprehensive mutation analysis for women seeking risk evaluation.

Paper 6

Location of BRCA1 in human breast and ovarian cancer cells

Authors

Scully R, Ganesan S, Brown M, *et al.*

Reference

Science 1996; **272**:123–125

Summary

In this paper, Scully *et al.* describe the nuclear localization of BRCA1 in breast and ovarian cancer cell lines. Immuno-staining with BRCA1-specific antibodies showed that endogenous BRCA1 migrates as a doublet of approximately 220 kDa and that BRCA1 localizes to discrete foci (dots) in the nucleus of all the cell lines tested, including breast cancer and ovarian cancer cell lines. This finding was in contrast to other studies, which suggested that BRCA1 was localized in the cytoplasm or secreted into the extracellular space (see related references 1–3). However, Scully *et al.* showed that the technique with which the cells were treated prior to staining with antibody greatly influenced the ability to accurately detect the location of BRCA1. Cytoplasmic staining of BRCA1 was only detected in alcoholic formalin-fixed cells, whereas nuclear BRCA1 signal was only apparent in cells that had been fixed in neutral-buffered formalin and exposed to microwave heating before staining. In a related publication, Wilson *et al.* further demonstrated that several antibodies were not BRCA1-specific and cross-reacted with p185HER2/*neu*, explaining the spurious finding of secreted protein.

These findings show that fixation conditions greatly influence the ability to detect nuclear BRCA1 signal.

Related references   **(1)**   Chen Y, Chen CF, Riley DJ, *et al.* Aberrant subcellular localization of BRCA1 in breast cancer. *Science* 1995; **270**:789–791.

   (2)   Scully R, Chen J, Plug A, *et al.* Association of BRCA1 with Rad51 in mitotic and meiotic cells. *Cell* 1997; **88**:265–275.

   (3)   Scully R, Chen J, Ochs RL, *et al.* Dynamic changes of BRCA1 subnuclear location and phosphorylation state are initiated by DNA damage. *Cell* 1997; **90**:425–435.

   (4)   Wilson CA, Payton MN, Pekar SK, *et al.* BRCA1 protein products: antibody specificity … *Nat Genet* 1996; **13**:264–265.

Key message

BRCA1 is a nuclear protein and is characterized by a 'nuclear dot' pattern. This finding has functional implications suggesting that BRCA1 acts solely in the nucleus, excluding the possibility that it functions as a paracrine hormone.

Why it's important

This paper proved definitively the cellular location of BRCA1.

Strengths

1. Multiple techniques were employed to determine the exact location of BRCA1.
2. Multiple cell lines and tissue preparations were tested to verify their results.
3. Technically flawless immunostaining clearly documents the BRCA1 nuclear foci.

Weaknesses

None

Relevance

This paper provided conclusive evidence that BRCA1 is a nuclear protein, resolving the controversy that had delayed functional study of BRCA1 for more than a year.

Paper 7

Tumorigenesis and a DNA repair defect in mice with a truncating Brca2 mutation

Authors

Connor F, Bertwistle D, Mee PJ, *et al.*

Reference

Nature Genetics 1997; **17**:423–430

Summary

BRCA2 function was investigated using murine models. A mutation in *Brca2* was introduced into the germline by homologous recombination in transfected embryonic stem cells. A *PGK-neo* cassette was introduced into exon 11 of *Brca2* that interrupts the open reading frame of the mouse protein. There had been several previous reports describing early embryonic lethality of homozygous mutations in *Brca2* null mice. However, in this case some of the homozygous *Brca2-/-*mutant mice survived to adulthood. Those that did survive had a wide range of defects, including small size, absence of germ cells and the development of lethal thymic lymphomas, which originate almost entirely from the immature double-positive thymocyte population. In addition, fibroblasts cultured from *Brca2-/-*embryos had a defect in proliferation in culture associated with the accumulation of *p53* and *p21*$^{Waf1/CIP1}$, which are known to mediate cell cycle arrest and are upregulated in response to DNA damage.

This paper was one of the first to describe a role for murine *Brca2* in DNA damage response and embryonic development. In addition, it was one of the first studies to generate homozygous *Brca2* null mice that survived to adulthood. Two other papers published almost simultaneously are worthy of mention. Sharan *et al.* (related reference 1) first documented the association of *Brca2* with Rad51, suggesting a role for *Brca2* in the Rad51-dependent repair of double-strand breaks. Patel *et al.* (related reference 2) reported that cells harboring a truncated *Brca2* gene have spontaneous accumulation of chromosomal abnormalities and chromatid breaks and arrest in G_1 and G_2/M accompanied by elevated p53 and p21 levels. This finding suggests that BRCA2 is important, not only in mediating the cellular response to DNA damage, but also in playing a role in maintaining genomic stability during cell division.

Related references (1)	Sharan SK, Morimatsu M, Albrecht U, *et al.* Embryonic lethality and radiation hypersensitivity mediated by Rad51 in mice lacking *Brca2*. *Nature* 1997; **386**:804–810.
(2)	Patel KJ, Yu VP, Lee H, *et al.* Involvement of *Brca2* in DNA repair. *Molecular Cell* 1998; **1**:347–357.

Key message

Brca2 appears to be essential for the maintenance of chromosomal integrity and efficient DNA damage repair.

Why it's important

This study was important since some of the knockout mice survived long enough to be investigated. As a result, this paper was one of the first to document the functional role of BRCA2 in DNA damage response and embryonic development.

Strengths

1. These were the first $Brca2^{-/-}$ mice to survive to adulthood.
2. A comprehensive description was given of the abnormalities these mice present, including small size, poor cell proliferation, aberrant development and thymic tumors.
3. This was the first evidence that *Brca2* is required for chromosomal integrity and efficient DNA repair.

Weakness

Key confirmatory experiments could not be performed due to the unavailability of reagents at the time these studies were conducted. Specifically the necessary antibodies had not yet been generated.

Relevance

This paper was the first in a series to describe a function for BRCA2 and its role in genome stability and DNA repair.

Paper 8

Ashkenazi Jewish population frequencies for common mutations in BRCA1 and BRCA2

Authors

Roa BB, Boyd AA, Volcik K, Richards CS

Reference

Nature Genetics 1996; **14**:185–187

Summary

A large population-based study was conducted to determine the frequency of Ashkenazi-specific founder mutations in *BRCA1* and *BRCA2*. Mutation screening was carried out on approximately 3000 Ashkenazi Jewish people and a carrier frequency of 1.09% was determined for the 185delAG mutations and 0.13% for the 5382insC mutation. *BRCA2* analysis on 3085 individuals from the same population showed a carrier frequency of 1.52% for the 6174delT mutation. This population-based study confirms that founder mutations in *BRCA1* or *BRCA2* are present in approximately 2.5% of unselected Ashkenazi Jews.

This study documents the high frequency of *BRCA1* and *BRCA2* founder mutations in the Ashkenazi Jewish population. In the same year, Struewing *et al.* (related reference 3) determined the frequency of the 185delAG in 858 Ashkenazim, and in 815 reference individuals not selected for ethnic origin. The frequency of 0.9% for this mutation among Ashkenazim and none in reference individuals suggested that one in a 100 women of Ashkenazi descent selected without regard to breast cancer history carry this mutation and may be at especially high risk of developing breast and/or ovarian cancer.

Related references (1) Tonin P, Weber B, Offit K, *et al.* Frequency of recurrent *BRCA1* and *BRCA2* mutations in Ashkenazi Jewish breast cancer families. *Nature Medicine* 1996; **2**:1179–1183.

(2) Offit K, Gilewski T, McGuire P, *et al.* Germline *BRCA1* 185delAG mutations in Jewish women with breast cancer. *The Lancet* 1996; **347**:1643–1645.

(3) Struewing JP, Abeliovich D, Peretz T, *et al.* The carrier frequency of the *BRCA1* 185delAG mutation is approximately 1 per cent in Ashkenazi Jewish individuals. *Nature Genetics* 1996; **11**:198–200.

Key message

Three Ashkenazi-specific mutations exist in *BRCA1* and *BRCA2*. The 185delAG mutation in *BRCA1* is seen at a frequency of approximately 1% of the Ashkenazi Jewish population. The 6174delT mutation in *BRCA2* is seen at a carrier frequency of approximately 1.5% but has a lower attributable risk than 185delAG, suggesting it is less penetrant.

Why it's important

This paper documented that there is a high frequency of founder mutations in *BRCA1* and *BRCA2* in the Ashkenazi Jewish population.

Strengths

1. This study is a population-based study of approximately 3000 Ashkenazi individuals, providing an accurate measure of allele frequency.
2. Comparisons were done on a mixed-ethnic reference group.

Weakness

Family history was not provided and the prevalence of other mutations in the Ashkenazi population was not determined; thus the attributable risk of other mutations in Ashkenazim cannot be estimated from this study.

Relevance

The frequency of these three mutations in the Ashkenazi Jewish population is at least 10 times that of *BRCA1* and/or *BRCA2* susceptibility alleles in non-Ashkenazi Jewish populations. Thus, models estimating the likelihood of finding mutations in specific patients must be modified in this ethnic group.

Paper 9

BRCA1 *mutations in women attending clinics that evaluate the risk of breast cancer*

Authors

Couch FJ, DeShano ML, Blackwood MA, *et al.*

Reference

New England Journal of Medicine 1997; **336**:1409–1415

Summary

This study defines the incidence of *BRCA1* mutations among patients seen in a clinically relevant population drawn from high-risk breast cancer evaluation clinics. Genomic DNA samples were obtained from 263 women with breast cancer and used for mutation screening. *BRCA1* mutations were identified in 16% of women with a family history of breast cancer, with the frequency of mutations significantly higher among women from families with a history of both breast and ovarian cancer. Among family members, an early average age of breast cancer diagnosis, the presence of ovarian cancer in the families, the presence of breast and ovarian cancer in a single individual, and Ashkenazi Jewish ancestry were all predictors of detecting a *BRCA1* mutation. No association was found between the presence of bilateral breast cancer or the number of breast cancers in a family and the detection of a *BRCA1* mutation, or between the position of the mutation in the *BRCA1* gene and the presence of ovarian cancer in the family.

Related references (1)	Shattuck-Eidens D, Oliphant A, McClure M, *et al. BRCA1* sequence analysis in women at high risk for susceptibility mutations. Risk factor analysis and implications for genetic testing. *Journal of the American Medical Association* 1997; **278**:1242–1250.
(2)	Parmigiani G, Berry D, Aguilar O. Determining carrier probabilities for breast cancer-susceptibility genes *BRCA1* and *BRCA2*. *American Journal of Human Genetics* 1998; **62**:145–158.
(3)	Frank TS, Manley SA, Olopade OI, *et al.* Sequence analysis of *BRCA1* and *BRCA2*: correlation of mutations with family history and ovarian cancer risk. *Journal of Clinical Oncology* 1998; **16**:2417–2425.

Key message

The overall frequency of *BRCA1* mutations is 16% among women attending a high-risk breast evaluation clinic, but may be as high as 70% in Ashkenazi Jewish women with both breast and ovarian cancer. Predictors of mutation status include an early average age of breast cancer diagnosis, the presence of ovarian cancer, the presence of breast and ovarian cancer in a single individual, and Ashkenazi Jewish ancestry. The percentage of site-specific breast cancer families with a *BRCA1* mutation is considerably lower than previously estimated.

Why it's important

This study was one of the first to evaluate the frequency of *BRCA1* mutations among women attending a high-risk breast evaluation clinic.

Strengths

1. The study population is truly representative of women attending a high-risk clinic and thus represents a model for providing risk estimates to these individuals.
2. The entire coding region and splice sites of *BRCA1* were screened for germline mutations.
3. The study identified predictors of mutation status.

Weaknesses

1. Not all mutations will be identified by conformation sensitive gel electrophoresis, the screening method used in this paper.
2. *BRCA2* mutation frequency was not determined.
3. The population studied was almost exclusively Caucasian.
4. The number of patients in some subsets is very small, leading in some cases to very wide confidence intervals.

Relevance

This paper provides guidelines for physicians counseling women about their risk assessment and suggests that *BRCA1* germline mutations account for less than 20% of site-specific breast cancer families.

Paper 10

Efficacy of bilateral prophylactic mastectomy in women with a family history of breast cancer

Authors

Hartmann LC, Schaid DJ, Woods JE, *et al.*

Reference

New England Journal of Medicine 1999; **340**:77–84

Summary

This was a retrospective study of 639 women with a family history of breast cancer who underwent bilateral prophylactic mastectomy at the Mayo Clinic between the years of 1960 and 1993. The women were divided into high-risk ($n = 214$) and moderate-risk ($n = 425$) on the basis of their family history. A non-surgical control group of sisters of those in the high-risk group and the Gail model were used to estimate the expected number of breast cancer cases in these two groups in the absence of prophylactic surgery. Following prophylactic surgery, there was an 89.5% ($p < 0.001$) reduction in risk of breast cancer in the moderate-risk group and a 90% reduction in risk in the high-risk group. These data suggest prophylactic mastectomy is extremely effective at reducing breast cancer risk, even in high-risk women.

Related references

(1)   Rebbeck TR, Levin AM, Eisen A, *et al.* Breast cancer risk after bilateral prophylactic oophorectomy in *BRCA1* mutation carriers. *Journal of the National Cancer Institute* 1999; **91**:1475–1479.

(2)   Eisen A, Rebbeck TR, Wood WC, Weber BL. Prophylactic surgery in women with a hereditary predisposition to breast and ovarian cancer. *Journal of Clinical Oncology* 2000; **18**:1980–1995.

Key message

This retrospective cohort study demonstrates the effectiveness of prophylactic mastectomy for reducing the risk of developing breast cancer in high- and moderate-risk women.

Why it's important

Prophylactic mastectomy is an option for breast cancer risk reduction among high-risk individuals but until this study, the effectiveness of this procedure was questioned in this group. The results suggested a highly significant reduction in the incidence of breast cancer and death from breast cancer following prophylactic mastectomy.

Strengths

1. This was a large, well-defined cohort.
2. The authors addressed ascertainment bias by including a sister sample set and Gail model analyses.

Weaknesses

1. This was a retrospective study with inherent biases.
2. No information on *BRCA1* and *BRCA2* mutation status was available. The family history information provided suggests that there will be few mutation carriers even in the high-risk group; thus a definitive study in *BRCA1* and/or *BRCA2* mutation carriers is needed.

Relevance

This study provides evidence that surgical prophylaxis is effective in reducing both an individual's risk for developing breast cancer and their mortality rate. These data are important for clinical decision-making.

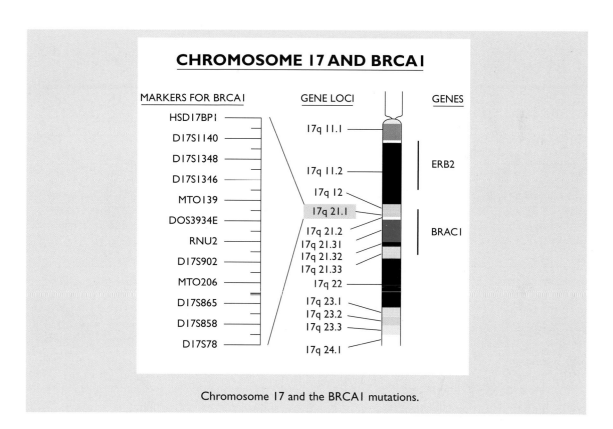

Chromosome 17 and the BRCA1 mutations.

CHAPTER 5

Molecular biology

MARC E LIPPMAN

Introduction

The selection of a small group of papers that are 'classics' in the cellular and molecular biology of breast cancer published in the last century is a daunting and humbling task. First and foremost, this has been an era of extraordinary promise. Breast cancer has moved from a nearly invariably lethal clinical entity to a disease in which the majority of women are cured. Furthermore, many of its most subtle aspects are beginning to be understood. The therapy has changed drastically with respect to both local and systemic therapy and, most importantly, we are now seeing the ushering in of a new era in which diagnosis, prognostication, treatment and prevention are all beginning to be placed upon the cellular and molecular biologic principles developed, in part, by the papers to be discussed here.

In reviewing the many wonderful publications of visionary colleagues, it is critical to offer apologies to any who believe that other papers ought to have been selected. There are many other worthwhile contenders for selection. My choices have been fundamentally based on two criteria: first, those papers which appear to have influenced thinking in such a fashion that a tremendous amount of downstream investigation has resulted; and second, those studies for which the tangible fruits are already largely in evidence in the clinical arena. Obviously, this creates a selection bias towards papers that have been published more than three or four years ago, a period of time that must elapse to see precisely what role these exciting new technologies and discoveries in molecular biology have in the approach to clinical breast cancer.

Finally, in re-reading some of these older studies, it is critical to understand how much these seminal findings influenced subsequent developments. Some of the studies from the 1970s, for example, appear so straightforward and obvious that it is hard now to appreciate how influential and important they were at the time and how much they contributed to the subsequent progress that we have seen in the field of breast cancer.

One paper which I will not cite as a 'classic', though it certainly began the biological understanding of breast cancer, is the paper by Beatson [1]. This exceptionally important paper published at the end of the nineteenth century demonstrated the relationship between the ovaries and the continued growth of some breast cancers. Beatson described several women with advanced breast cancer who experienced remissions following removal of their ovaries. While the elucidation of the biological mechanisms underpinning these tumor regressions would have to wait more than half a century for the development of the field of steroid endocrinology, nonetheless, Beatson's inductive thinking based on studies done in farm animals was insightful and crucial.

Reference

[1] Beatson GT. On the treatment of inoperable cases of carcinoma of the mamma: suggestions for a new method of treatment, with illustrative cases. *Lancet* 1896; **ii**:104–107, 162–165.

Paper 1

Estrogen receptor interactions. Estrogenic hormones effect transformation of specific receptor proteins to a biochemical functional form

Authors

Jensen EV, DeSombre ER

Reference

Science, 1973; **182**:126–134

Summary

In this influential paper, Jensen and DeSombre summarized their early findings on the interactions of estrogenic hormones with the estrogen receptor protein to whose identification they had contributed so significantly. Their work pointed out critical structure–activity relationships between estrogenic hormones and binding to the receptor and their studies characterize a series of steps that hormone receptors undergo following initial ligand binding. Their studies showed that these transformation and activation steps altered nuclear affinity of the receptor and led to interactions with nuclear components that changed RNA transcription.

Related reference (1)

Wyld DK, Chester JD, Perren TJ. Endocrine aspects of the clinical management of breast cancer – current issues. *Endocrine-Related Cancer* 1998; **5**:97–110.

Key message

Critically, these observations established the necessary role of estrogen receptor mediation in all estrogenic effects. As this paper began to explore subsequent events following receptor binding, the notion that receptor alone would be an insufficient condition for hormone-responsive tissue was also established. Our current view of steroid hormones as activators of nuclear transcription factors was begun by these groundbreaking studies.

Why it's important

Until significant investigations by this and other groups had been accomplished, the fundamental notion of how steroids interacted with target tissue was generally believed to be through allosteric regulation of peptide activity. Literally hundreds of papers had earlier appeared proposing that direct interaction between a variety of putative target proteins in steroids explained the biological effects observed. Most of this literature was deeply flawed because of the absence of appreciation of the actual physiologic concentrations of hormones required to induce phenotypic effects *in vivo*. This paper began a long process that would eventually result in the characterization of estrogen receptors as nuclear transcription factors, and place on a firm footing the measurement and quantification of estrogen receptors as a means of determining hormone responsivity.

Strength

The critical awareness of the central role of the estrogen receptor and the changes that would occur to it following hormone binding, which in turn would enable it to alter RNA expression.

Weakness

Following publication of this study much attention was given to so-called 'nuclear translocation of the receptor' and a variety of receptor size analyses by such means as sucrose gradient analysis. Many investigators were involved in years of study which eventually proved to be relatively non-germane to the central thesis of how estrogen receptors actually interact with the genome.

Relevance

To this day, the determination of the estrogen receptor as a means of both prognosticating human breast cancer and determining hormone dependence remains essential. The availability of the estrogen receptor (in crystal form) as described in subsequent papers has allowed a molecular unraveling of the mechanisms of antiestrogen and selective estrogen receptor modulator (SERM) activity.

Paper 2

The antitumor effect of antioestrogen ICI46474 (tamoxifen) in the DMBA-induced rat mammary carcinoma model

Author

Jordan VC

Reference

Journal of Steroid Biochemistry 1974; **5**:354–359

Summary

In this paper, Jordan was able to demonstrate that tamoxifen treatment of rats previously exposed to dimethylbenzanthracene (DMBA, a carcinogen that induced hormone-dependent breast cancers with a high degree of regularity), could prevent or delay the appearance of tumors. The effect required the continuous presence of tamoxifen begun shortly after the carcinogenic event.

Related references (1) Fisher B, Powles TJ, Pritchard KJ. Tamoxifen for the prevention of breast cancer (Current Controversies in Cancer). *European Journal of Cancer* 2000; **36**:142–150.

(2) Delmas PD, Bjarnason NH, Mitlak BH, *et al.* Effects of raloxifene on bone mineral density, serum cholesterol concentration, and uterine endometrium in postmenopausal women. *New England Journal of Medicine* 1997; **337**:1641–1687.

Key message

At the time this paper appeared, there were several model systems in existence for provoking breast cancer in experimental animals. The DMBA system was one of the best studied because of well-known hormone dependence of the majority of tumors produced. Previous work had shown that castrated animals or sexually immature animals would not develop breast tumors when treated with DMBA. It was also known that pregnancy would greatly reduce the carcinogenic effect of DMBA. It was already just becoming known that tamoxifen could treat metastatic breast cancer in women. This paper clearly showed that the chronic administration of tamoxifen could have a substantial preventive effect as well.

Why it's important

This and related work by Jordan and others is of critical importance because it placed the prevention of hormone-dependent breast cancers by SERM-like drugs on a firm biologic footing. In fact, these studies together with the previously well-known hormone-dependent nature of metastatic human breast cancer (as well as a series of epidemiologic studies that had suggested that hormonal factors contributed to the etiology of breast cancer including length of menstrual life, exposure to exogenous hormones, etc.), all suggested that antiestrogen intervention could potentially prevent breast cancer. These studies, combined with safety and efficacy studies in women with previously diagnosed breast cancer, were the critical underpinnings for the successful breast cancer prevention trials that have occurred during the past few years. Jordan's work led directly to the first trials of tamoxifen in the adjuvant setting in the highly influential NATO, Scottish National and NSABP trials. Their success in turn was directly responsible for the BCPT trial showing that tamoxifen administration could reduce breast cancer by nearly 50% in women at somewhat increased risk of the disease.

Strength

The great strength of this article was the simplicity of the system and the unequivocal experimental results obtained.

Weakness

The only weakness was the question of the relevance of the DMBA model system to human breast cancer. Subsequently, this theoretical weakness has been refuted, with tamoxifen demonstrating greater than a 50% ability to prevent breast cancer when administered for 5 years to women with an average risk of the disease. More recently, a different SERM, raloxifene, has also demonstrated substantial ability to prevent breast cancer in a lower risk population of postmenopausal women selected for study because of pre-existent osteoporosis.

Relevance

Tamoxifen is now one of the most widely prescribed drugs in the world. Its very acceptable toxicity profile has continued to be maintained and it is now being used to treat many thousands of women at risk for developing breast cancer. Much of that success and clinical utility can and should be traced to these original observations.

Paper 3

Oestrogen-responsive human breast cancer in long term tissue culture

Authors

Lippman ME, Bolan G

Reference

Nature 1975; **256**:592–593

Summary

This paper demonstrated that a human breast cancer cell line, MCF-7, maintained in long-term tissue culture could be made to respond to estrogens and antiestrogens in a reversible and mutually inhibitable fashion.

Related reference (1)   Wistuba II, Behrens C, Milchgrub S, *et al.* Comparison of features of human breast cancer cell lines and their corresponding tumors. *Clinical Cancer Research* 1998; **4**:2931–2938.

Key message

Until this paper was published, all previous work on estrogen action had been confined to isolated biochemical systems of questionable relevance or intact animal studies. By providing data that an isolated, clonal cell culture system could be made to respond in physiologically relevant ways to estrogens and antiestrogens, a model system was provided which would allow detailed subsequent studies to outline both the affector and effector limb of hormone responsivity; that is, steps following the interaction of estrogen with its receptor leading to alterations in gene expression and an analysis of downstream gene products influenced by activated estrogen–receptor complexes.

Why it's important

Isolated cell culture systems used to study estrogen action are critical because of the ways in which these systems were subsequently able to be manipulated. First, because of the ability to move such cells back and forth between athymic nude mice and cell culture, *in vivo* effects could be evaluated concurrently with effects seen in cell culture. Isolated cell culture systems allowed for genetic analysis in the form of mutagenic studies and variant cell lines derived under selection pressure. Thus, a multiplicity of hormone and drug resistant variants were obtained which were critical to the elucidation of pathways of drug and hormone resistance. More recently, with gene transfer and gene knockouts (with ribozymes and antisense strategies), very detailed analysis of the steps in hormone action have occurred.

Strength

The establishment of a convenient and relevant model for studying estrogen action.

Weaknesses

What was not fully appreciated when this paper was published was the critical effect of ambient estrogen concentrations in the cell culture medium and their influence on the ability to see estrogenic effects. In fact, there was a great deal of controversy shortly afterwards, with multiple groups either replicating or failing to replicate the results. It was not until later that the work of John Katzenellenbogen showed that at least one of the factors contributing to the discrepant results was the phenol red used as a pH indicator in the medium, which could function as a weak estrogen. This debate over whether or not estrogens could directly affect cells in culture preoccupied many investigators fruitlessly for some years.

Relevance

The human cell culture system for studying mechanisms of estrogen action remains a critically useful model system. Virtually all of the systemic therapies used in the management of breast cancer eventually have explored these estrogen-dependent cell culture systems both *in vitro* and in nude mouse experimentation.

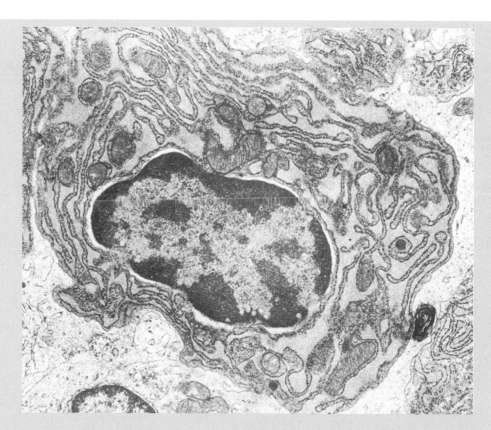

Electron microscope view of the nucleus and endoplasmic reticulum.

Paper 4

Predicting response to endocrine therapy in human breast cancer: a hypothesis

Authors

Horwitz KB, McGuire WL, Pearson OH, Segaloff A

Reference

Science 1978; **189**:726–727

Summary

This paper suggested that the progesterone receptor was an estrogen-inducible function in hormone-dependent tissue. As a result of this observation, it was posited that measurement of the progesterone receptor would serve as a surrogate not only for the presence of the estrogen receptor, but as a functional hormone response system and thus accurately predict which patients would respond to endocrine therapy.

Related reference (1) Lydon JP, DeMayo FJ, Conneely OM, O'Malley BW. Reproductive phenotypes of the progesterone receptor null mutant mouse. *Journal of Steroid Biochemistry and Molecular Biology* 1996; **56**(1–6):67–77.

Key message

Previous work had demonstrated the critical role of the estrogen receptor in mediating estrogen action. However, it was clear that many patients whose tumors were positive for the estrogen receptor failed to respond to hormone therapy. A variety of flaws in estrogen response systems had already been hypothesized, including defective estrogen receptors, that might lead to the presence of an estrogen-binding moiety without a functional hormone response. By measuring an estrogen-inducible protein (the progesterone receptor), it became possible to predict hormone dependence more accurately.

Why it's important

This critical paper vastly improved the ability to predict hormone responsivity in human breast cancer. Based on the fact that the progesterone receptor is an estrogen-inducible protein, one would hypothesize that it would virtually never be expressed in breast cancers in the apparent absence of the estrogen receptor. This has been observed in study after study in which breast cancers that are positive for the progesterone receptor, which are also estrogen receptor-negative, make up less than 5% of the total population. The majority of these few cases probably represent errors in the determination of one receptor or the other. Furthermore, when the population of breast cancers that is estrogen receptor-positive is divided into those which are progesterone receptor-positive and those which are progesterone receptor-negative, there is more than a 2½-fold difference in hormone responsivity favoring those containing both receptor proteins. Thus, patients whose tumors express both estrogen and progesterone receptors respond to endocrine therapy approximately 75% of the time. This has permitted vastly more precise treatment decision-making for patients with metastatic disease, as well as for those given adjuvant therapy. Furthermore, it provided a critical and straightforward system for studying mechanisms of estrogen induction of gene expression and thus the critical interplay between liganded estrogen receptor and both specific and non-specific transcriptional machinery, including co-activators and co-repressors essential to an understanding of SERM action.

Strengths

1. This paper presented a straightforward hypothesis which has been validated by ever-increasing amounts of data that have emerged ever since.
2. This paper revolutionized the selection of patients for endocrine therapy and provided a basis for the fact that, in most studies, the progesterone receptor is an even more powerful prognostic variable than the estrogen receptor.

Weaknesses

None

Relevance

This paper continues to provide the basis for rational selection of patients for endocrine therapy, and is the precursor of future molecular targeting attempts.

Paper 5

Differentiation of the mammary gland and susceptibility to carcinogenesis

Authors

Russo J, Tay LK, Russo IH

Reference

Breast Cancer Research and Treatment 1982; **2**:5–73

Summary

It has long been appreciated that early pregnancy acts as a critical protective factor for breast cancer both in human epidemiologic studies as well as rodent model systems with exogenous carcinogens. In this paper, hormonal effects of exogenous hormones as well as pregnancy on breast differentiation are explored. It is shown that pregnancy differentiates the terminal end buds into secretory units which are substantially more resistant to carcinogenic effects. Furthermore, pregnancy-induced morphogenetic events persisted indefinitely following parturition, providing lifetime risk reduction.

Related reference (1)   Russo J. Differentiation and pathogenesis of breast cancer. *Women and Cancer* 1998; **1**(Suppl 1):14–21.

Key message

One of the significant paradoxes in understanding the etiology of breast cancer in humans is provided by the apparently contradictory facts that while early menarche is associated with a significant increased risk of breast cancer, early first full-term pregnancy protects against breast cancer, whereas delayed pregnancy, particularly after age 30 is associated with an increased risk of breast cancer. Pathogenetic studies of human breast cancer demonstrate that terminal ducts and/or the intralobular terminal ducts are the sites of origin for breast cancer. During full differentiation of the mammary gland as induced by pregnancy and lactation, these structures are replaced by fully differentiated lobular units. This paper provided the first descriptive and biologic basis for understanding how differentiation of the mammary gland can alter risk for breast cancer.

Why it's important

The importance of this paper lies in a full appreciation of the critical role that hormones play in breast cancer risk. It is well appreciated that there is up to a 20-fold difference in risk of breast cancer amongst women living in different countries. Studies of migratory populations prove that these differences in risk are not due to genetic factors. In fact, these differences in risk can largely be explained by alterations in the hormonal milieu resulting from differences in three critical dates in a woman's life: first, age at menarche, which is controlled by height, weight, which in turn becomes largely regulated by diet; second, age at first full term pregnancy, which is commonly influenced by many social factors; and third, age at menopause. Height and weight also play a critical role in controlling time of menopause. Obviously, the molecular changes induced in the breast by these hormonal influences could provide critical data that might alter our ability to prevent the disease. For example, given that early pregnancy is protective against human breast cancer and, as this paper shows, there are morphologic changes in breast lobules which mirror breast cancer risk, then it might be possible to design exogenous hormone replacement systems that mimic early pregnancy, and by this means induce terminal differentiation of the breast. Thus the induction of the critical changes in lobules might even be used as a surrogate for evaluating breast cancer risk as well as the impact of a chemopreventive strategy.

By identifying and subcategorizing lobules with various risks of progression to malignancy, one can begin the molecular analysis of these different lobules in order to understand their differing biology. With more modern technologies such as gene array methodologies and laser capture microdissection, it will be possible to analyze in detail patterns of gene expression and cell–cell interaction in lobules at varying degrees of risk for breast carcinogenesis.

Strengths

1. This paper provides a biologic and morphologic surrogate for breast cancer risk in both rodent and human breast cancer.
2. The ability to link so strongly the well-defined rodent systems to human morphologic changes is an additional strength.

Weakness

The only weakness of these observations lies in the failure to as yet understand the precise circumstances required to safely induce breast lobule differentiation and the lack of a formal demonstration that this differentiation *per se* can prevent human breast cancer.

Relevance

As stated above, it cannot yet be concluded that these morphologic changes, while associated with varying degrees of breast cancer risk, are, in and of themselves, the source of protection. Additional work providing a clear understanding of the genomic and proteomic basis for 'differentiation' will hopefully allow for a better understanding of mechanisms by which breast lobular differentiation protects against cancer and also, hopefully, mechanisms of inducing that degree of differentiation safely.

Paper 6

Cloning of the human estrogen receptor cDNA

Authors

Walter R, Green S, Greene G, *et al.*

Reference

Proceedings of the National Academy of Sciences of the USA 1985; **82**:7889–7893

Summary

In this paper, the cloning of the human estrogen receptor cDNA is reported. The nucleotide sequence and the derived amino acid sequence permit division of the receptor into a variety of domains, including hormone binding, activation, DNA binding, and transcriptional regulation.

Related references **(1)** Couse JF, Korach KS. Estrogen receptor null mice: What have we learned and where will they lead us? *Endocrine Reviews* 1999; **20**:358–417.

(2) Norris JD, Paige LA, Christensen DJ, *et al.* Peptide antagonists of the human estrogen receptor. *Science* 1999; **285**:744–746.

(3) Murphy LC, Dotzlaw H, Leygue E, Douglas D, Coutts A, Watson PH. Estrogen receptor variants and mutations. *Journal of Steroid Biochemistry and Molecular Biology* 1997; **62**:363–372.

(4) Speirs V, Malone C, Walton DS, Kerin MJ, Atkin SL. Increased expression of estrogen receptor β-mRNA in tamoxifen resistant breast cancer patients. *Cancer Research* 1999; **59**:5421–5424.

Key message

The determination of the nucleotide sequence of the estrogen receptor provides the basis for critical analysis of receptor mutations and functional domains. It affords the ability to prepare large quantities of receptor for crystallographic analysis. Its three-dimensional structure would permit definitive analysis of mechanisms of action of hormones and anti-hormones, including SERMs.

Why it's important

The cloning of the estrogen receptor together with other steroid hormone receptors led directly to a clear understanding of their role as transcription factors. By understanding the domain structure of the receptor, it was possible to understand the preservation of ligand binding in the absence of a receptor which could promote gene transcription. Analysis was now possible on a multiplicity of human tumors and tissues for mutational events which might either inactivate the receptor or create a dominantly acting oncogene. The availability of the cDNA permitted both gene transfer and inactivation studies which allowed for significant analysis of mechanisms of receptor action.

Of additional importance, these studies led directly to the ability to make recombinant receptor which could in turn be crystallized. The crystal structure of the receptor clearly demonstrates how hormone binds to the receptor and how partial agonists such as antiestrogens alter the conformation of the receptor structure leading to altered recruitment of transcriptional coactivators and corepressors. These discoveries have finally unraveled the mystery of how the same ligand can function as an agonist in one tissue and an antagonist in another.

Strength

The great strength of this article lay in the development of a recombinant receptor critical for innumerable chemical and mechanistic studies. The exact definition of receptor function became possible by gene transfer to receptor-negative cells.

Weaknesses

For many years, it was thought that all of the estrogen receptor was a product of a single gene. Recently, this area has been revisited and a second estrogen receptor, now termed ERβ has been discovered, whose exact role in stimulating or inhibiting estrogen-dependent processes has not yet been fully elucidated. Thus some attributions of function were likely incorrect.

Relevance

The cloning of the estrogen receptor is critical to developing future methods of either creating (or recreating) hormone-dependent cells as well as abrogating hormone dependence. It is likely that the structural analysis of the receptor derived directly from its nucleotide sequence will eventually lead to the creation of new classes of pharmacologic agents able to antagonize or selectively agonize hormone effects in different tissues, thus avoiding toxicities of most currently available endocrine therapies.

Paper 7

Human breast cancer: correlation of relapse and survival with amplification of the HER-2/neu oncogene

Authors

Slamon DJ, Clark GM, Wong SG, Levin WJ, Ullrich A, McGuire WL

Reference

Science 1987; **235**:177–182

Summary

This article reports levels of genome amplification of the HER-2/*neu* (*erbB2*) oncogene in breast cancer and shows that high amplification levels are associated with an increased rate of relapse and decreased survival in a data set of women with early-stage breast cancer.

Related references (1)	Hung M-C, Lay Y-K. Basic science of HER-2/*neu*: a review. *Seminars in Oncology* 1999; **26**(4):51–59.
(2)	Shak S, for the Herceptin Multinational Investigator Study Group. Overview of the trastuzumab (Herceptin) anti-HER2 monoclonal antibody clinical program in HER2-overexpressing metastatic breast cancer. *Seminars in Oncology* 1999; **26**(4):71–77.
(3)	Sliwkowski MX, Lofgren JA, Lewis GD, Hotaling TE, Fendly BM, Fox JA. Nonclinical studies addressing the mechanism of action of trastuzumab (Herceptin). *Seminars in Oncology* 1999; **26**(4):60–70.
(4)	Ross JS, Fletcher JA. The HER-2/*neu* oncogene: prognostic factor, predictive factor and target for therapy. *Seminars in Cancer Biology* 1999; **9**: 125–138.

Key message

This paper demonstrates that the *erbB2* oncogene is commonly amplified in breast cancer and, furthermore, that amplification is associated with altered prognosis. While not necessarily proving a pathogenic relationship, the potential implication of the data is that this amplicon and its presumably overexpressed derived protein product contribute directly to disease pathogenesis.

Why it's important

The critical importance of this paper lies in documenting the role of the *erbB2* oncogene in human breast cancer. A variety of subsequent studies established the nearly perfect relationship between gene amplification and overexpression, whether measured by western blot, immunohistochemistry or other assay methodology. A wealth of follow-up studies subsequently demonstrated that over-expression of *erbB2* reliably predicted worse outcome for women with stage II breast cancer, although the data for women with stage I breast cancer remain somewhat more controversial. A critical subsequent experiment based on these studies linked overexpression to changes in the biology of the tumor. Initial observations demonstrated that overexpression was associated with an altered sensitivity to anthracycline-containing regimens as demonstrated by critical studies performed by the CALGB and the NSABP. Both cooperative groups demonstrated that patients receiving anthracycline-containing regimens, whose tumors also overexpressed *erbB2*, had substantially more benefit from the anthracycline-containing regimen compared to treatments without it.

However, overwhelmingly, the most important aspect of this work is the linkage of oncogene overexpression directly to disease pathogenesis. This work led directly to the exploration of means of blocking ErbB2 signaling in breast cancer. The first of these approaches to reach clinical practice involves the monoclonal antibody trastuzumab (Herceptin) which has been demonstrated both alone and in combination with either doxorubicin or paclitaxel, to increase the response rate to metastatic breast cancer, although the combination with anthracycline also very significantly increases the risk of cardiotoxicity. These clinical data provide a firm basis for a novel form of bio-logic therapy of breast cancer based upon interference with the function of a pathogenetic protein product and, as such, represents the creation of a remarkable and new paradigm for subsequent treatment of breast cancer based fully on disease pathogenesis.

Strength

This paper presents a straightforward hypothesis and verification of an association between ampli-fication of an oncogene and disease prognosis.

Weakness

Because of the heterogeneity of breast cancer and its many treatments, it still remains an area of some degree of controversy as to exactly how *erbB2* overexpression contributes to a worsened prognosis for patients with breast cancer.

Relevance

It is likely in the foreseeable future that virtually all breast cancers will be molecularly subtyped with therapies specifically directed against case-specific molecular causes rather than morphologic or other features and as such, this paper underlies the establishment of this approach. Because *erbB2* overexpression is common in other tumors as well (ovarian, gastric, bladder), this paper opened the door to the idea that tissue-specific diagnosis might be less important in choosing therapy than molecular profiling.

Paper 8

Tumor angiogenesis and metastasis – correlation in invasive breast carcinoma

Authors

Wiedner N, Semple JF, Welch WR, Folkman J

Reference

New England Journal of Medicine 1991; **324**:1–8

Summary

In this paper, microvessel density was measured in primary human breast cancers and this surrogate for angiogenesis was correlated with overall survival for patients with early stage breast cancer. A very high degree of correlation was seen between microvessel density and a worse prognosis.

Related references (1)   Giavazzi R, Taraboletti G. Angiogenesis and angiogenesis inhibitors in cancer. Forum. *Trends in Experimental and Clinical Medicine* 1999; **9**:261–272.

(2)   Brewer GJ, Dick RD, Grover DK, *et al.* Treatment of metastatic cancer with tetrathiomolybdate, an anticopper, antiangiogenic agent: phase I study. *Clinical Cancer Research* 2000; **6**:1–10.

(3)   Brower V. Angiogenesis inhibitors could represent a powerful adjunct to traditional cancer treatments, but the most effective routes for therapeutic intervention remain unclear. *Nature Biotechnology* 1999; **17**:963–968.

Key message

The critical point of this paper is the establishment of a relationship between the ability of a tumor to mount an angiogenic response in normal stroma and the ability of that tumor to metastasize to distant sites. By establishing the first link between angiogenesis and outcome in breast cancer, this paper provided crucial evidence supporting anti-angiogenic approaches for the management of breast cancer.

Why it's important

The work of Folkman and others has long emphasized the critical nature of stromal–epithelial interactions, particularly as they pertain to angiogenesis. It had been appreciated that the endothelium which makes up tumors, while abnormal in gross morphologic appearance, is nonetheless made up of non-malignantly transformed endothelial cells. Clearly, responses must be elicited in normal endothelial cells to stimulate their migration and growth, which represent either positive trophic stimuli from tumor cells or the relief of growth inhibitory signals that block endothelial proliferation. In this landmark study, areas within the tumor showing increased levels of angiogenesis as measured by the density of capillaries was highly correlated with distant metastatic disease. Therefore, the suggestion was created that such angiogenic activity is directly linked to the metastatic process – not an intuitively obvious notion. Because endothelial cells are themselves non-transformed, one might argue that they would be unlikely to change genetically in response to selective pressure and the number of signals responsible for their proliferation might be limited and therefore means of inhibiting their proliferation might on the one hand be more universally applicable, and on the other, less prone to the appearance of resistance. Thus, the demonstration that angiogenesis was linked to prognosis places anti-angiogenic therapy on a far stronger basis.

Strength

This paper establishes a link between morphologic evidence of angiogenesis and metastatic disease.

Weaknesses

1. The methodology used by these authors to measure microvascular density remains to this day controversial and difficult to replicate. It is based on 'hot spots' of angiogenesis within non-randomly selected portions of the tumor for which judgement is required.
2. The observation itself provides no obvious explanation as to why proliferation of blood vessels in hot spots necessarily is associated with an increased or decreased risk of metastasis.

Relevance

One of the most exciting areas of anticancer therapy investigation at this time is the development of anti-angiogenic agents. There are now emerging data that a variety of approaches including vascular endothelial growth factor (VEGF) receptor antibodies and tyrosine kinase inhibitors of the VEGF receptor may have antitumor activity in human beings. Thus, we appear to be on the verge of developing generic therapies for many forms of cancer based not on defeating the cancer cells themselves but targeting the evoked proliferative responses induced in normal endothelium.

Paper 9

The development of a functionally relevant cell culture model of progressive human breast cancer

Authors

Weaver VM, Howlett AR, Langston-Webster B, Peterson OW, Bissell MJ

Reference

Seminars in Cancer Biology 1995; **6**:175–184

Summary

In this paper, Mina Bissell and her colleagues describe a three-dimensional *in vitro* culture system in which normal and cancerous mammary cells are able to proliferate and develop three-dimensional interactions with themselves and defined basement membrane components which lead to a dramatically altered program of gene expression, far more reminiscent of gene expression patterns in fresh *in vivo* materials as compared to long-term cell culture.

Related references (1) Hosick HL, Inaguma Y, Kusakabe M, Sakakura T. Morphogenesis of mouse mammary epithelium in vivo in response to biomatrix prepared from stimulatory fetal mesenchyme. *Developmental Growth and Differentiation* 1988; **30**:229–240.

(2) Schroder JA, Lee DC. Dynamic expression of ERBB receptors in the developing mouse mammary gland. *Cell Growth and Differentiation* 1998; **9**:451–464.

(3) Neuenschwander S, Schwartz A, Wood TL, Roberts CT Jr, Henninghausen L. Involution of the lactating mammary gland is inhibited by the IGF system in a transgenic mouse model. *Journal of Clinical Investigation* 1996; **97**:2225–2232.

Key message

The critical message of this paper is that the *context* in which cells grow has much to do with their patterns of differentiation and response to a variety of agents. Though the standard 'dogma' of gene expression indicates that the products of genes eventually lead to proteins that are responsible for phenotypic effects, these data unequivocally show that influence through the extracellular matrix on cell shape remarkably alters the patterns of gene expression.

Why it's important

Work prior to this report had attempted to develop simple cell systems to model both normal mammary gland development and breast cancer *in vitro*. In fact, it has often been a major shortcoming of culture systems *in vitro* that many patterns of gene expression involving the breast – including milk protein synthesis, morphologic differentiation and response to exogenous agents – is very different from that seen *in vivo*. The seminal observation of this laboratory was that cell shape and interaction with either other identical cells in which three-dimensional structures could form or, in more simplified systems, interactions with basement membrane components can drastically alter patterns of gene expression. Thus, using novel culture conditions, Bissell and colleagues have been able to replicate normal mammary gland morphogenesis, milk protein production and other aspects of the lactogenic response as well as drastically altered patterns of gene expression in breast cancer cells. All of these changes are induced by imaginative culturing mechanisms in which cells, rather than being made adherent to tissue culture dish surfaces, are allowed to assume a three-dimensional configuration which recalls their normal duct structure and relationship to basement membranes.

Strength

Overwhelmingly, the greatest strength of this paper is the defining of a mechanism for growing cells in biologically relevant conditions which drastically changes their patterns of gene expression. These models are likely to be important to the normal human differentiation process as well as the process of human malignancy.

Weakness

The methodology used is quite technologically demanding and does not lend itself well to the availability of large amounts of cellular material for biochemical analysis.

Relevance

This paper partially reverses the classical dogma of information flow from the nucleus to the exterior of the cell. The data show conclusively that signals generated by the extracellular matrix that are conveyed back to the nucleus can profoundly alter patterns of gene expression. Not only are these observations fascinating in their own right, but their eventual elucidation at the molecular level is likely to suggest new forms of anticancer therapy.

Paper 10

Loss of heterozygosity in normal tissue adjacent to breast carcinoma

Authors

Deng G, Lu Y, Zlotnikov G, Thor A, Smith H

Reference

Science 1996; **274**:2057–2060

Summary

In this article, breast cancer and surrounding normal mammary epithelium was microdissected from patients with cancer. Malignant cells as well as morphologically normal cells at a distance from the primary tumor were analyzed for loss of heterozygosity (LOH). A significant degree of LOH (a surrogate for genetic alteration) was identified in apparently normal tissue. The conclusion of the work is that genetic changes in the breast precede morphologic evidence for malignant transformation.

Related reference (1)   Trent JM, Weber B, Guan XY, *et al.* Microdissection and microcloning of chromosomal alterations in human breast cancer. *Breast Cancer Research and Treatment* 1995; **33**:95–102.

Key message

Our current belief is that 100% of breast cancer is genetic; that is, all of breast cancer is caused by the accumulation of successive lesions in DNA which eventually result in changes in gene expression that reflect the malignant phenotype. The current study suggests that these changes occur before traditional morphologic or pathologic examination of tissue is able to detect evidence of malignancy.

Why it's important

The most fundamental question underlying the generation of all malignant tumors is what specific genetic changes are responsible for the disease. Subsidiary questions derived from this include whether or not these genetic changes are reversible and whether or not they can provide the basis for improved prognostication, diagnosis, therapy or prevention. The most traditional thinking concerning breast cancer is that a single mammary cell undergoes malignant transformation through a series of genetic events eventually resulting in a cell that completely reflects the malignant phenotype. The current work strongly suggests that changes may occur early in the breast with apparent growth advantages provided to such cells creating a so-called 'field' effect due to either the increased proliferation of cells or increased survival of affected cells by developing means of escaping apoptotic cell death. Thus, cyclic hormonal changes may greatly amplify the number of cells at risk for subsequent genetic damage which may result in further progression towards malignancy. The study further suggests that genetic analysis of apparently normal tissue in the breast may provide some indicator of cumulative DNA damage and the general risk to the individual for the subsequent development of breast cancer. One may also imagine that such analyses may provide some kind of measure of lifetime exposure to carcinogenic events within the breast. What this paper does not fully address, which has been the subject of significant additional research, is the product–precursor relationship between genetic events seen in normal or minimally abnormal tissue compared with fully transformed malignancies. Those studies tend to suggest that for the most part, genetic changes seen in normal tissue or benign hyperplasias are not truly benign in that they are preserved in the more transformed clones of cells seen within the same tissue. Thus, these studies may give important insights into the earliest genetic changes which underlie breast cancer.

Strength

This work is significant in helping to identify the earliest genetic changes which cause breast cancer.

Weaknesses

1. An original objection to this study was whether or not some of the LOHs seen in normal mammary cells might have represented errors in microdissection and come from neighboring contaminating tumor cells. This seems to have been ruled out by multiple studies replicating these results.

2. The general question of a small area in the breast that has undergone clonal expansion versus a true field effect involving much of the breast has not been fully addressed and would require multiple biopsies and analyses for LOH in multiple sectors of the breast.

3. The general technology of LOH is now rapidly advanced and a far more exhaustive genome-wide survey of areas of genetic change seen early in the breast can and should be undertaken. The critical problem will be identifying the specific genes involved in malignant change not just their chromosomal 'address'.

Relevance

As common sites of either amplification or loss of heterozygosity in the breast are mapped reproducibly to early lesions, more effective strategies of prevention will undoubtedly develop as will a more precise molecular classification of breast cancer. The latter will lead to far more accurate treatment selection and prognostication than can possibly be achieved by crude measures of cellular morphometry.

CHAPTER 6

Pathology

DAVID L PAGE

Introduction

In clinical medicine in general, and particularly in breast disease, the pathologist guides assignment of prognosis, prediction of therapeutic responsiveness, and choice of therapy with laboratory evaluation of tissues along with other evaluations of blood, radiology, etc. Indeed, although the word 'pathology' indicates any study of disease, it is the laboratory-based clinical role that has been the focus of pathologists evolving throughout the twentieth century. In the earlier part of the century, much clinical work in histopathology related to surgical therapy was done by surgeons. All of those early textbooks that were termed 'surgical pathology' were indeed the study of disease as presented by surgeons. An important and currently relevant example of fundamental anatomic principles, the radiating anatomy of the duct system of the breast, deserves note. Although clearly identified by a surgeon, Sir Astley Cooper [1], in the first half of the nineteenth century (Figure 6.1) the segmental approach to excision of breast lesions was utilized in the Milan trials [2], but largely ignored elsewhere until the few years prior to the twenty-first century, and is now fundamental to the surgical approach to most breast carcinomas.

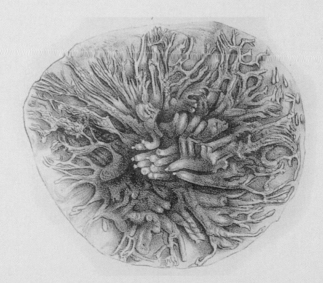

Figure 6.1   A drawing of the breast duct injection preparations of Sir Astley Cooper clearly presents the radiating anatomy of the system from the central duct into the various quadrants.

The evolution to our current level of understanding and clinical practice has been as it should be, balancing an overall classification scheme of biologic and anatomic plausibility integrated with adaptation to meet changing therapeutic capabilities and efficacies.

A continuing debate in the categorization of breast disease is whether to use terms in general use and modify them with current understanding and verifiable knowledge, or to create new schemes of classification. We feel very firmly that utilization of the current terms and modifying them with verifiable criteria linked to disease outcome is the proper approach. Our current categories began in the latter half of the twentieth century with a separation of the ordinary, or usual, types of breast cancers from those with special features [3,4]. The other two major influences on categories have been histologic grading and biologic markers.

These classic papers in breast pathology have been chosen because they have relevance to the current medical practice of breast disease. Most of them are involved in the evolution from description to verifiable criteria for case assignment, and the ability to predict outcomes presents a continuing challenge.

References

[1] Cooper AP. *The Anatomy and Diseases of the Breast.* Philadelphia: Lea and Blanchard, 1845.
[2] Veronesi U, Luini A, Galimberti V, Zurrida S. Conservation approaches for the management of stage I/II carcinoma of the breast: Milan Cancer Institute trials. *World Journal of Surgery* 1994; **18**:70–75.
[3] Elston CW, Ellis IO. *The Breast.* Edinburgh: Churchill Livingstone, 1998.
[4] Page DL, Jensen RA, Simpson JF. Premalignant and malignant disease of the breast: the roles of the pathologist. *Modern Pathology* 1998; **11**:120–128.

Paper 1

The diagnosis of tumors by aspiration

Author

Stewart FW

Reference

American Journal of Pathology 1933; **9**:801–813

Summary

Needle aspiration at the Memorial Hospital for Cancer and Allied Diseases in New York City was found to be an expeditious, practical method of tumor diagnosis in approximately 2500 cases. No untoward clinical results followed its use. The interpretation of smears of aspirated material often requires competent clinical assistance. Diagnosis by aspiration is as reliable as the combined intelligence of the clinician and pathologist makes it. The pathologist who ventures to interpret the material obtained by aspiration will have to revise or relearn many criteria. The clinician must appreciate how far the pathologist can logically go in interpreting the smear. Both must maintain a sympathetic attitude toward a new procedure. It is safe to state that in their own institution, the method so established its usefulness that it acquired a permanent place as a means of diagnosis.

Related references (1)   Barrows GH, Anderson TJ, Lamb JL, Dixon JM. Fine-needle aspiration of breast cancer. Relationship of clinical factors to cytology results in 689 primary malignancies. *Cancer* 1986; **58**:1493–1498.
(2)   Frable WJ. Needle aspiration of the breast. *Cancer* 1984; **53**:671–676.

Key message

There are many papers central to the establishment and evaluation of fine needle aspiration cytology in breast cancer diagnosis and management. This is chosen because of its early presentation and clear message of the necessity of clinical information in the interpretation of these samples.

Why it's important

This paper provides an example of the integration of laboratory, and clinical data that evolved into the so-called 'triple test' that integrates physical examination, mammographic appearance and cytologic interpretation in assessing the overall level of diagnostic certainty. This embodies clinical diagnosis by balancing probabilities – an approach long central to the art and science of medicine.

Strength

The concept of likelihood, intrinsic to evaluation of these samples, can be extended to indicate the types of cancers less likely to be clearly identified by needle aspiration. The clinical 'false negatives' of needle aspiration are usually small cancers, also of low malignant potential [1–3].

Weaknesses

1. The utility and breadth of relevance of needle aspiration is limited by the current technology of core needle biopsies that provide tissue samples [4] and the lack of experience of many pathologists in this demanding technique outside of specialty-directed clinics and centers.

2. This dependence on breadth of experience is also evident in that the adequacy of samples is operator dependent (related reference 1).

Relevance

While the continuing central role of cyto/histopathologic data in cancer diagnosis remains strong, its relevance is interwoven into the background and requirements of the individual clinical setting [4].

References

[1] O'Malley F, Casey TT, Winfield AC, Rodgers WH, Sawyers J, Page DL. Clinical correlates of false-negative fine needle aspirations of the breast in a consecutive series of 1005 patients. *Surgery, Gynecology and Obstetrics* 1993; **176**:360–364.

[2] Page DL, Johnson JE, Dupont WD. Probabilistic approach to the reporting of fine-needle aspiration cytology of the breast [see comments]. *Cancer* 1997; **81**:6–9.

[3] Lamb J, Anderson TJ. Influence of cancer histology on the success of fine needle aspiration of the breast. *Journal of Clinical Pathology* 1989; **42**:733–735.

[4] Pisano ED, Fajardo LL, Tsimikas J, *et al.* Rate of insufficient samples for fine-needle aspiration for nonpalpable breast lesions in a multicenter clinical trial: the Radiologic Diagnostic Oncology Group 5 Study. The RDOG5 investigators. *Cancer* 1998; **82**:679–688.

Paper 2

Comedo carcinoma (or comedo-adenoma) of the female breast

Author

Bloodgood JC

Reference

American Journal of Cancer 1934; **22**:843–849

Summary

In 1908 Bloodgood first described the comedo tumor of the breast and classified it among the adenocarcinomas as 'adenocarcinoma, comedo'. None of the 12 cases of the pure type had metastasis in the axilla, and there were no deaths from breast cancer. The only positive cure after local recurrence of carcinoma belonged to this group.

The pure comedo tumor (not mixed with fully developed cancer) takes its place among the borderline tumors of the breast. It must be recognized in frozen and permanent sections if progress is to be made in diagnosis and treatment. Comedo ductal carcinoma *in situ* was recognized as special because no patients had metastasis.

| **Related references (1)** | Bloodgood JC. Borderline breast tumors. *American Journal of Cancer* 1932; **16**:103–114. |
| **(2)** | Tod MC, Dawson EK. The diagnosis and treatment of doubtful mammary tumours. *Lancet* 1934; **ii**:1041–1045. |

Key message

The 'comedo adenoma' as opposed to comedo carcinoma (*in situ*) can be locally excised for cure. The former are examples of intermediate grade ductal carcinoma *in situ* (DCIS) (Figure 6.2), with 'adenoma' indicating benignancy.

Why it's important

This observation remains important today with the growing acceptance of the ability to locally excise small and lower grade DCIS lesions with defined, negative margins, and the related necessity of classifying subsets of DCIS.

Strength

At about the same time Bloodgood emphasized histologic examination of DCIS, he had identified some of the cases in Halsted's early series of breast cancers as examples of complex cysts of 'cyst-adenomatous changes' (related reference 1).

Weakness

Despite Bloodgood's strong support for a histologic definition of malignancy and the acceptance of borderline categories of malignancy, the former was not sufficiently clear to attain general understanding.

Many continued for decades to believe that there was a sharp line between benign and malignant, and continued gross examination as a diagnostic standard. In the same year, two prominent women physicians – one a pathologist and one a surgeon – stated that during surgery if a mass appearing as a cancer was found by the surgeon 'that mastectomy should be undergone immediately in the best interest of the patient's welfare'. That general approach was certainly the standard of care for surgeons and pathologists for the next 20 or 30 years despite the comments of Dr Bloodgood.

Relevance

The abiding importance of this article is a clear mandate for the histologic stratification of borderline categories indicating lesser treatment than the complete radical (Halsted) mastectomy.

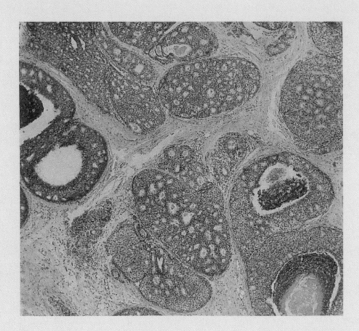

Figure 6.2   Histologic image from this classic paper by Bloodgood. This is an intermediate-grade ductal carinoma *in situ* with cribiform pattern and foci of necrosis. Bloodgood separated this from the higher-grade comedo lesions by terming it 'comedo adenoma'.

Paper 3

Lobular carcinoma in situ. *A rare form of mammary cancer*

Authors

Foote FW Jr, Stewart FW

Reference

American Journal of Pathology 1941; **17**:491–496

Summary

The mode of infiltration of these lobular cancers is peculiar and somewhat obscure and often has wide infiltration within the breast. Large numbers of isolated, loose cells of rather uniform size might be readily confused with large mast cells. When they metastasize to nodes, their form and distribution are such that they might be confused with cells of a lymphoma. The *in situ* lobular carcinoma occurred in multiple lobules and often was associated with invasion in multiple foci.

This first description of lobular carcinoma *in situ* (LCIS) and invasive lobular carcinoma (ILC) was quite complete descriptively, defining a special category of both infiltrating carcinoma and an associated variety of *in situ* carcinoma.

Related references (1)	McDivitt RW, Hutter RV, Foote FW Jr, Stewart FW. *In-situ* lobular carcinoma. A prospective follow-up study indicating cumulative patient risks. *Journal of the American Medical Association* 1967; **201**:82–86.
(2)	Hutter RV, Snyder RE, Lucas JC, Foote FW Jr, Farrow JH. Clinical and pathologic correlation with mammographic findings in lobular carcinoma *in situ*. *Cancer* 1969; **23**:826–839.
(3)	Hutter RV, Foote FW Jr. Lobular carcinoma *in situ*. Long term follow-up. *Cancer* 1969; **24**:1081–1085.

Key message

Foote and Stewart recognized the major special pattern of *in situ* and invasive breast cancer other than the general, catchall category of 'ductal' or no special type. Most of the major features relevant to mammographic correlation and oddities of behavior were also noted: diffuse infiltration in the breast, lymphoma-like involvement of metastatic sites and distant metastases with often subtle involvement of the breast.

Why it's important

Subsequent follow-up from Memorial Hospital in New York of women with biopsies of LCIS only, indicated a strong association with the later development of invasive carcinoma, often of the single cell infiltrative, lobular type (see related references 1–3).

This study provided the stimulus for later stratification of the premalignant changes of the lobular series [1–3].

Strength

This was a clear presentation of a distinct type of infiltrating breast cancer with special histologic features and a presumed precursor lesion for an infiltrating carcinoma of similar cytology and special histologic features.

Weakness

The lesions of LCIS were termed 'carcinoma' with no evidence other than circumstantial co-existence with a special pattern of invasive cancer.

Relevance

This paper provides a special set of premalignant and malignant phenotypes with distinct associations with long-term survival, and late failure, often with bony and/or gastrointestinal metastases. These are probably distinct molecular biological associations, beginning with alterations in E-cadherin.

References

[1] Marshall LM, Hunter DJ, Connolly JL, *et al*. Risk of breast cancer associated with atypical hyperplasia of lobular and ductal types. *Cancer Epidemiology, Biomarkers and Prevention* 1997; **6**:297–301.

[2] Page DL, Dupont WD, Rogers LW. Ductal involvement by cells of atypical lobular hyperplasia in the breast: a long-term follow-up study of cancer risk. *Human Pathology* 1988; **19**:201–207.

[3] Page DL, Kidd TE Jr, Dupont WD, Simpson JF, Rogers LW. Lobular neoplasia of the breast: higher risk for subsequent invasive cancer predicted by more extensive disease. *Human Pathology* 1991; **22**:1232–1239.

Paper 4

An atlas of subgross pathology of the human breast with special reference to possible precancerous lesions

Authors

Wellings SR, Jensen HM, Marcum RG

Reference

Journal of the National Cancer Institute 1975; **55**:231–273

Summary

One hundred and ninety-six whole human breasts were examined by a subgross sampling technique with histologic confirmation. The method permitted the enumeration and identification of essentially all the focal dysplastic, metaplastic, hyperplastic, anaplastic, and neoplastic lesions. Completely suitable for analysis were 67 breasts obtained by autopsy, 29 cancerous breasts obtained by mastectomy, and 23 contralateral to those with cancer. All lesions, photographed subgrossly, were subsequently confirmed and correlated histologically. Morphologic evidence supported the hypothesis that lesions traditionally grouped as mammary dysplasia or fibrocystic disease arose in terminal ductal-lobular units (TDLU) with the probable exception of papillomas of ducts larger than terminal ones. Of the contralateral breasts, 60% with clinical cancer contained such lesions. An atypical lobule (AL) of type A (ALA) had the following characteristics: (a) it was more common in cancerous breasts or in those contralateral to cancer than in breasts not so identified; (b) it was a terminal structure on the mammary tree; (c) it tended to persist after the menopause, whereas normal lobules usually atrophied; and (d) as ALA progressed to DCIS, the unfolded lobule resembled a duct which gave the false impression that DCIS was a ductal lesion. The morphologic evidence supported the hypothesis that the lesions herein called AL were derived from TDLU and were precancerous.

Many of our current concepts of premalignant lesions in the breast began in this first attempt to catalog the many singly identified lesions and their associations with breast cancer in the host.

Related references (1) Jensen HM, Rice JR, Wellings SR. Preneoplastic lesions in the human breast. *Science* 1976; **191**:295–297.

(2) Jacobs TW, Byrne C, Colditz G, Connolly JL, Schnitt SJ. Radial scars in benign breast-biopsy specimens and the risk of breast cancer. *New England Journal of Medicine* 1999; **340**:430–436.

(3) Jensen RA, Page DL, Dupont WD, Rogers LW. Invasive breast cancer risk in women with sclerosing adenosis. *Cancer* 1989; **64**:1977–1983.

(4) Page DL, Schuyler PA, Dupont WD, Jensen RA, Plummer WD Jr, Simpson JF. Atypical lobular hyperplasia as a unilateral predictor of breast cancer risk: a retrospective cohort study. *Lancet* 2003 **361**:125–129.

(5) Allred D, Mohsin SK, Fugua SA. Histological and biological evolution of human premalignant breast disease. *Endocrine Related Cancer* 2001; **8**:47–61.

Key message

Wellings and Jensen gave attention to precise patterns of lobular units and a clear differentiation of 'lobular' and 'ductal' lesion groups thay they called atypical lobules type B (ALB) and A (ALA) respectively. Later epidemiologic studies have used individual lesions and groupings of lesions to define cancer risk groups (related references 2 and 3).

Why it's important

Their definitions of lesions guided later epidemiologic, follow-up studies that gave attention to individual lesions and their associations (related reference 4).

The most common lesion that was positively associated with cancer, although weakly, was the ALA1. This is an unfolded, enlarged lobular unit with active-appearing columnar cells (related reference 5). The ALA1 may be a useful target for the appearance of premalignant molecular markers.

Strength

This paper drew attention to the importance of the differences between lobular units and terminal ducts (the TDLU) and the true ducts.

Weaknesses

1. The cancer associations are concurrent ones that provide circumstantial evidence only.
2. The primary definition of lesions was from subgross evaluation that provided the TDLU observation, with histologic analysis being secondary.

Relevance

The TDLU became the proper focus of attention as the likely sites for cancer development because they were the sites of benign proliferative lesions other than ductal papillomas.

Paper 5

Medullary carcinoma of the breast: a clinicopathologic study with 10 year follow-up

Authors

Ridolfi RL, Rosen PP, Port A, Kinne D, Miké V

Reference

Cancer 1977; **40**:1365–1385

Summary

Primary breast carcinomas from 192 patients treated between 1955 and 1965 for medullary carcinoma or duct carcinoma with medullary features were reviewed and reclassified using strictly defined pathologic criteria. Tumors that fulfilled requirements for medullary carcinoma were identified in 57 patients. Another 79 tumors that varied slightly from these criteria were termed 'atypical' medullary carcinoma and 56 were characterized as non-medullary carcinoma. When compared with the patients with non-medullary infiltrating duct carcinoma, patients with medullary carcinoma had a significantly higher survival rate at 10 years (34% versus 63%), similar frequency of axillary lymph node metastases, and a more favorable prognosis when nodal metastases were present. Within the medullary carcinoma group, patients had a significantly better survival rate if their primary tumors were smaller than 3 cm in diameter. The average size of medullary carcinomas was 2.9 cm and that of non-medullary carcinomas 4.0 cm. Bilaterality was not more common in patients with medullary carcinoma, but the interval between diagnosis of the tumors was twice as long when one lesion was medullary (8.8 years) than when both were infiltrating duct carcinomas (4.6 years). Bilaterality was significantly more common among patients with medullary carcinoma who had a positive family history. The medullary lesion was most often the second one to be diagnosed. The 79 patients with atypical medullary carcinoma had a 10-year survival rate of 74%. Patients in this group whose tumors had a sparse lymphoid infiltrate had a relatively poor prognosis. Intraductal carcinoma at the periphery of the lesion was not associated with a less favorable prognosis. It was concluded that intraductal carcinoma was consistent with the diagnosis of medullary carcinoma if all other criteria for the diagnosis were satisfied. With these exceptions, the authors were unable to draw any firm conclusions about favorable or unfavorable effects of other morphologic features on survival in the group with atypical medullary carcinoma. Until further study of this group reveals that some or all of the lesions form a distinct clinicopathologic entity they are best included under the heading of infiltrating duct carcinoma. When the criteria described in this report were used, medullary carcinoma proved to be a specific lesion associated with a significantly better prognosis than ordinary infiltrating duct carcinoma.

Related references (1)   Cooper HS, Patchefsky AS, Krall RA. Tubular carcinoma of the breast. *Cancer* 1978; **42**:2334–2342.

(2)   Dixon JM, Anderson TJ, Page DL, Lee D, Duffy SW. Infiltrating lobular carcinoma of the breast. *Histopathology* 1982; **6**:149–161.

Key message

Special histologic types or subtypes of breast cancer can be linked to clinical outcome parameters. This represents one of the earliest and best attempts to link special clusters of anatomic features to outcome. This approach seeks to accept that some clustering of features are rare, and best evaluated by beginning the inquiry with as precise case definition as possible. The credibility and utility of these exercises are advanced by designing a comparison population that is similar, but not precisely the same. Cooper *et al.* did this with tubular carcinoma and Dixon *et al.* did it for invasive lobular carcinoma (see related references 1 and 2).

Why it's important

We continue to search for precise definitions and biologic associations that may well become molecular.

Strength

This paper remains the key reference for studies seeking appropriate histologic definition of this special type of breast cancer.

Weakness

The uncertainties continue to derive from the rarity of this tumor type (about 4% of breast cancers maximally), and there are several defining variables, making precise testing of each possible combination a daunting task.

Relevance

There are specific clusterings of histologic elements that have special clinical relevance. Besides the seeming unlikely association of high nuclear grade and high proliferation rate with an improved prognosis, these features are associated with the cancers appearing within the *BRCA1* hereditary breast cancer families.

Paper 6

Intraductal carcinoma of the breast: follow-up after biopsy only

Authors

Page DL, Dupont WD, Rogers LW, Landenberger M

Reference

Cancer 1982; **49**:751–758

Summary

Twenty-eight women with ductal carcinoma *in situ* (DCIS) of the breast treated by biopsy only were identified in a histologic review of 11 760 biopsies performed between 1950 and 1968. Seven of the 25 women followed for more than three years developed invasive breast carcinoma, all in the same breast with a previously detected DCIS. Average follow-up interval for the 18 women not developing invasive carcinoma was 16 years. The invasive carcinomas presented clinically from three to ten years (average 6.1) after the biopsies demonstrating DCIS. Four women with invasive carcinoma developed distant metastases following mastectomy. This study suggests that 28% of women treated with biopsy only for DCIS presenting as an incidental histologic finding will develop invasive carcinoma in a follow-up period of approximately 15 years.

Related references (1) Betsill WL Jr, Rosen PP, Lieberman PH, Robbins GF. Intraductal carcinoma. Long-term follow-up after treatment by biopsy alone. *Journal American Medical Association* 1978; **239**:1863–1867.

(2) Page DL, Dupont WD, Rogers LW, Jensen RA, Schuyler PA. Continued local recurrence of carcinoma 15–25 years after a diagnosis of low grade ductal carcinoma *in situ* of the breast treated only by biopsy. *Cancer* 1995; **76**:1197–1200.

Key message

The natural history of small, low-grade DCIS is to recur after inadequate local resection in the same place in the same breast. This information comes from two important studies (this paper and related reference 1) often misquoted in the literature as representing surgical excision of DCIS. Actually, they represented biopsies done during the 1950s and 1960s with the dominant indication of palpability.

The two studies are strikingly similar in showing an incidence of these minimal DCIS lesions of 0.3% in breast biopsies reported as benign in this premammographic era and subsequent evolution of invasive carcinoma at the same site in the same breast extending over at least 20 years (related reference 2) largely confirming the unicentric nature of this disease in the majority of cases, also shown by three dimensional reconstruction studies [1].

Why it's important

The separation of specifically defined atypical ductal hyperplasia from smaller examples of DCIS is central to our evolution of understanding of minimal examples of DCIS. Despite some histologic similarities, atypical ductal hyperplasia (ADH) describes a totally different natural history, implicating a moderate increase in risk of later invasive breast cancer anywhere in either breast, importantly initially derived from this same cohort of women [2,3] (see also Paper 10 in this chapter).

Strength

Halsted, whose beliefs of breast cancer biology and treatment dominated much of the twentieth century, did not speak of the concept of 'carcinoma *in situ*'. However, this group of diseases are fulfilling a major concept of his approach to therapy – and that is that there are lesions within the breast that may be locally removed and controlled prior to the (highly likely to happen) development of metastatic capacity.

Weakness

Despite the consistency of information from the Memorial study (related reference 1) and the Vanderbilt study (related reference 2), their derivation from the pre-mammographic era, with necessaary restricted sampling of tissue, limits relevant information. Follow-up of these women was without the aid of mammography, limiting early diagnosis of advancing residual disease in the breast, and leading to most of the local recurrences as invasive cancer in the pre-mammographic era [2,3].

Relevance

There is now wide and growing acceptance of lower grades and smaller examples of DCIS as having the capability of successful local excision for cure, avoiding the implications of local residual disease having the capacity to evolve into more extensive DCIS as well as invasive cancer if not excised.

References

[1] Holland R, Hendriks JH, Vebeek AL, Mravunac M, Schuurmans Stekhoven JH. Extent, distribution, and mammographic/histological correlations of breast ductal carcinoma *in situ*. *Lancet* 1990; **335**:519–522.

[2] Page DL, Dupont WD. Anatomic markers of human premalignancy and risk of breast cancer. *Cancer* 1990; **66**:1326–1335.

[3] Page DL, Jensen RA. Ductal carcinoma *in situ* of the breast: understanding the misunderstood stepchild. *Journal of the American Medical Association* 1996; **275**:948–949.

Paper 7

Cell turnover in the 'resting' human breast: influence of parity, contraceptive pill, age and laterality

Authors

Anderson TJ, Ferguson DJ, Raab GM

Reference

British Journal of Cancer 1982; **46**:376–382

Summary

Morphological identification of cell multiplication (mitosis) and cell deletion (apoptosis) within the lobules of the 'resting' human breast is used to assess the response of the breast parenchyma to the menstrual cycle. The responses are shown to have a biorhythm in phase with the menstrual cycle, with a 3-day separation of the mitotic and apoptotic peaks. The study fails to demonstrate significant differences in the responses between groups defined according to parity, contraceptive-pill use or presence of fibroadenoma. However, significant differences are found in the apoptotic response according to age and laterality. The results highlight the complexity of modulating influences on breast parenchymal turnover in the 'resting' state, and prompt the investigation of other factors as well as steroid hormones and prolactin in the promotion of mitosis. The factors promoting apoptosis in the breast are still not clear.

Related references (1) Battersby S, Robertson BJ, Anderson TJ, King RJ, McPherson K. Influence of menstrual cycle, parity and oral contraceptive use on steroid hormone receptors in normal breast. *British Journal of Cancer* 1992; **65**:601–607.

(2) Pike MC, Spicer DV, Dahmoush L, Press MF. Estrogens, progestogens, normal breast cell proliferation. *Epidemiology Reviews* 1993; **15**:17–35.

Key message

The integration of histopathologic alterations with disease prediction also involves identification of normality, and the problems of identifying 'normality' in a system as complex as the human breast defies imagination. Any attempt to do so must first recognize the usual variables of age, puberty, menstrual cycling, pregnancy, lactation and involution.

Why it's important

These observations inaugurated a paradigm shift of broad importance. First, it indicated that the proliferative events in the human breast related to the menstrual cycle were quite different from that of the endometrium, previously assumed to be analogous.

Strength

The epidemiologic evidence has been relatively strong and consistent that the 'estrogen augmented by progestogen' in breast cancer risk is true, and that prostogens do not protect the breast from carcinogenesis as it does the endometrium [1]. The cancer risks of menopausal replacement with low doses of estrogen are small in any case and may not be equal in all women [1].

Weakness

Basic observations about the biology of human tissues are difficult to obtain, and even clear observations like this one awaited confirmation in the setting of epidemiologic studies [1].

Relevance

Progesterone has a different role in breast epithelial cell regulation than in the endometrium, progesterone probably grants a greater stimulatory effect to the breast epithelium in combination with estrogen than with estrogen alone.

Reference

[1] Schairer C, Lubin J, Troisi R, Sturgeon S, Brinton L, Hoover R. Menopausal estrogen and estrogen–progestin replacement therapy and breast cancer risk. *Journal of the American Medical Association* 2000; **283**:485–491.

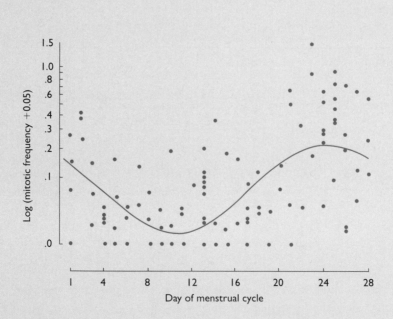

Figure 6.3 Frequency of mitoses on each day of the menstrual cycle, peaking in the latter half of the luteal phase.

Paper 8

Pathologic findings from the National Surgical Adjuvant Project for Breast Cancers (protocol no. 4). X. Discriminants for tenth year treatment failure

Authors

Fisher ER, Sass R, Fisher B

Reference

Cancer 1984; **53**:712–723

Summary

A search for prognostic discriminants of treatment failure in the tenth postmastectomy year was undertaken in 614 patients enrolled in protocol no. 4 of the National Surgical Adjuvant Project for Breast Cancers treated by radical mastectomy. Exploratory analysis of 38 pathologic and 6 clinical features disclosed 16 and 13 variables significantly related to nodal status and treatment failure, respectively. However, multivariate analyses with life tables adjusted or controlled for nodal status revealed that patients whose tumors measured less than 2 cm had a more favorable clinical course. All of the characteristics were also explored when patients were stratified according to numbers of nodal metastases, the most significant prognostic discriminant for disease-free survival in the tenth year. High histologic grade according to the authors' conventional grading method were observed to adversely influence disease-free survival in patients with negative nodes. Histologic grade and tumor size were significantly recognized as discriminatory in patients with 4+ nodes. It was therefore concluded that nodal category, histologic grade, and tumor size, in the contexts noted, represent strong prognostic discriminants exerting a rather constant influence on disease-free survival at least to the tenth postmastectomy period. The prognostic value of categorizing those patients with 4+ positive nodes into subgroups with 4 to 6, 7 to 12 and 13+ was reaffirmed. The actual disease-free survival of patients in the tenth year was not strikingly different from that observed previously by the authors at 5 years in this cohort.

Related references (1)	Fisher ER, Gregorio RM, Fisher B, Redmond C, Vellios F, Sommers SC. The pathology of invasive breast cancer. A syllabus derived from findings of the National Surgical Adjuvant Breast Project (protocol no. 4), *Cancer* 1975; **36**:1–85.
(2)	Fisher ER, Redmond C, Fisher B. A perspective concerning the relation of duration of symptoms to treatment failure in patients with breast cancer. *Cancer* 1977; **40**:3160–3167.

Key message

Among many 'firmaments' in the manner in which we now approach the classification of breast disease, perhaps the most important was the recognition that histologic grading and special histologic categories could co-exist to recognize the range of determinable histologic features.

Why it's important

This paper introduced the modern methodology of rigorous assessment of prognostic indicators in a multicenter trial setting. It also contained the important concept that most breast cancers could be best recognized histologically as 'not otherwise specified' because they did not fit in within a special histologic type (see related reference 1).

Strength

This paper provided a guideline for later assessment of predictors within other subsets, such as the different utility of some elements in node-negative as opposed to node-positive disease.

Weakness

It did not provide adequate guidance for the use of histologic grading, despite indicating its clinical usefulness.

Relevance

This study provided the verification of many of the strata used subsequently in clinical trials, particularly the grouping of lymph node involvement by numbers of nodes involved by cancer.

Paper 9

Pathologic predictors of early local recurrence in Stage I and II breast cancer treated by primary radiation therapy

Authors

Schnitt SJ, Connolly JL, Harris JR, Hellman S, Cohen RB

Reference

Cancer 1984; **53**:1049–1057

Summary

Thirty-four gross and histologic features of the primary tumor in 231 cases of clinical stage I and II invasive breast cancer were reviewed in an attempt to identify features which might correlate with an increased risk of local recurrence within the breast following biopsy and primary radiation therapy. Local recurrence risk at 5 years was calculated for each feature studied. While results are reported in terms of 5-year actuarial local recurrence risk, not all patients were followed for 5 years (median follow-up period, 44 months). Patients with cases in which the biopsy was less than excisional had a considerably greater actuarial risk of local recurrence at 5 years than those in which the biopsy was excisional (36% versus 8%; $p = 0.0005$). Among 154 infiltrating ductal carcinomas treated by excisional biopsy prior to radiotherapy, histologic features associated with a significantly increased local recurrence risk at 5 years were the combination of extensive intraductal involvement by carcinoma and high nuclear grade and/or high mitotic index. Twenty-seven tumors demonstrated this constellation of features, and there was a 5-year actuarial local recurrence risk of 39% among this group. The local recurrence risk for the remainder of the population was only 4% ($p < 0.0001$). Thus, through pathologic examination of the primary, the authors identified a subgroup of patients with a considerably increased risk of local recurrence following biopsy and primary radiotherapy.

Related references (1) Harris JR, Connolly JL, Schnitt SJ, *et al.* The use of pathologic features in selecting the extent of surgical resection necessary for breast cancer patients treated by primary radiation therapy. *Annals of Surgery* 1985; **201**:164–169.

(2) Schnitt SJ, Abner A, Gelman R, *et al.* The relationship between microscopic margins of resection and the risk of local recurrence in patients with breast cancer treated with breast-conserving surgery and radiation therapy. *Cancer* 1994; **74**:1746–1751.

Key message

The likelihood of recurrence in the preserved breast can be largely predicted by pathologic analysis of the excised tissue.

Breast preservation after diagnosis of breast cancer presented new challenges for pathologists and clinicians in the evaluation of the likelihood of successful preservation without recurrence in the preserved breast.

Why it's important

Clinical practice was changed by these observations, inaugurating the realization that failure in the preserved breast was largely the result of leaving ductal carcinoma *in situ* behind.

Weakness

Early papers in the series did not completely separate the importance of extensive in situ component from other features such as grade of the invasive component, accomplished later [1].

Relevance

The careful ascertainment of margins in resected specimens of breast cancer has become central to assessment by surgical pathologists [2,3].

References

[1] Nixon AJ, Schnitt SJ, Gelman R, Gage I, Bornstein B, Hetelekidis S, Recht A, Silver B, Harris JR, Connolly JL. Relationship of tumor grade to other pathologic features and to treatment outcome of patients with early stage breast carcinoma treated with breast-conserving therapy. *Cancer* 1996; **78**:1426–1431.

[2] Connolly JL, Boyages J, Nixon AJ, Peiro G, Gage I, Silver B, Recht A, Harris JR, Schnitt SJ. Predictors of breast recurrence after conservative surgery and radiation therapy for invasive breast cancer. *Modern Pathology* 1998; **11**:134–139.

[3] Fitzgibbons PL, Connolly JL, Page DL. Updated Protocol for the Examination of Specimens From Patients With Carcinomas of the Breast. *Archives of Pathology and Laboratory Medicine* 2000; **124**:1026–1033.

Paper 10

Risk factors for breast cancer in women with proliferative breast disease

Authors

Dupont WD, Page DL

Reference

New England Journal of Medicine 1985; **312**:146–151

Summary

To assess the importance of various risk factors for breast cancer in women with benign proliferative breast lesions, the authors reevaluated 10 366 consecutive breast biopsies performed in women who had presented at three Nashville hospitals. The median duration of follow-up was 17 years for 3303 women, 1925 of whom had proliferative disease. This sample contained 84.4% of the patients originally selected for follow-up. Women having proliferative disease without atypical hyperplasia had a risk of cancer that was 1.9 times the risk in women with non-proliferative lesions (95% confidence interval (CI) 1.2–2.9). The risk in women with atypical hyperplasia (atypia) was 5.3 times that in women with non-proliferative lesions (95% CI 3.1–8.8). A family history of breast cancer had little effect on the risk in women with non-proliferative lesions. However, the risk in women with atypia and a family history of breast cancer was 11 times that in women who had non-proliferative lesions without a family history (95% CI 5.5–24). Calcification elevated the cancer risk in patients with proliferative disease. Although cysts alone did not substantially elevate the risk, women with both cysts and a family history of breast cancer had a risk 2.7 times higher than that for women without either of these risk factors (95% CI 1.5–4.6). This study demonstrated that the majority of women (70%) who undergo breast biopsy for benign disease are not at increased risk of cancer. However, patients with a clinically meaningful elevation in cancer risk can be identified on the basis of atypical hyperplasia and a family history of breast cancer.

Related references

(1)   Page DL, Dupont WD, Rogers LW, Rados MS. Atypical hyperplastic lesions of the female breast. A long-term follow-up study, *Cancer* 1985; **55**:2698–2708.

(2)   Fitzgibbons PL, Henson DE, Hutter RVP, for the Cancer Committee of the College of American Pathologists. Benign breast changes and the risk for subsequent breast cancer – an update of the 1985 consensus statement. *Archives of Pathology and Laboratory Medicine* 1998; **122**:1053–1055.

Key message

The performance of a breast biopsy does not meaningfully increase a woman's later risk of breast cancer unless tissue changes are present that have been verified in follow-up studies to be linked to increased risk.

Why it's important

Distinguishing between limited lesions which had previously been called ductal carcinoma *in situ* (DCIS) and recognizing them as having a minor to moderate degree of general increased cancer risk avoided unnecessary mastectomies. Identification of the diagnostic lesion of atypical ductal hyperplasia (ADH) also provided a focal point for understanding the anatomical underpinnings of premalignant breast disease. This provision of a diagnosis without the word 'carcinoma' for minimal lesions previously regarded as small examples of DCIS reduced both overdiagnosis of carcinoma *in situ* and overtreatment of minimal lesions.

Recognition and evaluation of different premalignant lesions with epidemiologically identified risk also dispelled the myth that cysts provided any meaningful indication of breast cancer risk when present by themselves.

Strength

Both histologic criteria and risk implications were widely accepted (related reference 2) and confirmed in other cohort studies [1].

Weakness

The importance of overall size as well as uniformity and extent of histologic change was emphasized by Tavassoli and Norris [2], who also used the same basic criteria of these 1985 studies.

Relevance

This study indicates the need for precise histologic assessment of breast tissue; and specifically the mandate to use these histologic, cytologic and extent criteria when citing the risk implications.

References

[1] London SJ, Connolly JL, Schnitt SJ, Colditz GA. A prospective study of benign breast disease and risk of breast cancer. *Journal of the American Medical Association* 1992; **267**:941–944.

[2] Tavassoli FA, Norris HJ. A comparison of the results of long-term follow-up for atypical intraductal hyperplasia and intraductal hyperplasia of the breast. *Cancer* 1990; **65**:518–529.

Paper 11

Comparison of immunocytochemical and steroid-binding assays for estrogen receptor in human breast tumors

Authors

King WJ, DeSombre ER, Jensen EV, Greene GL

Reference

Cancer Research 1985; **45**:293–304

Summary

An estrogen receptor immunocytochemical assay which uses monoclonal antibodies to the estrogen receptor protein was applied to several human tissues, including human breast tumors, and the results were compared to those of steroid-binding assays performed on cytosol extracts of the same tissues. Specific immunoperoxidase staining in fixed, frozen sections was confined to the nucleus of selected cell populations within each tissue examined. In 117 human breast cancers, the presence or absence of nuclear staining was significantly associated with the concentration of cytosolic estrogen receptor. Thirty-eight estrogen receptor immunocytochemical assay-positive tumors were further assessed for several quantifiable features of the staining, including intensity, cellularity, and the proportion of tumor cells stained. Of these, epithelial cellularity showed the highest degree of correlation with the results of steroid-binding assays.

Related references (1)	McCarty KS Jr, Miller LS, Cox EB, Konrath J, McCarty KS Sr. Estrogen receptor analyses. Correlation of biochemical and immunohistochemical methods using monoclonal antireceptor antibodies. *Archives of Pathology and Laboratory Medicine* 1985; **109**:716–721.
(2)	Parl FF, Posey YF. Discrepancies of the biochemical and immunohistochemical estrogen receptor assays in breast cancer. *Human Pathology* 1988; **19**:960–966.

Key message

This paper provided verification of a tissue and immunologic-based assay of the estrogen receptor. With papers that followed soon in the 1980s, the evaluation of the estrogen receptor in breast cancer became based on specific antibodies.

Why it's important

The availability of tissue-based and individual cell localization allowed for the correct identification as negative of some tumors found to be falsely positive by previous techniques because of the inclusion of normal cells (positive for estrogen receptor) in the samples. Thus, false positives were avoided, particularly for smaller breast cancers. Proper identification of tumors with positive nuclear staining but low cellularity also allowed proper identification of estrogen receptor-positive carcinomas that had previously been thought negative because of the low cellular content in the samples (see related reference 2).

Strengths

1. This work was soon followed by studies validating this method in predicting response to therapy by antiestrogens (related reference 1 and [1,2]).
2. Allowed for specific evaluation of tumor cells, avoiding evaluating normal breast or the misinterpretation of low cellularity cancers as negative for estrogen receptor (related reference 2).

Weakness

Development of the important fine points of evaluation and cutpoints continue to evolve.

Relevance

The presence of tissue-based, cytologically identified estrogen receptor positively facilitated the availability of this important clinical test, since it can be done in fixed tissue. The precision of estrogen receptor status in breast cancers was enhanced, and this is the prototype of indicators of therapeutic responsiveness in breast cancer.

References

[1] McClelland RA, Berger U, Miller LS, Powles TJ, Jensen EV, Coombes RC. Immunocytochemical assay for estrogen receptor: relationship to outcome of therapy in patients with advanced breast cancer. *Cancer Research* 1986; **46**:4241S–4243S.
[2] Harvey JM, Clark GM, Osborne CK, Allred DC. Estrogen receptor status by immunohistochemistry is superior to the ligand-binding assay for predicting response to adjuvant endocrine therapy in breast cancer. *Journal of Clinical Oncology* 1999; **17**:1474–1481.

Paper 12

Comparative pathology of prevalent and incident cancers detected by breast screening. Edinburgh Breast Screening Project

Authors

Anderson TJ, Lamb J, Alexander F, *et al.*

Reference

Lancet 1986; **i**:519–523

Summary

In the Edinburgh Breast Screening Project, 210 cancers were detected from commencement in 1979 up to December 1984. By this time the full initial cohort had completed at least three visits and a proportion had attended for up to five visits, so pathological characteristics for prevalent and incident cancers could be compared. The main differences were in distribution of histological type of cancer, detection of occult invasive disease, and lymph-node positivity among incident tumors. Only the first of these was statistically significant. This evaluation showed that cancer detection by screening in Edinburgh conformed with screening theory, in which detection of good prognosis tumors is favored at the prevalence screens, and faster growing, aggressive tumors are found at the incidence screens. Qualitative histopathology may provide a better measure than standard quantitative judgments of size and lymph node status to compare the varieties of cancer detected by screening programmes and to understand the biology of the disease.

Breast cancer screening by mammography has been validated as a method capable of saving lives. Further, it has long been evident that cancers detected at first screen (prevalence cancers) differ in many ways from those ascertained at the next planned screen intervals (incidence cancers) and from cancers appearing between screening mammograms.

Related references

(1) Anderson TJ, Lamb J, Donnan P, *et al.* Comparative pathology of breast cancer in a randomised trial of screening. *British Journal of Cancer* 1991; **64**:108–113.

(2) Alexander FE, Anderson TJ, Brown HK, *et al.* 14 years of follow-up from the Edinburgh randomised trial of breast-cancer screening [see comments]. *Lancet* 1999; **353**:1903–1908.

Key message

Any intervention such as screening gives us an opportunity to further evaluate the associations of biologic and clinical behavior in the heterogeneous elements of breast cancers – in this case carefully defined and rigorously applied criteria for special histologic types of breast carcinoma.

Why it's important

Feinstein and colleagues [1] have indicated that there is something important beyond stage of detection that should characterize the tumors found in different screen settings. Unfortunately, these authors have not revealed the indictors from histopathology or elsewhere where such information may be found, as is related clearly in the paper discussed here.

Strengths

The evaluation of the histopathologic patterns was a prospective portion of the screening program in Edinburgh so that this information was completely and consistently collected. Later follow-up information is available [1,2]. Detection bias as well as tumor biology figure into these interactions of pathology with screen detection [2,3].

Weakness

The major weakness of this paper is that its clear message of the importance of histologic evaluation of breast cancer has not been more widely adopted.

Relevance

This work indicates that further evaluation of subsets identified by screening parameters will reveal indicators of biologic potential [2,3].

References

[1] Moody-Ayer SY, Wells CK, Feinstein AR. 'Benign' tumors and 'early detection' in mammography-screened patients of a natural cohort with breast cancer, *Archives of Internal Medicine* 2000; **160**:1109–1115.
[2] Groenendijk RPR, Bult P, Tewarie L, *et al.* Screen-detected breast cancers have a lower mitotic activity index. *British Journal of Cancer* 2000; **82**:381–384.
[3] Gilliland FD, Joste N, Stauber PM, *et al.* Biologic characteristics of interval and screen-detected breast cancers. *Journal of the National Cancer Institute* 2000; **92**:743–749.

Paper 13

Mammographically detected duct carcinoma in situ. Frequency of local recurrence following tylectomy and prognostic effect of nuclear grade on local recurrence

Authors

Lagios MD, Margolin FR, Westdahl PR, Rose MR

Reference

Cancer 1989; **63**:618–624

Summary

Seventy-nine patients with mammographically detected foci of duct carcinoma *in situ* (DCIS) of histologically confirmed extents of 25 mm or less were treated by tylectomy without irradiation or axillary dissection. Adequacy of excision was confirmed histologically, by radiographic–pathologic correlation and by postoperative mammographic examination. Eight patients (10.1%) recurred locally in the immediate vicinity of the biopsy site. Four patients developed recurrent *in situ* disease identified mammographically, and all were initially treated by reexcision. One of these patients subsequently elected to undergo mastectomy; no residual *in situ* or invasive disease was detected in the breast or in axillary lymph nodes. Four patients developed recurrent invasive disease; 50% of these recurrences were detected mammographically. All patients were treated by mastectomy with node dissection. Three had confirmed minimal invasive carcinomas and were N0; one patient had a 13 mm invasive lobular carcinoma with a single group I micrometastasis. All patients, including those treated for a recurrence, were free of disease at the time of this report but three patients had died of heart disease. Nuclear grade would appear to identify subsets of DCIS more likely to produce local failure after tylectomy alone. DCIS with high-grade nuclear morphology and comedo-type necrosis was associated with a 19% local recurrence rate after an average interval of 26 months; only one of ten patients with intermediate-grade DCIS developed a local recurrence at 87 months; and none of 33 patients with DCIS of micropapillary/non-necrotic cribriform type and low-grade nuclear morphology developed local recurrence in the follow-up period.

Related references (1)   Patchefsky AS, Schwartz GF, Finkelstein SD, *et al.* Heterogeneity of intraductal carcinoma of the breast. *Cancer* 1989; **63**:731–741.

(2)   Silverstein MJ, Lagios MD, Groshen S, Waisman JR, Lewinsky BS, Martino S, Gamagami P, Colburn WJ. The influence of margin width on local control of ductal carcinoma in situ of the breast. *New England Journal of Medicine* 1999; **340**:1455–1461.

Key message

Mammographically detected lesions of DCIS may be satisfactorily treated by surgery with careful attention to margins and continued follow-up by mammography, supported by the three-dimensional studies of Holland *et al.* [2] indicating unicentricity of the great majority of DCIS lesions.

Why it's important

This study documents the successful excision of low-grade, mammographically detected DCIS.

These studies inaugurated the modern era of surgery for DCIS, replacing the mythology that DCIS must be managed by treating the entire breast by mastectomy or excision plus radiotherapy to the whole breast. A few cases previously reported by Millis and Thynne [1] also documented apparent successful surgical excision of DCIS.

Strength

This work gave increased practical meaning to the observations of Patchefsky *et al.* (related reference 2) that different types of DCIS are more extensive within the breast.

Weakness

This has often been criticized for not being a multicenter trial-based study – however, the strength of large numbers is balanced by precise case definition, often lacking in larger, multicenter trials.

Relevance

Silverstein *et al.* (related reference 2) give important details in establishing the local curability of DCIS by surgery alone, following strict case definitions and precise guidelines. Thus, within 10 years, precise guidelines as to the types of DCIS amenable to local excision without treatment of the entire breast by radiation had been developed and widely accepted.

References

[1] Millis RR, Thynne GSJ. *In situ* intraduct carcinoma of the breast: a long term follow-up study. *British Journal of Surgery* 1975; **62**:957–962.
[2] Holland R, Hendriks JH, Vebeek AL, Mravunac M, Schuurmans Stekhoven HJ. Extent, distribution, and mammographic/histological correlations of breast ductal carcinoma *in situ*. *Lancet* 1990; **335**:519–522.

Paper 14

Pathological prognostic factors in breast cancer. I. The value of histological grade in breast cancer: experience from a large study with long-term follow-up

Authors

Elston CW, Ellis IO

Reference

Histopathology 1991; **19**:403–410

Summary

Morphologic assessment of the degree of differentiation has been shown in numerous studies to provide useful prognostic information in breast cancer, but until recently histologic grading has not been accepted as a routine procedure, mainly because of perceived problems with reproducibility and consistency. In the Nottingham/Tenovus Primary Breast Cancer Study the most commonly used method, described by Bloom and Richardson, was modified in order to make the criteria more objective. The revised technique involved semiquantitive evaluation of three morphologic features – the percentage of tubule formation, the degree of nuclear pleomorphism and an accurate mitotic count using a defined field area. A numerical scoring system was used and the overall grade was derived from a summation of individual scores for the three variables: three grades of differentiation were used. Since 1973, over 2200 patients with primary operable breast cancer had been entered into a study of multiple prognostic factors. Histologic grade, assessed in 1831 patients, showed a very strong correlation with prognosis: patients with grade I tumors had a significantly better survival than those with grade II and III tumors ($p < 0.0001$) (Figure 6.4). These results demonstrated that this method for histologic grading provides important prognostic information and, if the grading protocol is followed consistently, reproducible results can be obtained. Histologic grade forms part of the multifactorial Nottingham prognostic index, together with tumor size and lymph node stage, which is used to stratify individual patients for appropriate therapy.

Related references (1)   Blamey RW, Davies CJ, Elston CW, Johnson J, Haybittle JL, Maynard PV. Prognostic factors in breast cancer – the formation of a prognostic index. *Clinical Oncology* 1979; **5**:227–236.

          (2)   Dalton LW, Pinder SE, Elston CE, *et al*. Histologic grading of breast cancer: linkage of patient outcome with level of pathologist agreement. *Modern Pathology* 2000; **13**:730–735.

Key message

While many analyses for prognostic indicators settled on size, nodal status, hormone receptors and sophisticated measures, including cell proliferation, a measured plan of testing combined histologic grade was begun in Nottingham, UK (NCHG). Blamey, Elston and their colleagues sought to refine and validate the use of a combined histologic grade that integrates scores from glandular differentiation, nuclear patterns and mitotic counts. This overall measure is then added to anatomic stage information of tumor size and nodal status to provide powerful prognostic information, rendered in an index.

Why it's important

Many other prognostic indicators have been tested, but none so consistently found useful, and additive to stage information. The Nottingham group [1] as well as others have indicated that low-stage, low-grade tumors rarely metastasize, and have shown that the prognostic difference between older and younger women (favoring survival for older women) is largely explained by the greater incidence of higher-grade cancers in younger women [2,3].

Strength

There are now good indications that the combined histologic grade is not only a reliable prognostic indicator, but also is a predictor of chemotherapeutic responsiveness [4–6].

Weakness

Any measure must be reliable and repeatedly verified; and so it will be with histologic grade. It is likely that it will be modified to have different cutpoints to serve different needs in the greatly heterogeneous diseases of breast cancer. For example, in node-positive disease, very low mitotic counts may be needed to identify an improved prognostic group.

Relevance

The robustness of the combined grade with proven predictiveness along with fostering observer agreement in case assignment has led to its formal adoption by many groups in many countries.

Perhaps the most important element in short-term consideration of survival is the mitotic count, verified in many other studies of cell proliferation [4–6].

References

[1] Galea MH, Blamey RW, Elston CE, Ellis IO. The Nottingham Prognostic Index in primary breast cancer. *Breast Cancer Research and Treatment* 1992; **22**:207–219.

[2] Kollias J, Elston CW, Ellis IO, Robertson JF, Blamey RW. Early-onset breast cancer – histopathological and prognostic considerations. *British Journal of Cancer* 1997; **75**:1318–1323.

[3] Kollias J, Murphy CA, Elston CW, Ellis IO, Robertson JF, Blamey RW. The prognosis of small primary breast cancers. *European Journal of Cancer* 1999; **35**:908–912.

[4] Pinder SE, Murray S, Ellis IO, *et al.* The importance of the histologic grade of invasive breast carcinoma and response to chemotherapy. *Cancer* 1998; **83**:1529–1539.

[5] Simpson JF, Gray R, Dressler LG, *et al.* Prognostic value of histologic grade and proliferative activity in axillary node-positive breast cancer; results from the Eastern Cooperative Oncology Group companion study, EST 4189. *Journal of Clinical Oncology* 2000; **18**:2059–2069.

[6] Page DL, Gray R, Allred DC, *et al.* Prediction of node-negative breast cancer outcome by histologic grading and S-phase analysis by flow cytometry: an Eastern Cooperative Oncology Group study (2192). *American Journal of Clinical Oncology* 2001; **24**:10–18.

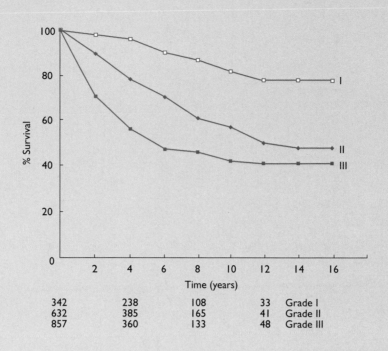

342	238	108	33	Grade I
632	385	165	41	Grade II
857	360	133	48	Grade III

Figure 6.4 Percentage of patients surviving to 16 years for combined histologic grade categories I (low), II and III (high). Note that the survival for the intermediate grade (II) approaches that of women in the high-grade category during the latter half of the follow-up period.

CHAPTER 7

Breast imaging

DANIEL B KOPANS

Introduction

The early detection of breast cancers by mammography has had a major impact on breast health care and the treatment of these malignancies. Randomized, controlled trials that eliminate lead time bias and length bias sampling have shown that earlier detection can reduce the death rate from these cancers. Prior to the development of mammography and subsequently the application of ultrasound, computed tomography (CT), and other imaging techniques, breast evaluation was limited to the clinical tools of palpation, needle aspiration, and ultimately surgical excision.

The development of mammography made it possible to detect cancers before they became clinically evident and permitted a conservative approach to local cancer control.

Since many of the lesions found by mammography proved to be benign at biopsy, it became clear that methods were needed to guide surgeons to lesions that they could not palpate. Dodd was the first to report placing needles in the breast to 'localize' clinically occult, mammographically detected lesions. The development of the 'spring hookwire' localizer by Kopans provided the first device that could be positioned to provide an anchored, three-dimensionally accurate guide to these lesions. This allowed for an aggressive approach to lesions found by mammography.

The adaptation of ultrasound for breast evaluation eliminated the need to aspirate or surgically remove cysts, and has altered the approach to breast biopsy. More recently, it has permitted the accurate guidance of needles into lesions in 'real time' that permit the removal of cores of tissue to establish a diagnosis with less trauma to the patient than surgical open biopsy.

With the application of CT to breast evaluation, it became apparent that management of breast problems was not simply through the use of mammography, but, increasingly, the breast was being evaluated using the other imaging modalities that were also being developed for other parts of the body. Radiologists became expert in interpreting the various images being obtained of the breast tissue, and the subspeciality of Breast Imaging was born.

With the demonstration that screening could reduce the rate of death came the realization that high-quality mammography was required to find small cancers. Tabar in Sweden was among the first to evaluate each step in the mammography imaging chain to develop the best approach to generating these high-resolution and high-contrast X-ray images. This was expanded upon by Eklund and others to try to systematically improve the positioning of the breast in the mammography device. In addition to the importance of positioning, exposure, and film processing, it became apparent that mammography was not simply obtaining images of the breast. Different practitioners had different levels of expertise. Thresholds for intervention were variable. Sickles was the first to review his service screening program in a systematic fashion and to establish, through an audit of the practice, goals for screening that included sensitivity, specificity, recall rates, and anticipated tumor sizes.

Efforts have been made in the USA to systematize reporting so that the results of the test could be conveyed to the referring physician and ultimately the patient in a clear, concise fashion with an unambiguous action-oriented conclusion. The American College of Radiology established the

Mammography Accreditation Program and soon followed with the American College of Radiology Breast Imaging Reporting and Data System (BIRADS).

Work by Kobayashi in ultrasound that defined the various shapes, echo textures, and effects on the transmission of sound have been refined as the technology has improved. Although ultrasound is still used primarily to differentiate cysts from solid lesions, Stavros, building on the observations made by Fornage and others, developed descriptors for breast lesions seen by ultrasound. These descriptors can be used to separate lesion characteristics on ultrasound into those that are usually found in benign lesions and those that raise concern of a malignancy.

As technology advances, it is very important that we do not lose sight of the fact that merely being able to image a lesion does not mean that it has true clinical value. The program defined by Moskowitz *et al.* some 20 years ago remains valid today. New technology should be evaluated in a blinded fashion to determine its independent contribution as a screening test to detect unsuspected cancer, or as a diagnostic test to differentiate benign lesions from malignant ones. Ultimately, because a screening test involves healthy asymptomatic individuals, and as such has the potential to cause harm (anxiety, unnecessary biopsies, and overtreatment), in order for a new test to be used for screening, its efficacy to reduce the rate of death must be shown in randomized, controlled trials.

Paper 1

Experience with mammography in a tumor institution: Evaluation of 1000 cases

Author

Egan RL

Reference

Radiology 1960; **75**:894–900

Summary

Egan reported on 1000 X-ray mammograms performed at the MD Anderson Hospital and Tumor Institute between 1956 and 1959. This was the first report of a blinded analysis of the mammograms. Egan intentionally did not have access to the clinical information, so that his interpretations of the mammograms were not biased. He also avoided the use of an indeterminate report to insure that he was fully committed to his interpretation. The study included a follow-up of all cases.

Related references   **(1)**   Warren SL. Roentgenographic study of the breast. *AJR* 1930; **24**:113–124.

     (2)   Leborgne R. Diagnosis of tumors of the breast by simple Roentgenography: calcifications in carcinomas. *AJR* 1951; **65**:1–11.

     (3)   Eklund GW, Cardenosa G. The art of mammographic positioning. *Radiological Clinics of North America* 1992; **30**:21–53.

Key message

Mammography should be performed using a standardized approach that is reproducible and can be transferred to other settings.

Why it's important

Others had defined the basic characteristics of breast cancers as seen on mammography. This paper has been considered the first description of a systematic approach to X-ray imaging of the breast. Although mammograms had been used to evaluate the breast in the early 1900s, Egan is credited with having developed an approach that was reproducible, and could be learned by others. He described how the breast should be positioned, and provided tables of X-ray technique settings. This paper describes the X-ray techniques to be used and approaches to positioning the breast that are the basis for modern mammography. Egan described the value of imaging the breast from two directions – the side, and top to bottom – to permit triangulating the lesion's location. He explained the relationship of calcifications to breast cancer, explaining that the coarser deposits were related to benign disease. His description of benign masses as having round or smoothly lobulated shapes with sharply defined margins, although not a certain diagnosis, has remained correct for 40 years. Although many of his other observations have not withstood the test of time, they provide an important foundation for modern mammographic interpretation.

Strengths

1. The techniques described in this paper form the basis of modern mammography. Although mammographic equipment has evolved significantly with the development of dedicated mammography devices with smaller focal spots, rigid compression, automatic exposure control, and constant-potential generators, the basic principles of the use of low-energy photons remains the same.

2. Positioning has evolved as well, to use the mediolateral oblique technique, but here too the basic principles remain the same. Egan described the importance of objective analysis of a new technique by using 'blinding' to the history and clinical information when interpreting the studies to learn the inherent value of the mammogram. This approach applies today when new technologies are suggested. Egan was also aware of the importance of long-term follow-up to evaluate the potential for false negatives.

3. His descriptions of benign and malignant lesions remain true today.

Weaknesses

1. Since this is an old paper, the actual techniques have been replaced, but the underlying issues remain the same.

2. Comments about breast changes with age are not as simple as Egan suggests. Although the basic concepts have changed little, the simplified differentiation of benign from malignant lesions does not hold up perfectly. There are some sharply circumscribed cancers, and many ill-defined lesions are benign.

Relevance

This analytical approach is important for any new technology that is developed for breast imaging. Standardization of the technique is necessary before a new test can be properly evaluated for its efficacy.

Most of Egan's observations have withstood the test of time. He championed rigorous, systematic analysis with initial blinded interpretation using the new technology, and the importance of long-term follow-up to establish 'truth'.

Strength

This paper describes a technique that is easily reproduced by any radiologist with a dedicated mammography system. It relies on the simple geometry of orthogonal (right-angle) views to position a guide in or alongside a lesion.

Weakness

This is a description of a technique that happens to work very well, but the paper did not provide any prospective documentation of its accuracy.

Relevance

Although many breast biopsies of clinically occult lesions are now accomplished using imaging-guided needle biopsy, this method of needle localization represents the safest, most accurate diagnostic approach. It continues to be useful for diagnosis as well as to guide the surgical removal of cancers diagnosed by needle biopsy.

Paper 4

Assessment of radiation risk from screening mammography

Author

Feig SA

Reference

Cancer 1996; **77**:818–822

Summary

This editorial was written in response to related reference (2). It clearly defines the issues related to the potential for X-ray carcinogenesis in the breast and its importance in mammographic screening. In 1976, Bailar (related reference 1) raised the concern that the X-rays from mammographic screening might cause as many breast cancer deaths as might be averted through early detection. Feig presents the issues in a succinct fashion.

Related references **(1)** Bailar JC. Mammography: a contrary view. *Annals of Internal Medicine* 1976; **84**:77–84.

(2) Mettler FA, Upton AC, Kelsey CA, Rosenberg RD, Linver MN. Benefits versus risks from mammography: a critical assessment. *Cancer* 1996; **77**:903–909.

(3) Feig SA, Hendrick RE. Radiation risk from screening mammography of women aged 40–49. *Monographs of the National Cancer Institute* 1997; **22**:119–124.

Key message

The benefits from screening mammography outweigh the risk from radiation carcinogenesis in the breast.

Why it's important

One of the major impediments to mammographic screening has been the concern that the X-ray imaging might cause the cancers that it is being used to find and that this might negate its value. This editorial provides a clear summary of the issues, and, in conjunction with related reference (2), reassurance that, for women over the age of 40, the benefits from early detection far outweigh even the theoretical risks.

Strength

This paper summarizes important evidence on both sides of the arguments.

Weakness

This is an editorial and not a scientific paper, so it is subject to the interpretations of the author.

Relevance

Theoretically, radiation-induced carcinogenesis could obviate the benefits from screening mammography. However, the preponderance of the evidence does not support that conclusion that this should be a concern with commonly used doses of radiation in women over the age of 40.

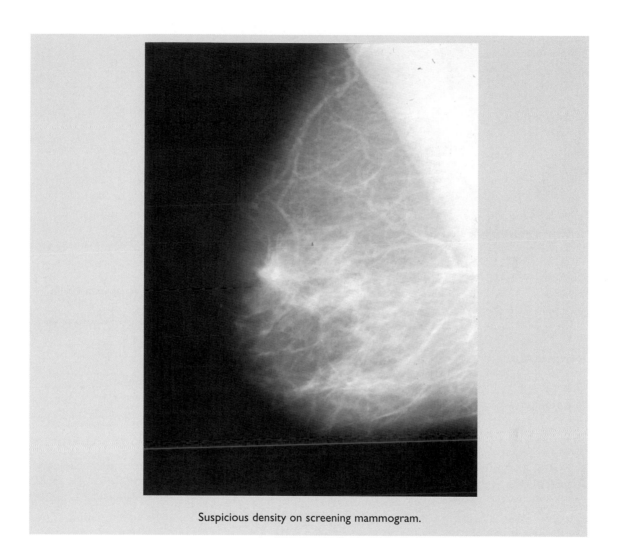

Suspicious density on screening mammogram.

Paper 5

Mammographic feature analysis

Authors

D'Orsi CJ, Kopans DB

Reference

Seminars in Roentgenology 1993; **27**:204–230

Summary

The Breast Imaging Reporting and Data System (BIRADS) of the American College of Radiology provides radiologists with precise definitions of mammographic findings for both benign and malignant lesions. This system is described in this paper. A framework for analysis is provided along with the five final assessment categories that are action-oriented and are required by MQSA. The goal is to more effectively communicate the implications of findings to physicians and patients as well as to better correlate mammographic findings with outcomes.

Related reference   (1)   The Breast Imaging Reporting and Data System of the American College of Radiology. Third edition. Reston, VA: American College of Radiology 1998.

Key message

This paper, and BIRADS, urge the systematic analysis and clear reporting of findings detected by mammography.

Why it's important

Prior to the introduction of BIRADS, referring physicians frequently complained that mammographic reports were often confusing, contradictory, and unintelligible. By providing a dictionary of terms so that all radiologists can use an identical terminology, a reporting format that requires an assessment of breast tissue density and a description of significant findings, and guidelines that link findings with recommendations for biopsy or follow-up, this paper and BIRADS have improed the reporting of mammographic studies.

Strength

This paper provides verbal, mammographic, and artistic descriptions of findings that appear on mammograms.

Weaknesses

1. A more structured presentation would be easier to learn, and this is provided in the ACR BIRADS.
2. No data are given to support the division of findings into the various levels of risk that are provided.

Relevance

BIRADS provides an important standardization for mammographic interpretation. The use of standardized terminology will also permit the pooling of large amounts of data to further refine the signs that indicate benign and malignant lesions.

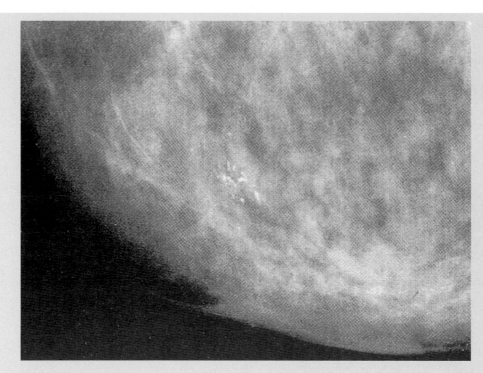

Microcalcifications seen on magnified view of a screening mammogram.

Paper 6

Evaluation of new imaging procedures for breast cancer: Proper process

Authors

Moskowitz M, Feig SA, Cole-Beuglet C, *et al.*

Reference

AJR 1983; **140**:591–594

Summary

The authors review successive phases in the evaluation of a new breast imaging technology. This starts with determining whether there is any potential for the new instrument, its proper operation, and criteria for interpreting the studies. The results need to be compared with a gold standard such as pathology. The second phase evaluates the new technology in a blinded fashion. The final phase is the use of the instrument as an independent screening test compared with the gold standards of clinical examination and mammography.

Related reference   (1)   Kopans DB. Recent issues in breast cancer detection and the premarket approval by the Food and Drug Administration of a US system for breast lesion evaluation: What happened to Science? *Radiology* 1997; **202**:315–318.

Key message

New technologies should be validated, scientifically, before they are used clinically.

Why it's important

Technological changes are occurring rapidly. In order to avoid major expenses and unnecessary risks to patients, new technologies should be carefully and properly evaluated and efficacy demonstrated in an objective and scientific fashion.

Strength

This is a broad overview that can be applied to any new technology for breast cancer screening.

Weaknesses

1. No data are provided to suggest the levels of sensitivity, and specificity that are required to prove efficacy.
2. There is no mention of cost/benefit analysis.

Relevance

Given the explosion in technology, this paper maintains its importance. All new technology should undergo proper scientific validation before it is promoted as efficacious.

Paper 7

Diagnostic ultrasound in breast cancer: Analysis of retrotumorous echo patterns correlated with sonic attenuation by cancerous connective tissue

Author

Kobayashi T

Reference

Journal of Clinical Ultrasound 1979; **7**:471–479

Summary

This is one of a series of reports that resulted in the development of the basic ultrasound criteria for analyzing breast masses. It summarized the use of the shape of the lesion, its boundary echoes (margins), and the influence of the lesion on the passage of sound (through-transmission).

Related references (1) Fornage BD, Lorigan JG, Andry E. Fibroadenoma of the breast: sonographic appearance. *Radiology* 1989; **172**:671–675.

(2) Stavros AT, Thickman D, Rapp CL, Dennis MA, Parker SH, Sisney GA. Solid breast nodules: use of sonography to distinguish between benign and malignant lesions. *Radiology* 1995; **196**:123–134 (Paper 8 in this chapter).

Key message

The author developed a method for classifying breast lesions seen with ultrasound, believing that benign lesions could be distinguished from malignant lesions.

Why it's important

Although subsequent studies have found that distinctions between benign and malignant criteria are less certain than suggested in this report, the approach described here has provided the framework for the future observations made by other investigators, including Fornage *et al.* and Stavros *et al.* (related references 1 and 2).

Strengths

1. The paper correlates the results from ultrasound examination with histology from subsequent biopsies.
2. Given the poor quality of the ultrasound images compared with those from modern systems, the observations are surprisingly accurate.

Weaknesses

1. Only a small number of lesions were studied, and these were limited almost entirely to malignant histology.
2. The quality of the images is poor relative to those obtained with more modern technology.

Relevance

The descriptive observations and terms defined in this paper remain in use today. Modern ultrasound still relies on an evaluation of the shape of a mass, its margins, its internal echo pattern, and the pattern of echoes behind the mass. The only thing that has changed is that the ultrasound detail has become much sharper and the tissue differences more distinct. The basic observations made by the early pioneers in breast ultrasound remain the same.

Paper 8

Solid breast nodules: Use of sonography to distinguish between benign and malignant lesions

Authors

Stavros AT, Thickman D, Rapp CL, Dennis MA, Parker SH, Sisney GA

Reference

Radiology 1995; **196**:123–134

Summary

This is a review of 750 breast lesions (mammographically detected as well as palpable) that were evaluated using hand-held ultrasound. The authors used a lesion classification scheme that allowed them to separate many of the benign lesions from the malignant lesions using features seen on ultrasound. Using their criteria, a lesion with benign characteristics had less than a 0.5% chance of being malignant.

Key message

Using rigorous criteria to interpret the findings from a high-frequency ultrasound examination of the breast, it is possible to differentiate many benign from malignant lesions.

Why it's important

The vast majority of lesions detected by mammography or clinical examination are benign. However, in many cases the only accurate method for differentiating benign solid lesions from malignant solid lesions is a tissue biopsy. If imaging can be used to accurately separate lesions that do not require biopsy from those that do, many biopsies with benign results may be avoided.

Strength

A large number of cases were evaluated by multiple investigators prospectively.

Weaknesses

1. In this report, palpable lesions are grouped with non-palpable ones, and the authors included lesions that were obviously malignant and were not diagnostic dilemmas. Since these all have 'non-benign' characteristics, the inclusion of these lesions augments the specificity of ultrasound.

2. The investigators were not blinded to the clinical and mammographic results, and the results were not segregated by age. The risk of breast cancer is extremely remote among women under the age of 30; including results from studying these women in the summary estimates also contributes to an overestimation of the specificity of this technique.

Relevance

A major hazard of breast cancer screening is the false-positive rate. Methods to reduce the number of biopsies with benign results reduce the trauma and cost induced by screening. This is beneficial if only a few cancers are missed as a result.

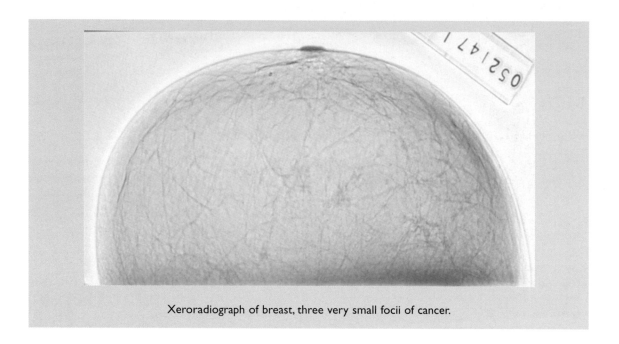

Xeroradiograph of breast, three very small focii of cancer.

Paper 9

Whole-breast US imaging: Four-year follow-up

Authors

Kopans DB, Meyer JE, Lindfors KK

Reference

Radiology 1985; **157**:505–507

Summary

This paper summarizes the experience of a blinded evaluation of breast cancer screening using whole-breast ultrasound. 1140 women underwent a clinical breast examination, X-ray mammography, and whole-breast ultrasound evaluation using state-of-the-art equipment. Each study was blinded to the results of the other so that the separate contribution of each could be established. It was demonstrated that ultrasound was less sensitive than mammography in detecting breast cancer and that ultrasound screening resulted in an unacceptably high false-positive rate with no increase in cancer detection.

Related reference **(1)** Kolb TM, Lichy J, Newhouse JH. Occult cancer in women with dense breasts: detection with screening US – diagnostic yield and tumor characteristics. *Radiology* 1998; **207**:191–199.

Key message

This paper demonstrated that early breast cancers could not be reliably detected by ultrasound.

Why it's important

From time to time, ultrasound is suggested as an alternative to mammography because it does detect some lesions (usually larger lesions) missed by mammography and does not utilize radiation with its theoretical risk of radiation-induced cancer. This paper is important not only for its findings, but also because it outlines methods that may be used to establish the efficacy of a new technology.

Strength

This was a blinded evaluation of a questionable technique: whole-breast ultrasound screening. This is the model that can be used for evaluation of other diagnostic modalities.

Weakness

The equipment being studied was state-of-the-art in 1983. The technology has undergone significant improvement and the conclusions may no longer be as applicable as they once were.

Relevance

Scanning the breast using ultrasound has been suggested for breast cancer screening (related reference 1). This study demonstrates that this is not an appropriate application of that technology.

Digital mammography, computer-aided diagnosis, and telemammography

Authors

Feig SA, Yaffe M

Reference

Radiological Clinics of North America 1995; **33**:1205–1230

Summary

This is an overview of digital mammography that provides insight into the potential advantages of this technology in which the display of the image does not dictate the imaging parameters. This means that the image exposure can be optimized to enhance the visualization of breast lesions. A very practical advantage of an electronic image is that storage costs can be substantially reduced by eliminating the space needed for film. Electronic images will not be as easily lost, can be copied perfectly, can be viewed simultaneously in as many locations as needed, and can be sent around the world in minutes to obtain consultation from experts.

The authors describe the major forms of digital detectors that are being developed, ranging from film digitization to the use of amorphous selenium. They describe scanning systems that image the breast using a mechanical sweep of the X-ray beam and detector, as well as large-area arrays to image the entire breast simultaneously.

Image display remains the greatest weakness for digital mammography, since the high resolution of the images cannot be displayed on ordinary monitors. The authors review the advantages of having a computer analyze the images as an aid in detecting cancers and assessing the risk of the tissue patterns.

Related reference   **(1)**   Niklason LT, Kopans DB, Hamberg LM. Digital breast imaging: tomosynthesis and digital subtraction mammography. *Breast Disease* 1998; **10**:151–164.

Key message

Having a computer image of the X-ray absorption characteristics of the breast offers the opportunity to improve detection and diagnosis of early breast cancers. Digital mammography is likely to replace conventional film/screen mammography for breast cancer detection and diagnosis.

Why it's important

Digital mammography, and the new approaches that will be developed using it, will extend the ability of mammography to detect early breast cancers. It will do this while reducing the number of women who are called back for what prove to be false alarms.

Strength

This is a detailed yet highly readable review that takes physics and makes it understandable for the average reader.

Weakness

Several of the techniques that are quite promising using digital mammography are not covered. These include digital tomosynthesis, and contrast subtraction angiography of the breast. These are covered in related reference (1).

Relevance

Digital imaging may replace analog imaging in all areas of medicine, including breast imaging.

CHAPTER 8

Screening

A PATRICK FORREST

Introduction

Before undertaking screening for any chronic disease, it is necessary that a number of principles be met. These were listed in a report commissioned by the World Health Organization in 1968, which is cited here (Paper 1). Important principles are that there should be an early asymptomatic stage of the disease which can be detected by a suitable test. These are considered in the next two citations, in the first of which 'minimal cancer' is defined as that which is non-invasive or which, if invasive, is 0.5 cm in diameter or less (Paper 3). Such tumours were shown to have an uncommonly low incidence of metastases in the axillary nodes, low recurrence rates and long survival following treatment as was confirmed in the large Breast Cancer Detection Demonstration Project in the USA, which expanded 'minimal size' to 1.0 cm. As tumour size and node metastases are time-dependent phenomena, detection at an earlier stage is bound to prolong life, even if the date of death remains the same. The success of screening in reducing deaths can only be measured by mortality rates in the population targetted.

Such 'minimal' tumours are rarely clinically evident. Although mammography is not an ideal test, it is the only practical one. In the 1960s the developments leading to the modern mammography were taking place, and much credit is due to Egan in the MD Anderson Center who meticulously examined every detail of the technique and validated its use in the multi-institutional study cited here (Paper 4). He also was consultant to the first randomized trial of the breast screening instituted by Shapiro and Strax in 1963 through the Health Insurance Plan Trial of New York State. The final report of this trial, indicating a 30% reduction in the mortality from breast cancer at 10 years in those offered screening, is cited here (Paper 5).

It was reports of this trial, a second randomized trial started in Sweden in 1971 (Paper 7) and two case–control studies from the Netherlands, which convinced the Working Group set up by the UK Ministers of Health in 1985 that there was a case for the mammographic screening of asymptomatic women. In their report, which is cited (Paper 6), each stage of the screening process was examined in detail as were benefits, costs and methods of quality assurance, leading to guidelines for the organization of a population screening service, which was subsequently implemented for women aged 50–64 years (now to be extended to 70) in the UK.

Naturally there was dissent, this including the opinion that the Working Group had acted with undue haste and should have awaited the results of further trials being carried out in Sweden, Edinburgh and Canada. The results of these trials, which include half a million women, have since been repeatedly analysed, one of greatest relevance being the overview of the five Swedish trials cited here (Paper 8). In women aged 50–69 years, mortality from breast cancer, which was validated by an independent committee, was reduced by 29% at 5–13 years follow-up. Meta-analyses of published results are in agreement, the only trial not showing benefit in this age group being that carried out in Canada, which had an unusual design.

There is great controversy about the benefit of mammographic screening in women of 40–50 years of age. A consensus conference (see Paper 9) was held in the National Cancer Institute (NCI) in 1997, at which the benfits and costs of screening in this age group were explored. Although the panel initially indicated that the data available did not warrant the introduction of mammographic screening in this age group, this was subsequently overturned, and the NCI now recommends that regular mammographic screening should start at the age of 40.

Screening is not a diagnostic test, and women in whom a mammographic abnormality is detected are required to undergo further tests, which may include a surgical biopsy. Due to developments in imaging techniques (Paper 8), this can, in suitable cases, now be performed by an automated biopsy gun which allows multiple sampling without removing the instrument. Also cited is the development of a model for determining the risk of breast cancer in women undergoing annual mammography, which has been modified to allow definition of risk in the general population to determine eligibility for inclusion in prevention trials (Paper 10).

Many doctors still advise women to regularly examine their own breasts 'by rote'. A report cited here (Paper 12) is of a large randomized trial of breast self-examination conducted in Shanghai which to date does not show any increase in detection of breast cancer or reduction in deaths. The detection of benign disease was increased 2.5 times.

Finally, an early paper (Paper 13) indicating dissent from the introduction of screening is presented. The reasons underlying subsequent criticisms of the validity of mammographic screening, particularly regarding costs and benefits, are considered.

Paper 1

Principles and practice of screening

Authors

Wilson JMG, Jungner G

Reference

World Health Organization Public Health Paper No. 34, Geneva, 1968

Summary

This paper sets out 10 principles which require to be met before introducing screening, which aims to 'discover those amongst the apparently well who are, in fact, suffering from disease'. A screening test is not necessarily diagnostic – those with positive or suspicious findings may be referred for further investigation. These principles can be summarized as follows:

- The disease must present an important health problem.

- Its natural history must be adequately understood, including the course of its development from 'latent' to 'declared' disease. This latent phase must be recognizable.

- There should be a suitable test or examination which can recognize this latent phase. This test must be acceptable to the population being screened.

- Facilities must be available for the diagnosis and treatment of those who prove to have a positive (abnormal) screening test. There must be an agreed policy on whom to treat as 'patients' for whom treatment must be acceptable and of greater benefit than when delayed to a later stage.

- The total cost of screening should be economically balanced in relation to expenditure on other health needs.

- A single episode of screening is unsuitable for a chronic disease, for which it must be a continuing process.

Related references **(1)** Moss S. General principles of cancer screening. In: *Evaluation of Cancer Screening* (Chamberlain J, Moss S, eds). London: Springer-Verlag, 1996: 1–13.

(2) Day NE, Baines CJ, Chamberlain J, Hakama M, Miller AB, Prorok P. Project on screening for cancer; report of the workshop on screening for breast cancer. *International Journal of Cancer*, 1986; **38**:303–308.

(3) Bears OH, Shapiro S, Smart C, McDivitt RW. Report of a working group to review the National Cancer Institute–American Cancer Society Breast Cancer Detection Demonstration Project. *Journal of the National Cancer Institute* 1979; **62**:639–709.

Key message

Screening for the early diagnosis of a disease is not an *ad hoc* process; there are general principles which must first be satisfied before embarking on a programme to test validity.

Why it's important

This report was commissioned by the World Health Organization, which had recognized that screening for chronic diseases was likely to become more prevalent in developed countries as communicable diseases were coming under control and less important as a cause of death. Screening for 'killer' diseases such as cardiovascular disease, stroke and cancer, was growing in importance, and knowledge of the underlying principles was an essential first step. The implications of putting screening for a chronic disease into practice on a population basis are great and must be understood before institution of a programme.

Before screening for any disease, including breast cancer, is introduced on a population basis, it must be established that there is an early treatable pre-clinical phase of the disease; that there is a suitable test to detect this pre-clinical phase, the sensitivity and specificity of which has been validated; that the effectiveness of screening has been evaluated, best by randomized trials, and that the cost is not out of line with that of other health needs. Although the early literature was supportive, including a review of the massive US Breast Cancer Detection Demonstration Project which included over 280 000 women, some people still doubt that these conditions have been met for breast cancer screening.

Strengths

1. This report was commissioned by World Health Organization as screening for chronic disease was becoming a subject of growing importance in developed countries.
2. It provides knowledge of principles of screening and what it entails to put a programme into practice.
3. It recognizes that the detection of disease by screening is not always economical of a country's resources and that the total load of medical diagnosis and therapeutic work may be increased.
4. It indicates that only a prospective survey to determine whether morbidity has been reduced and working life improved can determine the saving or increase in cost to the community.

Weaknesses

1. Insufficient information is given on psycho-social aspects of screening.
2. Ethical issues are insufficiently addressed, but Moss (related reference 1) stresses the responsibility to provide full information to all those who were given a screening test, so that undue concern following notification of a positive test, and false re-assurance should the screening test be negative, can be avoided.

Relevance

'Screening' must be differentiated from 'case-finding', which is the testing of those who, as patients, have consulted their doctor for an unrelated condition – for example, estimating blood pressure in a patient with a sore ear. Screening is the application of a test to those who are well and without symptoms, and who only become patients should their screening test prove positive, requiring further investigations for diagnosis and possible treatment. Screening can cause anxiety, particularly when the test is falsely positive, and it is essential that its sensitivity (its ability to detect true cases of the disease), its specificity (its ability to detect true negatives correctly) and its positive predictive value (the probability that those with a positive test have the disease in question) are within acceptable limits.

The effectiveness of screening must be evaluated before instituting a programme, preferably by randomized trials in which the mortality or other adverse effect of the disease in those allocated for screening is compared with those who receive only normal health care. It is critical that possible adverse effects on the well-being of well persons are recognized and included in the costs.

Fundamental to these considerations is that the disease itself is of such importance that it warrants the considerable cost of screening. This generally requires that the disease has high prevalence in the population and that the potential yield of cases detected by screening also is high.

Paper 2*

Statistical power in breast cancer screening trials and mortality reduction among women 40–49 with particular emphasis on the National Breast Screening Study of Canada

Authors

Kopans DB, Halpern E, Hulka CA

Reference

Cancer 1994; **74**:1196–1203

Summary

Statistical power lies at the heart of any trial. This paper summarizes the important issues involved in breast cancer screening and the trials used to validate its efficacy. The paper focuses on the controversy that persists concerning the screening of women aged 40–49. It explains the fundamental statistical issues involved in screening trials and the analysis of their results, pointing out that the studies and the data that were acquired were never designed to be analysed by age groups. This resulted in misinterpretation and misrepresentation of the results.

Related references (1)	Miller AB, Baines CJ, To T, Wall C. Canadian National Breast Screening Study: 1. Breast cancer detection and death rates among women aged 40–49. *Canadian Medical Association Journal* 1992; **147**:1459–1476.
(2)	Fletcher SW, Black W, Harris R, *et al.* Report of the International Workshop on Screening for Breast Cancer. *Journal of the National Cancer Institute* 1993; **85**:1644–1656.

Key message

There are factors involved in breast cancer screening trials that are fundamental to their interpretation. The basic statistical issues, including the underlying power of the data, cannot be ignored – or false conclusions may be drawn. The authors point out how trials can be compromised by their design and execution (related reference 1) and how data can be used inappropriately to draw conclusions that are not justified (related reference 2).

---

* This review was written by DB Kopans.

Why it's important

Screening for breast cancer is an expensive approach to its control. Extremely large, properly designed and executed trials are required to demonstrate that earlier detection actually leads to fewer deaths. The failure of most involved in the issues of breast cancer screening to understand the fundamental issues in screening trials lies at the heart of the controversies that have arisen. This paper dissects the issues and demonstrates the problems that have occurred in the analysis of the trials.

Strength

This is a clearly written review that makes statistical issues understandable to the average physician.

Weaknesses

1. A prospective trial with sufficient power is needed to prove a benefit for any group of women.
2. This article can only summarize the available information and the problems with trial design, execution and data analysis.

Relevance

Large amounts of time and money are being spent on screening. There are significant 'harms' that are the result of screening (anxiety, time away from work and breast biopsies). Physicians should be aware of the pros and cons, and understand the rationale behind screening and the justification for doing it.

Paper 3

An orientation to the concept of minimal breast cancer

Authors

Gallagher HS, Martin JE

Reference

Cancer 1971; **28**:1505–1507

Summary

This was a study of the mammographic and histopathological features of 209 cancers in radical mastectomy specimens. The objectives were to determine factors which might improve the accuracy of mammography and whether there was an upper limit of size, measured radiologically, at which local treatment might be curative, as indicated by the absence of axillary node metastases. The authors reported that when the volume of the tumour was 0.125 ml (diameter 0.5 cm) or less the incidence of node involvement was less than 10%, applying the term 'minimal cancer' to those which were non-invasive, or, if invasive, were 0.5 cm or less in diameter. In a subsequent follow-up study of 415 women with such minimal tumours treated by radical mastectomy in four centres, survival over 1–26 (median 5) years was 97%. This threshold of size was subsequently increased to 1 cm.

Related references
(1) Gallager HS. Minimal breast cancer: results of treatment and the long-term follow-up: In: *Breast Carcinoma: Current Diagnosis and Treatment* (Feig SA, McLelland R, eds). New York: Masson, 1983: 291–294.
(2) Kolscienzy S, Tubiana M, Le MG, Valleron AJ. Breast cancer: relationship between the size of the primary tumour and the probability of metastatic dissemination. *British Journal of Cancer* 1984; **49**:709–715.
(3) Tabar L, Duffy SW, Vitak B, Chen H-H, Prevost TC. The natural history of screen-detected breast cancer: what have we learned. *Cancer* 1999; **86**:449–462.
(4) Anderson TH, Alexander FE, Lamb J, Smith A, Forrest APM. Pathological characteristics that optimise outcome prediction of a breast screening trial. *British Journal of Cancer* 2000; **83**:487–492.

Key message

There may be a radiological size of tumour at which cure can be achieved following local treatment alone.

Why it's important

The concept that there may be a critical size of breast cancer at which local treatment is curative is basic to early detection by mammographic screening.

Evidence for a linear relationship between tumour size and lymph node metastases is well established. This is also true for systemic spread of tumour cells to form micrometastases. Kolsciesny (related reference 2) recorded tumour size in 2648 women with invasive breast cancer treated by mastectomy who were then followed-up over a period of 25 years to map the development of overt systemic disease. When the volume of the tumour was 1 ml (diameter 1 cm) or less, this did not exceed 20%.

Cancers detected by mammographic screening are smaller and more commonly node-negative than those which are detected symptomatically, but these parameters alone are inadequate surrogates for mortality. Small node negative tumours may be rapidly fatal; node involvement does not preclude long-term survival. The aggressiveness of the tumour, as indicated by its pathological type and histological grade, requires to be taken into account as does the possibility that micrometastases may remain dormant for many years. The relationship of these factors to eventual cure is still not understood.

Strengths

1. This paper established the concept of 'minimal' breast cancer which could be cured by local therapy alone.
2. The concept was validated by follow-up data from four US centres.

Weaknesses

1. Non-invasive cancer is included in the group classified as minimal. As many may not become invasive during the patient's life-time, unnecessarily radical treatment is a matter of concern.
2. This study related cancers only to radiological size and node status; no information was given on tumour type or grade.
3. This was a study of symptomatic cancers.

Relevance

It is a recognized principle of screening for cancer that there must be an early 'latent' phase which can be detected by a suitable test and cured by appropriate treatment. It has been assumed that the small node-negative breast cancers come into this category, but recent data from screen-detected cancers in the Two County and Edinburgh trials (related references 3 and 4) suggest that histological type and grade must also be taken into account. As small tumours increase in size they become less differentiated – so-called 'phenotypic drift'. The earlier detection of small grade III (aggressive) invasive cancers may give short-term mortality reduction but for long-term benefit these small cancers must be detected while still of favourable grade.

Paper 4

Experience of mammography in a tumour institution: Evaluation of 1000 studies

Author

Egan RL

Reference

Radiology 1960; 75:894–900

Summary

It was Egan's original report of 1000 breasts in 634 women (which engendered 15 000 requests for reprints) using standard diagnostic X-ray units and industrial film which gave credibility to the techniques in the USA. Two hundred and forty lesions were malignant of which all but two were correctly coded. Twenty of 435 benign lesions were falsely coded as malignant. Cancers were also detected in 19 breasts without a clinical abnormality. Following his findings, a multi-institutional study was reported in which 1580 breasts were examined radiologically prior to a biopsy for clinical disease (related reference 2). The radiologist was not aware of the clinical findings. The sensitivity was 7.9% and specificity 90.1%.

Related references **(1)** Egan RL, Historical perspective. In: Egan RL. *Breast Imaging, Diagnosis and Morphology of Breast Diseases.* Philadelphia: WB Saunders, 1988: 1–11.

(2) Clark RL, Copeland MM, Egan RL, *et al.* Reproducibility of the technique of mammography [Egan] for cancer of the breast. *American Journal of Surgery* 1965; **109**:127–133.

(3) Ingleby H, Gershon-Cohen J. *Comparative Anatomy, Pathology and Roentgenology of the Breast.* Philadelphia: University of Pennsylvania Press, 1960.

(4) Shapiro S, Venet W, Strax P, Venet L. *Periodic Screening for Breast Cancer. The Health Insurance Plan Project and Its Sequelae, 1963–1986.* Baltimore: Johns Hopkins University Press, 1988 (Paper 5 in this chapter).

Why it's important

Before mammography could be used to screen the breasts of well women it was essential to ensure that quality was high and the risk of radiation low. Although it was in 1913 that a German surgeon, Salomon, first described X-ray imaging of mastectomy specimens, and in 1930 that Warren first reported its application to living patients, it was only in the 1950s that technical improvements and radiological–pathological studies allowing the establishment of mammography as a diagnostic aid were introduced by Leborgne in Montvideo, Gros in Paris and Egan and Gershon-Cohen in the USA. It was necessary to develop a system with a resolution that would allow detection of the smallest of calcifications within the breast while contrasting fibrous and glandular components. This demanded a particular spectrum of X-ray photons, compression of the breast into a slice to avoid scatter and blurring of the image, and highly sensitive film–screen systems to reduce the dose of radiation to acceptable levels. The development of the first dedicated mammography unit, the Senograph, by Gros in association with Compagnie Generale L'Electrique in France, which incorporated a molybdenum rather than a tungsten anode and a compression device independent of the X-ray tube was a landmark for modern mammography. But it was Egan's studies and his painstaking attention to detail that gained international credibility. The Egan technique was adopted for use in the 23 medical care groups participating in the Health Insurance Plan trial of screening (related reference 4).

Initially, there were concerns that the dose of radiation was too great, but with the development of highly sensitive film–screen combinations this was reduced to an acceptable level. Two standard projections were first employed – medio-lateral and cranio-caudal – but with Lundgren's demonstration that a medio-lateral oblique projection would include a large proportion of breast tissue including the axillary tail, this single view was used as a sole screening test in Sweden and the UK. But it is now accepted that for the initial screen a cranio-caudal view should also be taken.

Strength

Technical developments have allowed the use of mammography for screening normal breasts.

Weakness

Mammography is not an ideal screening test.

Relevance

Mammography is generally regarded as the optimal test for breast screening, in that it can detect masses as small as 5 mm in diameter and also those impalpable tumours causing architectural distortion or microcalcifications. However, it is not an ideal screening test, which should be precise, quick, simple and cheap. In the Swedish Two County trial its sensitivity was estimated at 87% for the detection of tumours expected to arise within 12 months of screening, but less than 50% for those expected to arise later. Specificity is in the order of 95%.

While film mammography is predominately used in screening programmes, digital imaging is gaining in popularity, particularly for incorporation into stereotactic units used for core biopsies, which allow immediate display. Magnetic resonance imaging has also been used for early detection, but is unlikely to be practical. Studies of nipple aspirates are also under investigation, but lack precision. Mammography, as a screening test, would appear to be here to stay for some time.

Paper 5

Periodic Screening for Breast Cancer. The Health Insurance Plan Project and Its Sequelae, 1963–1986

Authors

Shapiro S, Venet W, Strax P, Venet L

Reference

Periodic Screening for Breast Cancer. The Health Insurance Plan Project and Its Sequelae 1963–1986. Baltimore: Johns Hopkins University Press, 1988

Summary

The Health Insurance Plan (HIP) project was the first trial ever to test the efficacy of screening for cancer at any site. It was initiated in December 1963 to determine 'whether periodic breast screening with mammography and clinical examination of the breast holds substantial promise for lowering mortality in the female population from breast cancer'. Sixty-two thousand women of 40–64 years of age receiving their medical care from the Health Insurance Plan of New York State were individually randomized either to be invited to participate in four annual screens or to form a control group. The trial ended in 1986 allowing breast cancer deaths to be ascertained during 15–20 years from entry. Early reports that screen-detected cancers were less likely to have involved lymph nodes and had longer survival when adjusted for lead-time were followed by mortality entry to the trial there was a reduction of breast cancer deaths of 30% in the study group, which at 18 years was still evident at 23%. This book presents full details of all aspects of this trial; additional studies confirmed that the analyses were free from bias.

Related references **(1)** Breslow I, Henderson B, Massey T, *et al.* Working group on the gross net benefits of mammography in mass screening for the detection of breast cancer. *Journal of the National Cancer Institute* 1977; **59**:473–478.

(2) Aron J, Prorok P. Analysis of the mortality effect in a breast cancer screening study. *International Journal of Epidemiology* 1986; **15**:36–43.

(3) Chu KC, Smart CR, Tarone RE. Analysis of breast cancer mortality and state distribution by age for the Health Insurance Plan trial. *Journal of the National Cancer Institute* 1988; **80**:1125–1132.

(4) Tabar L, Fagerberg CJG, Gad A, *et al.* Reduction from mortality from breast cancer after mass screening with mammography: randomised trial from the Breast Cancer Working Group of the Swedish National Board of Health and Welfare. *Lancet* 1985; **i**:829–832 (Paper 7 in this chapter).

Key message

This, the first randomized trial screening for breast cancer by mammography and clinical examination, reported a significant reduction in deaths from breast cancer in women invited to be screened.

Why it's important

This trial provided the first indication that the screening of the breasts of normal women by clinical examination and mammography reduced deaths from breast cancer. It set standards for screening: clinical examinations were carried out by dedicated physicians; radiographers were specially trained, films were double-read, first by the group radiologist and then independently by two of three staff radiologists in the central office. The quality of films was monitored and a sample externally reviewed. A major effort was made to indoctrinate group surgeons and radiologists in the significance of non-palpable mammographic lesions and the indications for biopsy. Record keeping was meticulous, project records were matched against the NY State Cancer Registry to ascertain completeness of identification of cancers and 100% follow-up completed over 18 years. Policies for determining cause of death were constructed and samples matched against national files.

Strengths

1. This was a meticulously conducted randomized trial which provided the first information that mammographic (and clinical) screening reduced death from breast cancer.
2. Every aspect of the trial was critically monitored and subject to external review.
3. Additional information was presented on factors affecting breast cancer risk and survival.
4. Results were confirmed by alternative methods of survival analysis in which lead-time and length analysis were obviated.
5. A pathological review was conducted by the National Cancer Institute.

Weaknesses

1. 45% of screen-detected cancers were detected by clinical examination alone; only 33% were non-palpable mammographic lesions. The quality of mammography was described as 'less than optimal'.
2. Data on tumour size and grade were lacking.

Relevance

The HIP trial provided the first evidence that screening reduced breast cancer mortality. It also established standards for conducting randomized trials of screening in a large population. There have been criticisms of the design and of the fact that only 33% of cancer detected through screening were not palpable; but the conduct of the trial has been subject to expert external review and the mortality analyses have been supported by alternative methods of survival analyses. Their results were confirmed in a report of a second randomized trial in Sweden in which 163 000 women over 40 years were randomized in clusters between 1971 and 1981 to be invited for screening or to form a control group. A seven-year mortality reduction of 31% was reported in 1985 (related reference 4).

Paper 6

Breast Cancer Screening: Report to the Health Ministers of England, Wales, Scotland and Northern Ireland

Authors

Working Group chaired by Sir Patrick Forrest

Reference

Breast Cancer Screening: Report to the Health Ministers of England, Wales, Scotland and Northern Ireland. London: Her Majesty's Stationery Office, 1986

Summary

The working group was appointed by the UK Ministers of Health in July 1985 to consider whether there was a need for a change in UK policy on the provision of mammographic facilities and the screening of symptomless women. It sought to suggest a range of policy options and set out the service planning, manpower, financial and other implications of implementing such options. The group presented an interim report in January 1986 indicating that the information available from overseas trials presented a convincing case, on clinical grounds, for such a change in UK policy; but that it would not be sensible to introduce mammographic screening without providing back-up diagnostic and treatment services. The report fully discussed four stages of mammographic screening: the basic screen (to detect an abnormality); assessment of the abnormality (to determine whether a surgical biopsy should be performed); biopsy and histological examination of removed tissue; and the treatment of screen-detected cancers. The organization of a screening service, the likely service requirements, estimates of cost and comparisons with other health service uses were discussed, and the need for quality assurance and continued research emphasized. The report recommended that mammographic screening should be available to women aged 50–64 years, each 3 years.

Related references (1) Forrest AP. *Breast Cancer: The Decision to Screen.* Fourth HM Queen Elizabeth the Queen Mother Fellowship. The Nuffield Provincial Hospitals Trust, 1990.

(2) Forrest APM. Breast cancer: the decision to screen *Journal of Public Health Medicine* 1991; **13**:2–12

(3) Roebuck, EJ. A personal approach to breast cancer screening in the UK. *Breast* 1994; **3**:60–68.

(4) Nystrom L, Rutqvist LE, Wall S, *et al.* Breast cancer screening with mammography: overview of screening trials. *Lancet* 1993; **341**: 973–978 (Paper 8 in this chapter).

(5) Skrabanek P. False premises and false promises of breast cancer screening. *Lancet* 1985; **ii**:316–320.

Key message

This report formed a 'blueprint' for mammographic screening in UK which was adopted as the standard working manual by several other countries setting up population programmes of screening.

Why it's important

The report of the UK working group was accepted by Government as justification for introducing mammographic screening for breast cancer as a national service in Great Britain and Northern Ireland. Its importance in terms of reducing deaths from breast cancer has still to be fully established, and although deaths from the disease are steadily falling in countries with established screening programmes, the contribution of earlier diagnosis is still uncertain. However, the recommendations that a National Programme of Breast Screening be established as a separate service to normal health care, that stringent standards should be applied to all aspects of the programme, and that these would be subject to intensive monitoring and quality control has provided a template for national population screening programmes which others have followed. Further, the principles of care applied to women attending for screening have spread into the symptomatic sector.

Strengths

1. The working group was impartial, relying on expert witnesses to provide data and opinions.
2. The programme suggested was comprehensive, providing for the assessment of screen-detected abnormalities by expert teams working within the screening service.
3. There was standardization of data collection and annual reporting of performance by the National Breast Cancer Screening Evaluation Unit.
4. Advice on quality assurance at all levels and of the need for central advisory bodies was put into effect and performance indicators formed.
5. The need for training of radiologists and radiographers was taken into account.
6. An economic appraisal was carried out.
7. There was recognition that the recommendations were based on current knowledge and of the need for coordinating research into optimum interval, age, risk factors, acceptability, natural history and screening methods with economic studies built in where appropriate.

Weaknesses

1. There has been criticism that the decision was based on inadequate evidence (see related reference 4).
2. There has also been criticism that inadequate attention was paid to adverse effects.

Relevance

The initiation of a screening programme for breast cancer in the UK has had a great impact on health services. The requirement that one mammographic screening unit (either in a static building or mobile van) be provided for each half-million of the population, each to perform 12 000 examinations each year, led to an immediate need for expertise in breast imaging, which at that time was limited. The development of designated multidisciplinary assessment teams, which serve several screening units, has provided expertise in techniques for assessment of mammographic lesions by ultrasound, fine needle aspiration, cytology and biopsy, which for occult lesions required special localizing techniques. Realization that there also should be a multidisciplinary approach to treatment has led to the establishment of specialized breast teams in the symptomatic sector. The insistence of quality control of all stages of the screening process has provided a model for other screening services, spinning over into routine health care. Because of the smaller size of tumours detected mammographically, treatment allowing preservation of the breast is more common; axillary lymph nodes are more often free of disease, so that adjuvant chemotherapy may be avoided. But there are also disadvantages, in that the screening of normal women may cause anxiety and may lead to unnecessary investigations and overtreatment of non-invasive cancer (related reference 5).

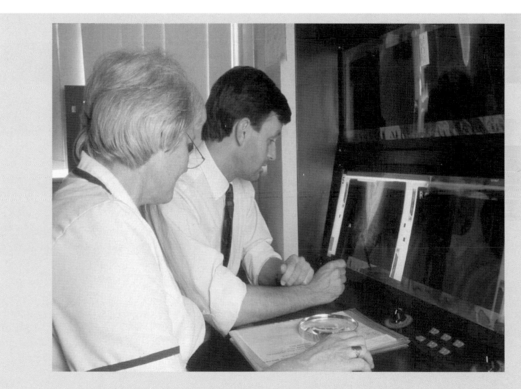

Screening assessment at work – the radiologist and radiographer as a team.

Paper 7*

Reduction in mortality from breast cancer after mass screening with mammography: Randomised trial from the Breast Cancer Working Group of the Swedish National Board of Health and Welfare

Authors

Tabar L, Fagerberg CJG, Gad A, *et al.*

Reference

Lancet 1985; **i**:829–832

Summary

The Swedish Two County randomized, controlled trial of breast cancer screening is acknowledged to be one of the best. 134 867 women aged 40–74 were randomly assigned to be invited for screening or to act as unscreened controls. This is the first report from the trial that demonstrated a mortality reduction for screening women aged 40–74 using mammographic screening.

Related references (1)	Shapiro S, Venet W, Venet L, Roeser R. Ten- to fourteen-year effect of screening on breast cancer mortality. *Journal of the National Cancer Institute* 1982; **69**: 349–355.
(2)	Shapiro S, Venet W, Strax P, Venet L. *Periodic Screening for Breast Cancer. The Health Insurance Plan Project and Its Sequelae, 1963–1986.* Baltimore: Johns Hopkins University Press, 1988 (Paper 5 in this chapter).
(3)	Baker LH. Breast Cancer Detection Demonstration Project: five-year summary report. *CA – A Cancer Journal for Clinicans* 1982; **32**: 194–202.

Key message

Mammographic screening of asymptomatic healthy women aged 40–74 can reduce the rate of death from breast cancer by approximately 25–30%.

---

* This review was written by DB Kopans.

Why it's important

The Health Insurance Plan of New York (HIP) (related references 1 and 2) was the first randomized controlled trial of breast cancer screening. The HIP demonstrated, in the most objective way possible, that screening (actually the invitation to screening) could lead to fewer breast cancer deaths. A randomized, controlled trial was the only way to avoid lead-time bias and length bias sampling. Since the primitive mammography in the HIP study was of poor quality, and since women were screened using clinical examination as well as mammography, the independent contribution of mammography could not be ascertained. The Breast Cancer Detection Demonstration Project (BCDDP) (related reference 3) demonstrated that large numbers of women could be screened fairly efficiently, and that mammographic screening could detect small, clinically occult cancers that had a more favourable prognosis. However, since the BCDDP was not a randomized, controlled trial, the true efficacy of screening was not proved. The Swedish trials were the first to scientifically confirm the independent benefit of mammography. Clinical breast examination was not employed in these trials. Thus, the mortality reductions could only be due to mammography.

Strength

This was a very large, randomized, controlled trial that eliminated the biases that make it impossible to use survival data to prove the benefit of screening.

Weaknesses

1. There are some who are concerned that the cluster randomization used in the Swedish Two County Trial may not be as balanced as individual randomization. Women in one geographic part of the county were invited for screening while women in another geographic area were not invited and were the unscreened controls. Some suggest that this might have resulted in an imbalance between the two groups.

2. Screening was accomplished using single-view oblique mammographic projections. This approach has been shown to miss up to 25% of cancers. The screening intervals were 2–3 years between screens. There are still no data from well-designed and well-performed trials that provide information on the benefit that may accrue from annual, high-quality, two-view mammography.

Relevance

The randomized, controlled trials of screening form the basis and rationale for modern breast cancer screening. This was the first 'proof' that mammographic screening, by itself, could reduce mortality.

Paper 8

Breast cancer screening with mammography: Overview of screening trials

Authors

Nystrom L, Rutqvist LE, Wall S, *et al.*

Reference

Lancet 1993; **341**:973–978

Summary

This article presents an overview of the five randomized trials in Sweden in which the mortality of those invited to screening by mammography alone was compared with those not invited. The overview was based on 282 777 women followed for 5–13 years in randomized trials in Malmö, Kopparberg, Ostergotland, Stockholm and Gothenburg. Unlike meta-analyses, the overview was not restricted to published reports, but the individual cohorts were linked to regional cancer registries to identify cases of breast cancer and with the Swedish Cause of Death Register to ascertain fatal cases. These were reviewed independently by an 'end-point committee' which included an oncologist, surgeon, radiologist and pathologist who reached a consensus on determining whether breast cancer was the 'underlying cause of death' or 'breast cancer present at death'. These two evaluations gave similar results, there being a consistent risk reduction in all studies which, in women of 50–69 years of age, was a significant 29%.

Related references **(1)** Wald NJ, Chamberlain J, Hackshaw A, on behalf of the Evaluation Committee. Report of the European Society of Mastology Breast Cancer Screening Evaluation Committee (1993). *Breast* 1993; **2**:209–216.

(2) Kerlikowske K, Grady D, Rubin SM, *et al.* Efficacy of screening mammography. A meta-analysis. *Journal of the American Medical Association* 1995; **273**:149–154.

(3) Fletcher SW, Black W, Harris R, Rimer BK, Shapiro S. Report of the International Workshop on Screening for Breast Cancer. *Journal of the National Cancer Institute* 1993; **85**:1644–1656.

(4) Gotzsche PC, Olsen O. Is screening for breast cancer with mammography justifiable? *Lancet* 2000; **355**:129–134.

(5) Alexander FE, Anderson TJ, Brown HK, *et al.* 14 years of follow-up from the Edinburgh trial of breast-cancer screening. *Lancet* 1999; **353**:1903–1908.

(6) Miller AB, Baines CJ, To T, Wall C. Canadian National Breast Screening Study: breast cancer detection and death rates among women ages 40–49 years. *Canadian Medical Association Journal* 1992; **147**: 1459–1476.

(7) Miller AB, Baines CJ, To T, Wall C. Canadian national breast screening study: breast cancer detection and death rates among women ages 50–59 years. *Canadian Medical Association Journal* 1992; **147**: 1477–1488.

(8) *Lancet*, 2000; **355**:744–752.

Key message

A combined overview analysis of five Swedish randomized trials of mammographic screening which included over 250 000 women indicated a significant reduction of mortality from breast cancer at 5–13 years in women over 50 years of age.

Why it's important

This paper was the first serious attempt to merge the results of individual trials of mammographic screening carried out in three cities and two counties in Sweden. With the inclusion of previously unreported data, longer follow-up and independent reviews of all fatal cases of breast cancer, a significant mortality benefit of 24% was observed for women of 40–74 years of age and of 29% for those over 50 years, providing strong evidence that in older women mammographic screening provided benefit. A sub-group analysis in women 40–50 years did not reveal significant benefit.

In 1993, further 'meta-analyses' of published results of all trials (including in addition to the Swedish trials the HIP trial in New York and the Edinburgh and Canadian trials) were reported by a European Evaluation Committee on Breast Screening and by other groups. An International Workshop was held in the National Cancer Institute in 1993 at which all trials were reviewed. It was concluded that for women of 50–69 years of age, screening reduced breast cancer mortality by about one-third.

Strengths

1. This was a carefully conducted overview of all women included in the five Swedish trials in which linkage with the Swedish Cancer Registry and Death Register was used to confirm cases diagnosed and fatalities.
2. An independent 'end-point' committee reviewed causes of death.
3. Two models were used to evaluate deaths from breast cancer – 'underlying cause of death' and 'breast cancer present at death', which gave equal assessments.

Weakness

The individual trials differed in design, for example, methods of randomization, and there was variable 'contamination' of the control groups by opportunistic mammography.

Relevance

The Swedish overview established a base for the conduct of further combined analyses of all randomized trials in which women who were randomly offered mammographic screening were compared with control women who were not offered screening. Although these further analyses merged the reported results of individual trials rather than, as in the Swedish overview, reviewed individual case findings, they represent 'stronger scientific evidence regarding the effectiveness of screening for breast cancer than for any other cancer (related reference 3).

Two Danish statisticians, Gotzsche and Olsen (related reference 4), have questioned the validity of four of these trials and that of two other trials (related reference 5), but not that of the Canadian trials (related references 6 and 7), on the grounds of faulty randomization and a lack of effect on all-cause mortality. Their criticisms were not accepted by others (related reference 8): one cannot expect that modern randomization procedures now used to test therapeutic procedure could at that time have been applied to these large population trials. Nor can all-cause mortality be regarded as a realistic end-point in screening trials. Despite imperfections, differences in favour of screening in women aged 50–74 years are seen in all but one of the seven studies which include over half a million women (related reference 2).

Paper 9

Consensus Statement, National Institutes of Health Consensus Development Panel

Author

National Institutes of Health Consensus Conference on Breast Cancer Screening for Women ages 40–49

Reference

Monographs of the National Cancer Institute **22**; 1997: vii–xvii

Summary

This statement followed a consensus conference at the National Cancer Institute in January 1997 to assess currently available data regarding the effectiveness of mammography screening for women aged 40–49 years. Presentations of updated results of all randomized trials of breast screening were reported with particular emphasis on subset analyses of benefit in women aged 49 years or less. The initial unanimous conclusions of the 13-member panel were 'that the data currently available do not warrant a universal recommendation for mammography for all women in their forties; and that 'a women should have access to the best possible relevant information regarding both risks and benefits, presented in an understandable and usable form,' so that they may decide whether to undergo mammography or not. Subsequently two members produced a minority report in which they recommended that there should be active encouragement for women in their forties to be routinely screened.

Key message

The majority view of the panel was that the available evidence did not support a universal recommendation for mammographic screening for women in their forties.

Related references (1) Kerlikowske K. Efficacy of screening mammography amongst women aged 40–49 and 50–59: comparison of relative and absolute benefit. *Monographs of the National Cancer Institute* 1997; **22**:79–86.

(2) Berry DA. Benefits and risks of screening mammography for women in their forties: a statistical appraisal. *Journal of the National Cancer Institute* 1998; **90**:1431–1439.

Why it's important

This consensus statement following a three-day conference attended by leading experts at the National Cancer Institute provided further evidence of the value of mammographic screening for breast cancer in women aged 50–69 years. However, the panel concluded that the smaller mortality benefit observed in younger women did not justify the risks of routine screening. Although initially unanimous, two members of the panel subsequently filed a minority report believing that the panel had underestimated benefit and overestimated risks. This view was subsequently supported by the US National Cancer Advisory Board, as a result of which the National Cancer Institute formally recommended that women should undergo routine screening by mammography each 1–2 years from age 40, concurring with the American Cancer Society which recommends annual screening from age 40.

It is important to appreciate that the conclusions of consensus conferences need not be automatically adopted by the agencies sponsoring them. But why go to the trouble and expense of seeking the opinions of experts in the field?

Strength

This was the most up-to-date review of randomized trials of mammographic screening carried out by experts which strengthened the evidence of a mortality benefit in women of 50–69 years of age, but did not provide convincing evidence of similar benefit in younger women.

Weakness

The conclusions of 11 members of a 13-member panel on the evidence available that routine screening of women aged 40–49 years was not justified was overturned following a minority report by a radiologist and obstetrician.

Relevance

The National Institutes of Health Consensus Development Program is a unique assessment process in American medicine which aims to clarify the state of art in a field of science. Since the first reports of the results of randomized trials of mammographic screening there has been controversy regarding its role in women aged 40–49 years. As only one of the eight trials which included women of this age did not also include older women, reliance has been placed on subset analyses. These have indicated that mortality benefit in women of 40–49 years is considerably less and, in some trials, occurred later than in women over 50. Although the majority opinion of the consensus panel was not acted upon, it does provide further support for the exclusion of such young women in national programmes of population screening, at least until the results of two large trials of mammographic screening in women of 40 years currently in progress in Europe are known.

Paper 10

Percutaneous large-core breast biopsy: A multi-institutional study

Authors

Parker SH, Burbank F, Jackman RJ

Reference

Radiology 1994; **193**:359–364

Summary

In 1988 two technologies were welded together in Denver, Colorado – a dedicated stereotactic breast biopsy system with the patient lying prone and an automated biopsy gun [14G] – which allowed any lesion of the breast visible on mammography to be biopsied without recourse to open surgery. This paper describes a retrospective assessment of its reliability in 20 institutions in which 6152 breast lesions, 984 malignant, were biopsied. The majority (92.7%) were not even vaguely palpable; of which 86.1% had an average diameter of 15 mm or less. High frequency ultrasound was used to localize 1008 of them while the remainder (4744) were localized by the stereotactic radiological system.

The objective of the study was to determine whether, with suitable training and following a standard protocol, the success of the method could be replicated throughout the world. In the event this was clear: only 15 of 4955 lesions diagnosed as benign were 'missed' cancers.

It was concluded that on economical, psychological and physical grounds, guided large core biopsy should supplant surgical biopsy in the vast majority of cases.

Related references **(1)** Ferzli GS, Hurwitz JB, Puza T, Vorst-Bilotti SV. Advanced breast biopsy instrumentation: a critique. *Journal of the American College of Surgeons* 1997; **185**:145–151.

(2) Jackman RJ, Marzoni FA. Needle localisation biopsy. Why do we fail? *Radiology* 1997; **204**:677–684.

(3) Parker SH, Burbank F. A practical approach to minimally invasive breast biopsy. *Radiology* 1996; **200**:11–20.

Key message

The sampling of non-palpable breast lesions using a dedicated system for stereotactic localization of automated biopsy gun is as accurate as an open surgical needle localization biopsy.

Why it's important

The importance of this paper lies in its evaluation of a dedicated system for core biopsy of mammographically detected lesion of the breast. Localization biopsy following the radiologically guided insertion of hooked wires has been regarded as the 'gold standard' but a recent survey of 49 reports including 12 563 cases reported a 'miss rate' for the diagnosis of cancer averaging 2.0% (related reference 2). This is greater than that reported in the multi-institutional survey cited here in which automated core biopsy guided by a dedicated stereotactic system using a prone table was used. Additional advantages are the lack of a scar, the absence of a deformity within the breast causing a future mammographic abnormality, the confident diagnosis of a benign lesion and the easier surgical field for a definitive operation should it prove to be a cancer.

A disadvantage of the automated biopsy gun used in this study is that multiple insertions and passes are necessary to obtain the 5–10 cores of tissue which are required for a satisfactory biopsy. This has been solved by the development of the Mammotome (Biopsys Medical, Irvine, California) which allows multiple samples of tissue to be obtained without removing the instrument. This is achieved by the incorporation of a vacuum which draws sequential samples into a cutting chamber and transports them along the probe for collection.

The Mammotome must not be confused with the Advanced Breast Biopsy Instrumentation (ABBI) system, a motorized unit which cuts a cylinder of tissue up to 2 cm in diameter from just below the dermis to, and including, the lesion. This is a quasi-surgical procedure, which advisably is carried out in the operating room in case conversion to an open surgical biopsy is required. Although it was suggested that the ABBI might be used therapeutically, approval by the American Food and Drug Administration (FDA) has only been given for its use as a diagnostic instrument.

Strength

This is a complete system for sampling tissue from a mammographically detected lesion of the breast without open surgery.

Weakness

The capital expense of a dedicated unit with a prone table, digital mammography and the Mammotome is forbidding.

Relevance

There is no doubt that being equipped with digital mammography and using the Mammotome, represents the 'state of art' for the biopsy of a non-palpable mammographically visible lesion of the breast. However, the capital expense is considerably greater than that for the 'add-on' units for stereotactic guidance of fine-needle aspiration cytology or core biopsy used in the UK screening service. But unquestionably, the prone table is more comfortable and less worrying for the patient. In skilled hands, 5–10 cores of tissue can be taken in 10–15 minutes at an operating cost that is considerably less than an open surgical biopsy.

Paper II

Projecting individual probabilities of developing breast cancer for white females who are being examined annually

Authors

Gail MH, Brinton LA, Byer DP, *et al.*

Reference

Journal of the National Cancer Institute 1989; **81**:1879–1886

Summary

This was a case–control study including 2852 white women whose breast cancers were detected on screening in the Breast Cancer Demonstration Project in the USA and 3136 matched controls. The objective was to predict the risk of breast cancer in women attending an annual programme of mammographic screening. The main factors emerging were age, age at menarche, age at first live birth, number of previous breast biopsies and a history of breast cancer in a first-degree relative. The relative risks for each factor alone in combination were used to construct a table from which an individual woman undergoing regular mammographic screening can be informed about her probable risk of developing breast cancer at 10, 20 and 30 years and be counselled on what action she might wish to take.

Related references (1)   Fisher B, Constantino JP, Wickermann DL, *et al.* Tamoxifen for the prevention of breast cancer: report of the National Surgical Adjuvant and Bowel Project P-1 study. *Journal of the National Cancer Institute* 1998; **90**:1371–1388.

(2)   Constantino JP, Gail MH, Pee D, *et al.* Validation studies for models projecting the risk of invasive and total breast cancer incidence. *Journal of the National Cancer Institute* 1999; **91**:1541–1548.

(3)   Madigan MP, Ziegler RG, Benichou J, Byrne C, Hoover RN. Proportion of breast cancer cases in the United States explained by well established risk factors. *Journal of the National Cancer Institute* 1995; **87**:1681–1685.

Why it's important

This attempt to predict breast cancer risk in women undergoing regular mammographic screening has gained great importance from its use to select women for inclusion in the NSABP tamoxifen prevention trial (related reference 1). Although the model over-predicted breast cancer risk in other populations of women such as the Nurses Health, Cancer and Steroid studies, its modification to define risk in women less than 50 years of age equivalent to that of a 60-year-old woman has been validated. The modified model substituted age-specific incidence rates of invasive cancer from national estimates from the Surveillance, Epidemiology and End Results Program of the National Cancer Institute for the total (including non-invasive cancer) breast cancer incidence rates recorded in the BCDP. Lobular but not ductal carcinoma *in situ* was included as an additional factor.

Strength

This was an attempt to define a simple method for determining risk of breast cancer in individual women undergoing mammographic screening which has subsequently been validated for other use.

Weaknesses

1. It included risk of both invasive and non-invasive cancer.
2. It takes no account of other established risk factors such as oestrogen and alcohol use.
3. It over-estimates risk in other populations of women not undergoing screening.
4. It does not allow for extended pedigree and is therefore weak in determining risk associated with germline mutations.

Relevance

Some of those who dissented from the introduction of mammographic screening suggested that it should be restricted to women at high risk. An effective discriminant should be able to detect 80% of breast cancer cases in 20% of the population, which is not possible using established risk factors. A recent report suggests that in the USA well-established risk factors (earlier age at menarche, late age at first birth, nulliparity, history of benign disease, higher family income and first-degree relative with breast cancer) may explain between 45–55% of all cases; an estimate considerably greater than those previously described, but not of sufficient size to allow selective screening.

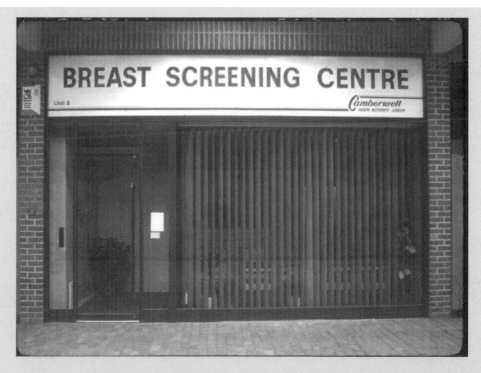

Breast screening center Camberwell South East London.

Paper 12

Randomized trial of breast self-examination in Shanghai: Methodology and preliminary results

Authors

Thomas DB, Gao DL, Self SG, *et al.*

Reference

Journal of the National Cancer Institute 1997; **89**:355–365.

Summary

This is a report of one of the only two randomized trials of breast self-examination (BSE) carried out in Shanghai, China; the other is the WHO trial in two cities (St Petersburg and Moscow) in Russia. In the Shanghai trial 267040 female employees in 520 factories in the Shanghai Textile Industry were assigned during 1989–1991 on the basis of the factory in which they were employed to a BSE instruction group or as controls. Training in BSE was rigorous using silicone breast models, personalized instruction, video re-enforcement sessions and frequent reminders. A high level of participation was documented in the BSE group, and randomly sampled women in this group demonstrated greater proficiency in detecting lumps in breast models than did randomly sampled controls. Yet the number of breast cancers detected in the two groups to the end of 1994 was equal: 331 in BSE; 332 in control groups. Cancers detected in the BSE group were no smaller than those in controls, and cumulative breast cancer mortality rates over 5 years were virtually the same (30.9 versus 32.7 per 100 000). More benign lesions were detected in the BSE group (1457 versus 623).

Related references **(1)**   UK Trial of Early Detection of Breast Cancer Group. Sixteen year mortality from breast cancer in the UK TEDBC. *Lancet* 1999; **353**:1909–1914.

(2)   Holmberg L, Ekbom A, Calle E, *et al.* Breast cancer mortality in relation to self-reported use of breast self-examination. A cohort study of 450,000 women. *Breast Cancer Research and Treatment* 1997; **43**:137–140.

(3)   Semiglazov WF, Moiseyenko VM, Bavli HJR, *et al.* The role of breast self-examination in early breast cancer detection [results of the 5 year USSR/WHO randomised study in Leningrad]. *European Journal of Epidemiology* 1992; **8**:498–502.

(4)   Haagensen CD. *Carcinoma of the Breast: A Monograph for the Physician.* New York: American Cancer Society, 1950.

(5)   Baxter N, with the Canadian Task Force on Preventative Health Care. Preventative Health Care 2001 Update: Should women be routinely taught self examination to screen for breast cancer? *Canadian Medical Association Journal* 2001; **164**:1837–1846.

Why it's important

Considerable pressure has been placed on women to practise BSE 'by rote' through widely distributed leaflets and other forms of communication – yet there is no evidence that it benefits. A number of retrospective studies have confirmed that in women practising BSE the cancers which they detect are more likely to be small and node-negative than those arising symptomatically; but only one cohort study from Finland has suggested that mortality is reduced. Two comparative studies of mortality have been published, one from the American Cancer Society, the other the UK trial of Early Detection of Breast Cancer – neither showed benefit.

The results from only the Leningrad portion of the Russian trial have been reported, and showed no benefit after 8 years of follow-up; but compliance dropped precipitously and by the fourth year only 18% of women still practised BSE. It is likely that the randomized trial in Shanghai, in which, compliance has been carefully monitored, will provide the best evidence on its value.

Strength

This was a large and well-controlled randomized trial of BSE.

Weakness

Continuing follow-up may prove difficult.

Relevance

The Health Ministers in the UK decided not to advocate BSE 'by rote' as part of the screening service, but launched a campaign of 'breast awareness' in which women should pay attention to any changes in their breasts, as in any other part of the body. If concerned they should consult their doctor. However, BSE is still actively promoted in other countries. It is important that, like other dogma, Haagensen's statement that 'from the point of view of the greatest possible gain in early diagnosis, teaching a woman to examine her own breasts is more important than teaching the technique of breast examination to physicians' is critically assessed.

A systematic review by the Canadian Task Force on Preventative Health led to the conclusion that 'because there is fair evidence of no benefit and good evidence of harm' routine teaching of BSE should not be included in the periodic health examination of women aged 40–69 (related reference 5).

Paper 13

False premises and false promises of breast cancer screening

Author

Skrabanek P

Reference

Lancet 1985; **ii**:316–320

Summary

This first paper by Skrabanek questioned the credibility of screening for breast cancer, disputing the evidence for the size of benefit observed in the recently published HIP (New York) and Two-counties (Sweden) randomized trials and case-control (Holland) studies. He regarded breast cancer as an incurable disease, indicating that as it may take 8–9 years for a tumour to reach 1 cm in size, 'early diagnosis' by mammography is unlikely to affect the chance of cure but increases the time of anxiety and fear. Although mammography is the only method to detect breast cancer before it is palpable, false-positive tests result in unnecessary investigations and the risk of over-treatment, particularly of non-invasive cancer, while false negative tests, by giving false re-assurance, may eventually delay diagnosis. He was concerned that informed consent had not been the rule in screening studies and condemned breast self-examination as dishonest.

Related reference	**(1)**	De Koning HJ, Coebergh JWW, van Dongen JA. Current controversies in cancer. Is mass screening for breast cancer cost effective? *European Journal of Cancer* 1996; **32A**:1835–1844.
	(2)	Baum M. Point of view. The breast screening controversy. *European Journal of Cancer* 1996; **32A**:9–11.
	(3)	Wright CJ, Mueller CB. Screening mammography and public health policy: the need for perspective. *Lancet* 1995; **346**:29–32.
	(4)	Steggles S, Lightfoot N, Sellick SM. Psychological distress associated with organized breast cancer screening. *Cancer Prevention and Control* 1998; **2**:213–235j.

Key message

This paper expresses doubts that population screening for breast cancer is justified, since its costs may exceed the benefits.

Why it's important

This was the first of a series of papers by Skrabanek and others in which the validity of the evidence that the benefits of screening outweighs its costs is doubted. There is no doubt that screening can have psychological consequences. A review of ten studies indicates that, of these, anxiety is the most prevalent, with a disproportionate impact on those recalled for further tests (related reference 4). But this is a normal reaction, and although its intensity and duration are uncertain there is no evidence for serious psychiatric morbidity.

The implications of false positive and false negative tests are clearly important; these depend upon the quality of the initial screening test, and also of the subsequent assessment procedures. So also is the risk of over-treatment real. The cost-effectiveness of screening is also debated, and although these are not considered excessive compared to other health needs, some express the belief that the money would be better spent on strengthening the symptomatic sector and on fundamental research.

Strength

This paper expresses a contrary opinion on the introduction of screening for breast cancer.

Weakness

Selective use of the literature and tendentious interpretation of scientific data weakened the author's arguments.

Relevance

It is correct that those opposing the introduction of screening for breast cancer should be able to express their views, but regrettable that their opinions should be taken out of the scientific arena and at times exaggerated by the popular press. This only can do harm as it increases the uncertainty of the majority of women who participate in screening programmes. There is no question that overdiagnosis, overtreatment and false reassurance must be minimized, that the quality of all steps in the screening process must be beyond reproach, and that women must be aware of benefits and costs before participating.

The key question to which we require an answer is whether the natural progression of breast cancer, particularly when non-invasive or 'minimally invasive', is modified by earlier diagnosis. From the evidence available it does appear that this is so, but, considering the heterogeneity of the disease, there is still much to learn about its natural history.

CHAPTER 9

Benign disease

ROBERT MANSEL

Introduction

Benign breast disease forms a large part of the breast problems encountered in clinical practice, with between 10 and 20 patients with benign symptoms being seen for every case of breast cancer in the average clinical practice. There is a huge literature extending back almost 300 years, much of which is devoted to differentiating benign disease from malignant disease. Clinical conditions such as bacterial mastitis, cyst formation, and breast pain have been known for centuries, so I have not included the original descriptions of each conditions in the classic papers, but rather, more recent papers that have changed practice. This has meant that classic descriptions such as Astley Cooper's description of cysts and Montgomery's description of areolar tubercles have not been included.

No papers relating to the risk of breast cancer have been included, since these are covered elsewhere in this volume.

The Cardiff Mastalgia Clinic was established in 1974 by Professor LE Hughes in response to the confusion in the literature relating to the various forms of so-called benign breast disease. The research programme first categorized mastalgia (chosen as the preferred term instead of mastodynia), and then systematically examined the value of treatments in controlled randomized trials. Bromocriptine, danazol, progestogens, and goserelin were examined in turn and the results published. This body of work forms the largest proportion of controlled trials in the world literature. The clinic continues today and is currently involved in the new international multicentre trial of tamoxifen gel in mastalgia.

Paper 1

The clinical picture of dilated ducts beneath the nipple frequently to be palpated as a doughy worm-like mass – the varicocele tumour of the breast

Author

Bloodgood JC

Reference

Surgery, Gynecology and Obstetrics 1923; **36**:486–495

Summary

This paper describes clearly the classic dilating type of duct ectasia and lists all the relevant clinical features. The point is made that most of the conditions described, such as cysts or duct ectasia, do not require operative intervention. Attention is also drawn to the other classic features of duct ectasia, such as nipple retraction and inflammatory episodes. Bloodgood also draws attention to the fact that duct ectasia with periductal mastitis can closely mimic the signs of cancer.

Related references **(1)** Haagensen CD. Mammary duct ectasia – a disease that may simulate cancer. *Cancer* 1951; **4**:749–761.

(2) Ewing M. Stagnation in the main ducts of the breast. *Journal of the Royal College of Surgeons of Edinburgh* 1963; **8**:134–142.

(3) Tedeschi L, Ouzouman G, Byrne JJ. The role of ductal obstruction and hormonal stimulation in main duct ectasia. *Surgery, Gynecology and Obstetrics* 1962; **114**:741–744.

Key message

There was a clear and comprehensive description of the clinical and pathological features of the various phases of duct ectasia.

Why it's important

This paper drew attention to the various modalities of duct ectasia that could cause clinical confusion, and made the point that most benign disease can be differentiated from cancer by careful clinical examination. This is relevant, even in these days of routine mammography and ultrasonography of the breast. The widely differing presentations of duct ectasia are beautifully described in detail, and these descriptions should be understood by today's clinicians, since duct ectasia can easily be misdiagnosed and it still is the cause of the occasional tragic mastectomy done for a hard craggy lump, which was clinically said to be an obvious cancer. This is a salutary warning never to perform ablative breast surgery without a prior cytological or histological diagnosis.

Strengths

1. Detailed descriptions were given that still stand the test of time.
2. Clear conclusions were reached based on great clinical experience.

Weaknesses

1. This was a series of collected case reports.
2. There were no control groups for the main observations.
3. The paper does not differentiate cystic change from duct ectasia.

Relevance

This paper provides useful descriptions of clinical entities that remain relevant in clinical practice today.

Paper 2

Fistulas of lactiferous ducts

Authors

Zuska JJ, Crile G Jr, Ayres WW

Reference

American Journal of Surgery 1951; **81**:312–317

Summary

This paper presents five cases of duct ectasia complicated by fistula formation, and reports that inflammation was a prominent feature in these cases. It describes the classic position of the mammary duct fistula opening at the areolar edge, and reports that a communication can be demonstrated between that opening and the lactiferous ducts using a probe and thus confirming the presence of a fistula. The authors also note that the patients are all relatively young for breast disease, which is a finding noted for inflammatory-type duct ectasia. A proposed pathogenesis is discussed that proposes that inflammation precedes the establishment of the fistula opening. The recommended treatment was excision of the fistula tract.

Related references **(1)** Tice GI, Dockerty MB, Harrington SW. Comedomastitis. A clinical and pathologic study of data in 172 cases. *Surgery, Gynecology and Obstetrics* 1948; **87**:525–540.

(2) Bundred NJ, Dixon JM, Chetty U, Forrest APM. Mammillary fistula. *British Journal of Surgery* 1987; **74**:466–468.

(3) Patey DH, Thackray AC. Pathology and treatment of mammary duct fistula. *Lancet* 1958; **ii**:871–873.

Key message

This paper alerted surgeons to the presence of inflammatory mammary duct fistula.

Why it's important

This was the first paper to outline the pathogenesis, clinical features, and treatment of mammary fistula, all of which are relevant today. The authors noted the key features of young age, inflammation and abscess formation, and the communication between the track and the major lactiferous ducts. This condition was difficult to treat effectively, and the principles laid down for treatment remain standard today, with only the addition of antibiotic cover during surgery.

Strengths

1. This was an accurate observational study of the key features of a previously poorly understood condition.
2. It laid down the correct principles of treatment.

Weakness

This was a small case report series.

Relevance

It defined the correct treatment of the condition, which remains the current standard.

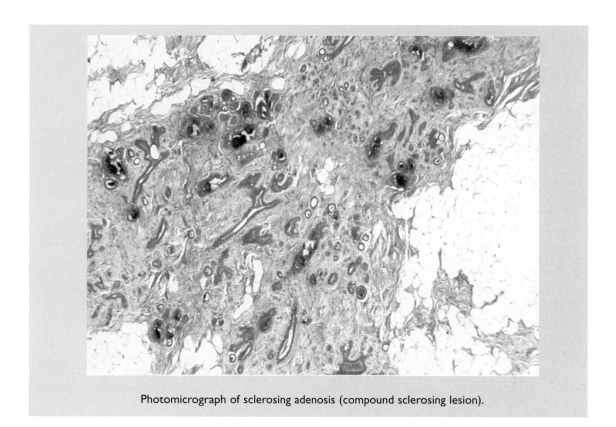

Photomicrograph of sclerosing adenosis (compound sclerosing lesion).

Paper 3

Natural history of cystic disease of breast treated conservatively

Authors

Patey DH, Nurick AW

Reference

British Medical Journal, 1953; **i**:15–17

Summary

This paper describes the management of breast cysts by David Patey in his private practice. Seventy-six cases of cysts were recorded between 1931 and 1950, whereas 260 cases of carcinoma were seen in the same time frame. This suggests selection, since cystic disease is known in routine NHS practice to be equally as common as breast cancer. The majority of the cysts were treated by aspiration (69 of 76), and were then followed for up to 16 years. Patey noted that only one case of carcinoma developed in the whole follow-up period, and this was a tumour in the opposite breast. He also noted that 20 patients out of the 55 aspirated at least 2 years previously presented with recurrent cysts.

Related references	**(1)**	Jones BM, Bradbeer JW. The presentation and progress of microscopic breast cysts. *British Journal of Surgery* 1980; **67**:669–671.
	(2)	Forrest APM, Kirkpatrick JR, Roberts MM. Needle aspiration of breast cysts. *British Medical Journal* 1975; **iii**:30–31.
	(3)	Bloodgood JC. The pathology of chronic cystic mastitis of the female breast with special consideration of the blue-domed cyst. *Archives of Surgery* 1921; **3**:445–452.

Key message

This paper suggested that it was safe to aspirate cysts rather than remove them surgically.

Why it's important

This paper supplied evidence that after aspiration of breast cysts, the incidence of subsequent cancer (even on long-term follow-up) was low, since only one case was recorded in 16 years of follow-up. Standard management at this time was surgical biopsy with frozen section, and this new approach offered a huge saving in terms of inconvenience and expense by managing cysts by aspiration. Also, the authors showed that around 40% of patients would have a recurrent cyst on follow-up, and this is very typical of current results. Subsequent work has shown that the cancer risk is actually related to the presence of associated hyperplasia and not due to the cyst itself.

Strengths

1. This was a personal observational study with close follow-up.
2. The paper offered a much simpler and effective form of management.

Weaknesses

1. These were highly selected patients in private practice, as shown by the preponderance of cancer patients.
2. Cancers from two sources and intracystic cancers were included in the data.

Relevance

This paper remains relevant today, since aspiration of cysts is now the standard management and the rate of recurrent cysts is very similar to that reported in this paper. The only addition in modern practice is the use of ultrasound to diagnose intracystic cancers.

Paper 4

Excision of the major duct system for benign disease of the breast

Author

Hadfield J

Reference

British Journal of Surgery 1960; **48**:472–477

Summary

A series of 31 patients were treated by total duct excision for nipple discharge, mammillary fistula, duct papillomas, and cysts. Hadfield advocates the operation for many of these benign conditions and notes that subsequent pregnancy is not a problem despite complete excision of the milk ducts. He also notes that the operation is curative for discharge related to duct papilloma.

Related references

(1) Urban JA. Excision of the major duct system of the breast. *Cancer* 1963; **16**:516–520.

(2) Atkins HJB. Mammillary fistula. *British Medical Journal* 1955; **ii**:1473–1474.

Key message

The major duct system can be excised for benign disease without any major cosmetic or functional problems.

Why it's important

This was the first paper to describe the specific technique of total duct excision, although Hadfield acknowledges that he learnt the technique at the Memorial Hospital in New York, where it had been developed by Urban and Adair. Urban published his own personal series of 167 cases 3 years after this paper. Hadfield described a periareolar incision (unlike the radial incision used by Urban), because this is cosmetically better. The operation described and the indications for it have not changed over the years, and it remains one of the standard operations on the nipple areolar region.

Strength

This was the first description of a new technique useful for several benign conditions.

Weaknesses

1. No report was given of the complications of the operation (e.g. infection, recurrent fistula, and loss of nipple sensation).
2. The entity of retention cyst of the duct system, which is an ill-defined diagnosis, was included.

Paper 5

Clinical syndromes of mastalgia

Authors

Preece PE, Hughes LE, Mansel RE, Baum M, Bolton PM, Gravelle IH

Reference

Lancet 1976; **ii**:670–673

Summary

A total of 232 patients with breast pain were studied with a structured pro forma measuring the type of pain, the periodicity and duration of pain, its distribution and radiation, and aggravating and relieving factors. In addition, the impact on lifestyle was described. Analysis showed that the pain could be classified into clear groups: the dominant pattern was cyclical pronounced pain (40%), while there was non-cyclical pain in 27% of cases. These patterns were easily defined in the clinic using simple pain charts.

Related references

(1) Dowle CS. Breast pain: classification, aetiology and management. *Australia and New Zealand Journal of Surgery* 1987; **57**:423–428.

(2) Bishop HM, Blamey RW. A suggested classification of breast pain. *Postgraduate Medical Journal* 1979; **55**:59–60.

(3) Preece PE, Mansel RE, Hughes LE. Mastalgia: psychoneurosis or organic disease? *British Medical Journal* 1978; **i**:29–30.

Key message

This was the first description of a prospectively studied group of patients with pure mastalgia, with resulting sorting of patients into clinically relevant subgroups. Previous work had included a variety of premenstrual syndromes as well as mastalgia.

Why it's important

This paper was the first to clearly define this symptom complex as a clear entity separate from the heterogeneous groups of premenstrual syndromes that had been previously described. The use of a simple pain chart allowed clinicians to categorize patients with breast pain using this classification. Subsequent work has shown that the subgroups so defined respond differently to therapy, and thus the classification has turned out to be useful for selecting patients for therapy.

Strengths

1. This was the first prospectively studied group of patients with breast pain.
2. It produced a clear classification that was clinically useful.
3. It described non-breast referred pain as a presentation of mastalgia.

Weakness

This was a questionnaire study with no correlation with biochemistry or pathology.

Relevance

The findings of this paper have been borne out by subsequent studies and the classification remains useful to current clinicians.

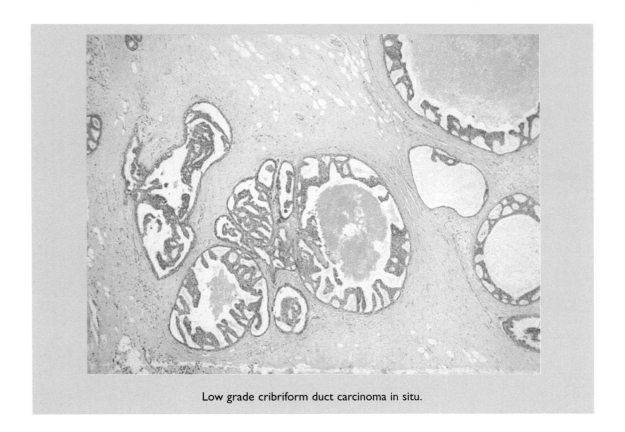

Low grade cribriform duct carcinoma in situ.

Paper 6

A double-blind trial of the prolactin inhibitor bromocriptine in painful benign breast disease

Authors

Mansel RE, Preece PE, Hughes LE

Reference

British Journal of Surgery 1978; **65**:724–727

Summary

This was a double-blind crossover trial of the prolactin inhibitor bromocriptine in painful benign breast disease, involving a total of 40 patients (29 with cyclical mastalgia and 11 with non-cyclical mastalgia). Six months' treatment was given, with a crossover with placebo therapy, and response was assessed using a visual analogue scale. The drug was shown to produce a significant improvement in symptoms in the cyclical patients, but not in the non-cyclical patients. The symptomatic responses were also correlated with significant depressions in prolactin levels.

Related references **(1)** Asch RH, Greenblatt RB. The use of an impeded androgen – danazol – in the management of benign breast disorders. *American Journal of Obstetrics and Gynecology* 1977; **127**:130–134.

(2) Fentiman IS, Caleffi M, Brame K, Chaudhary MA, Hayward JL. Double-blind controlled trial of tamoxifen therapy for mastalgia. *Lancet* 1986; **i**:287–288.

(3) Minton JP, Foecking MK, Webster DJT, Mathews RH. Response of fibre cystic disease to caffeine withdrawal and correlation of cyclic nucleotides with breast disease. *American Journal of Obstetrics and Gynecology* 1979; **135**:157–158.

Key message

The trial showed that treatment targeted at reducing hormone levels in cyclical mastalgia effectively reduced the symptoms of breast pain.

Why it's important

This was the first of many new studies in breast pain that used a controlled trial format with a placebo control and semi-objective measurements of breast symptoms. Prior to this study, the literature consisted of open observational studies with no controls, and suffered from the usual high placebo responses in subjective symptoms. In this study also, biochemical measurements of relevant hormones were correlated with changes in symptoms. Although bromocriptine is now seldom used as therapy for breast pain, this trial was the forerunner of a format that has now become standard in the study of therapy in breast pain. The study of new therapies for breast pain also led to exploration of new ideas for management, such as the restriction of caffeine and essential fatty acid therapy, not all of which have stood the test of time.

Strengths

1. This study employed a controlled trial crossover format against placebo.
2. Patients were predefined into symptomatic pain patterns.
3. Correlations were made with biochemistry.

Weakness

There was a relatively small number of patients.

Relevance

The trial established the necessity for studying the subjective symptom of breast pain in a controlled manner, and led to subsequent trials using several other agents, but with a similar trial structure.

Paper 7

Accumulation of hormones in breast cyst fluid

Authors

Bradlow HL, Schwartz MK, Fleisher M, *et al.*

Reference

Journal of Clinical Endocrinology and Metabolism 1979; **49**:778–782

Summary

Bradlow and his group measured several immunoreactive peptide hormones in breast cyst fluid from 47 patients and compared the levels with those in the serum. Luteinizing hormone (LH) and follicle-stimulating hormone (FSH) levels were higher in the serum than in cyst fluid, but the reverse was true of prolactin. Aspirations of multiple cysts in the same patient showed a high degree of agreement of hormone levels in cysts in individual patients. The greatest variability was seen with human chorionic gonadotrophin (hCG) levels. On the basis of the hCG levels, it was possible to split the patients into two separate subgroups.

Related references **(1)** Haagensen DEG, Mazoujian VG, Dilley CE, Pederson CE, Kisler SJ, Wells SA. Breast gross cystic disease fluid analysis I: Isolation and radio immunoassay for a major component protein. *Journal of the National Cancer Institute* 1979; **62**:239–244.

(2) Dixon JM, Miller WR, Scott WN. Natural history of cystic disease: the importance of cyst type. *British Journal of Surgery* 1985; **72**:190–192.

(3) Miller WR, Humeniuk V, Kelley RW. DHAS in breast secretions. *Journal of Steroid Biochemistry* 1980; **13**:145–151.

Key message

This paper showed two essential facts: that the concentration of peptide hormones was remarkably different in cyst fluid compared with serum, and that there appeared to be two populations of breast cysts.

Why it's important

This paper established that the fluid in breast cysts was not formed by a passive process but in fact by an active process requiring secretion of hormones against established gradients. This work then led on to the discovery that simple molecules such as ions and indeed the pH of breast cysts seem to divide cysts into two widely different subpopulations. This work led to a great deal of further research trying to establish whether these different subpopulations as defined biochemically could in fact act as markers of future risk of breast cancer.

Strengths

1. This paper came from an extremely strong steroid biochemistry laboratory.
2. It addressed a common clinical problem with prospects for great utility in terms of measuring cancer risk.
3. It showed clear differences in biochemical measurements in apparently similar patients.

Weakness

The patient population was not clinically well defined, and the basis of selection for the study was unclear but was probably retrospective and opportunistic.

Relevance

It established that cyst formation is an active process and not simply due to degeneration, but the hope of establishing a simple biochemical test of risk has not materialized.

Paper 8

ANDI – A new perspective on benign breast disorders

Authors

Hughes LE, Mansel RE, Webster DJT

Reference

Lancet 1987; **ii**:1316–1319

Summary

This paper was the culmination of many years' work from the Cardiff group on the topic of benign breast disease, and attempted to bring an ordered framework to the confusing terminology and varied physiology of the condition known variously as 'chronic mastitis', 'fibrocystic mastitis', and 'benign disease'. The paper sought to classify common but low-risk breast conditions as variants of normal physiology, rather than true breast disease leading to breast cancer. In so doing, it attempted to place common breast symptoms in a category of aberrant physiology, which could be treated in terms of quality of life, but also removed them from the high-risk category, thus giving reassurance to the patients.

Related references	(1)	Love S, Gelman RS, Silen W. Fibrocystic disease of the breast. A nondisease. *New England Journal of Medicine* 1982; **307**:1010–1014.
	(2)	Atkins HJB. Chronic mastitis. *Lancet* 1938; **i**:707–712.

Key message

Most women seeking medical attention for breast symptoms were suffering from aberrant physiology rather than true disease of the breast.

Why it's important

This paper led to a lot of discussion and was timely since it coincided with a large body of work showing that the long-term risk of breast cancer for the vast majority of the pathological conditions associated with benign symptoms was low or at the level of the population risk. This allowed clinicians to treat such symptoms on their merits to improve quality of life while being able to reassure patients that they remained at the population risk for breast cancer. Although the headline term ANDI has not achieved wide usage, there has been a general trend for the term 'benign breast disease' to be replaced by 'benign breast change' or 'fibrocystic change', and this was the primary purpose of the paper.

Strengths

1. This paper brought together multiple concepts and pathologies into one conceptual framework.
2. It addressed a current need to rationalize terminology.

Weaknesses

1. This was a conceptual paper rather than a data-driven hypothesis.
2. In the view of some pathologists, it removed too many true pathologies into the aberrant physiology classification.

Relevance

This work has helped to clarify the management of patients with benign symptoms and reduce the anxiety derived from cancer risk. It has also informed the development of clinical guidelines for referral for breast symptoms.

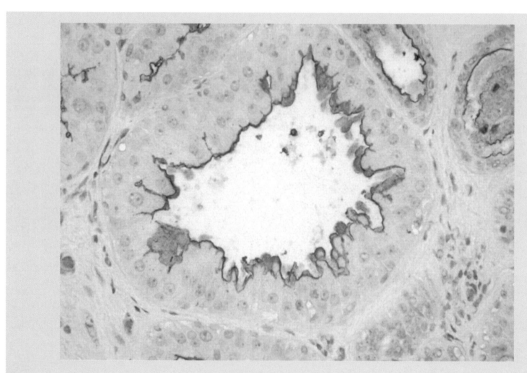

High grade duct carcinoma in situ.

Paper 9

Case for conservative management of selected fibroadenomas of the breast

Authors

Cant PJ, Madden MV, Close PM, Learmonth GM, Hacking EA, Dent DM

Reference

British Journal of Surgery 1987; **74**:857–859

Summary

This paper argued that the increasing sensitivity of fine-needle aspiration and ultrasonography allowed a preoperative diagnosis of fibroadenoma with a high degree of confidence. The risks of missing a cancer when a diagnosis of fibroadenoma had been made were calculated to be 1 in 3313 for ages 20–24, and 1 in 229 for ages 25–29. The authors thus recommended only triple assessment in patients up to the age of 25 years.

Related references **(1)** Wilkinson S, Anderson TJ, Rifkind E, Chetty U, Forrest APM. Fibroadenoma of the breast: a follow up of conservative management. *British Journal of Surgery* 1989; **76**:390–391.

(2) Morrow M, Wong S, Venta L. The evaluation of breast masses in women younger than forty years of age. *Surgery* 1998; **124**:634–640.

(3) Hindle WH, Alonzo LJ. Conservative management of breast fibroadenomas. *American Journal of Obstetrics and Gynecology* 1991; **164**:1647–1650.

Key message

Non-surgical management of fibroadenomas is reasonable in younger patients.

Why it's important

This paper brought together the modern diagnostic method of triple assessment and argued that it was no longer necessary to perform diagnostic excision biopsies in young patients for this benign lesion. The authors showed the rarity of cancer formation in young patients, and thus that it was not necessary to remove fibroadenomas 'just in case'. The non-operative management of fibroadenoma is now standard, with core biopsy replacing fine-needle aspiration in many centres.

Strengths

1. This paper crystallized the concept of non-operative management of benign lesions in the way that Patey did for cysts.
2. It gave clear and quantifiable figures for the risk of missing cancer.

Weaknesses

1. The risk calculations were based on cancer occurrence on follow-up (which is liable to bias due to patients lost to follow-up).
2. The index lesions were not confirmed histologically to be fibroadenomas.

Relevance

It has led to the acceptance of the concept of non-operative management for fibroadenoma, which is now standard practice.

CHAPTER 10

Surgical treatment

J MICHAEL DIXON

Introduction

In the 17th and 18th centuries, breast cancer was considered to occur as a result of stagnation or coagulation of one of the bodily humours. Bloodletting was believed to drain off these excessive humours and restore the proper balance. Initially, all breast lumps were treated in a similar manner, but in 1829 Astley Cooper (Paper 1) identified that they could be either benign or malignant, and he was the first to differentiate cysts from breast cancer, although it was over 50 years later that the first comprehensive description of breast cysts occurred. After Cooper's description, cysts were treated by surgical excision, but Cooper demonstrated that they could be treated successfully by simple drainage. In the early 19th century, a number of physicians began to favour a more aggressive surgical approach, and surgery was initially performed without the benefits of anaesthesia. In the second half of the 19th century, the ancient practice of surgery began to offer new hope derived from two revolutionary innovations: the introduction of anaesthesia and the adoption of antiseptic principles.

By the last decades of the 19th century, the radical mastectomy developed by William Halsted at Johns Hopkins University became the standard procedure for breast cancer (Paper 2). Halsted and his fellows routinely removed the entire breast, lymph nodes and pectoralis major muscle with its connecting ligaments and tendons. Retrospective studies suggested that patients undergoing a Halsted radical mastectomy had a significantly better survival than those who underwent a less radical operation. Halsted's radical mastectomy prevailed as the standard procedure for the next 50 years, but by the middle of the 20th century, it was gradually replaced by the modified radical mastectomy proposed by Patey and colleagues (Paper 3). This operation removes all the breast and axillary nodes but leaves the underlying pectoralis major muscle intact. There are some who believed that the problems with radical mastectomy was that it was not radical enough, and the supraradical mastectomy was developed, which extended the radical mastectomy to include removal of the internal mammary nodes. A trial of radical mastectomy versus supraradical mastectomy reported by Labour and colleagues (Paper 4) showed no advantage for the supraradical mastectomy over a standard radical mastectomy. Radical mastectomy was later formally compared with the less radical standard mastectomy with or without chest wall irradiation by Fisher and colleagues (Paper 6). In this study, there was no significant difference in outcome between any of the treatments. In the early 1970s, it became clear that certain cancers had poor outcomes when treated by local radical surgery alone, and Haagensen (Paper 5) identified a series of clinical characteristics that now define locally advanced breast cancer and that are associated with a high rate of local recurrence after mastectomy alone.

Having failed to demonstrate a significant survival advantage for more radical operations, the next question was whether patients with breast cancer did in fact need a mastectomy. The first study comparing a breast conservation procedure with mastectomy was performed by Veronesi and colleagues in Milan (Paper 7). Patients with small operable breast cancers were randomized to either a radical mastectomy alone or an extensive local resection known as quadrantectomy combined with axillary dissection and radiotherapy to the whole breast. In this study, breast conserving treatment produced equivalent local control and survival rates to mastectomy. This was subsequently confirmed in an NSABP (National Surgical Adjuvant Breast Project) study reported by Fisher and colleagues (Paper 8) comparing segmental mastectomy with or without radiation and total mastectomy for localized breast cancer. The NASABP did demonstrate the need for postoperative radiotherapy after segmental excision.

The axillary nodes are the most common metastatic site for breast cancer. In recent years, there has been interest in how the axilla in breast cancer should be managed. Veronesi and colleagues (Paper 9) demonstrated that axillary spread occurs in a stepwise manner, with the majority of patients who have axillary node involvement having lower axillary nodes involved first. In 1994, Guiliano and colleagues (Paper 10) showed that it was possible to identify the first node or sentinel node draining a breast cancer using a blue dye. Following these initial studies, combining blue dye and radioisotope techniques, sentinel nodes can be identified in over 95% of patients, and ongoing trials are evaluating this approach further.

As well as differentiating cysts, Astley Cooper carefully demonstrated the anatomy of the breast tree and identified 12–15 major ducts that emptied onto the surface of the nipple. These ducts are affected by the conditions of periductal mastitis and duct ectasia. Periductal mastitis is a disease mainly of smokers, and although the lesions of periductal mastitis were initially considered sterile, Bundred and colleagues (Paper 12) demonstrated that inflammatory lesions around the nipple harbour a mixture of both aerobic and anaerobic organisms. Mammary duct fistula is a complication of periductal mastitis, and Atkins (Paper 11) noted that it had much in common with fistula *in ano*. Atkins demonstrated that a mammary duct fistula can be treated successfully by opening the fistula, which cured the problem and stopped the troublesome purulent discharge, which if left untreated can last for many years.

Paper I

Diseases of the Breast, Part 1

Author

Cooper AP

Reference

Diseases of the Breast, Part 1. Longmans: London, 1829

Summary

Cooper described a series of patients with what he called 'hydatid disease of the breast'. He described four types of these swellings, three of which he considered benign. The first type of hydatid is what we now recognize as a simple cyst lined by flat epithelium. The second type was an apocrine cyst, the third was a cluster of cysts and the fourth type of hydatid he describes as a vascular and malignant cystic lesion. Cooper describes patients who he treated with different types of cysts and their outcomes. He quite clearly distinguishes benign cysts from intracystic cancers.

Related references	(1)	Reclus P. La maladie kystique des mammelles. *Revue de Chirurgie* 1883; **3**:761–776.
	(2)	Brissaud E. Anatomie pathologique de la maladie kystique des mammelles. *Archives de Physiologie Normale et Pathologique* 1884; **3**:98–113.
	(3)	Dixon JM. Cystic disease and fibroadenoma of the breast: natural history and relation to breast cancer risk. In: *Breast Cancer – New Approaches* (Stewart HJ, Anderson TJ, Forrest AP, eds). Edinburgh: Churchill Livingstone, 1991: 258–271.

Key message

Cooper describes breast cysts and was the first to separate these lesions from breast cancer.

Why it's important

Fifty years before the first comprehensive clinical and pathological description of cystic disease, Astley Cooper recognized that cysts were independent new formations which were unrelated to breast cancer.

Strengths

1. From looking at pathology specimens and describing each patient, Cooper managed in detail to describe four categories of breast cysts.
2. Although Cooper noted that cysts and cancers could co-exist, careful observation of mastectomy specimens convinced him that these were separate entities.

Weakness

His observations were based on relatively few patients.

Relevance

Cysts are benign conditions and are totally separate from breast cancer. They are now recognized to be aberrations of normal breast involution rather than a neoplastic condition. Cooper was the first to recognize that cysts and cancers are separate conditions.

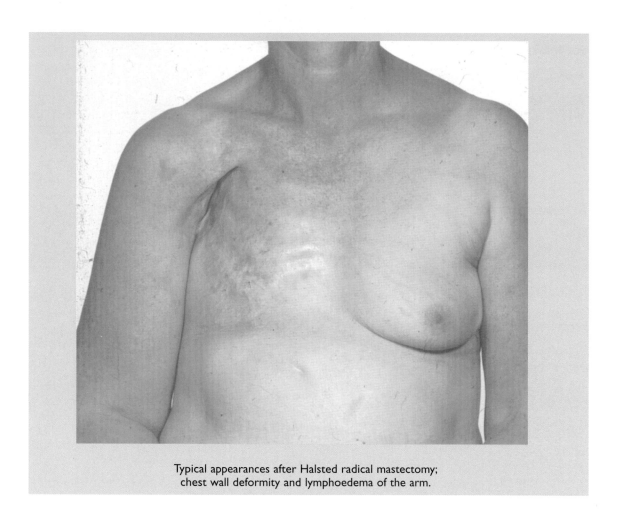

Typical appearances after Halsted radical mastectomy;
chest wall deformity and lymphoedema of the arm.

Paper 2

The results of operations for the cure of cancer of the breast performed at the Johns Hopkins hospital from June 1889 to January 1894

Author

Halsted WS

Reference

Annals of Surgery 1894; **20**:497–556

Summary

This paper describes 50 patients undergoing a Halsted radical mastectomy and at the time of publication the author reported only three local recurrences. Halsted describes his method of mastectomy widely excising skin, subcutaneous fat and the pectoralis major muscle. The pectoralis minor muscle was divided and all the lymphatics and vessels below the subclavian vein to the apex of the axilla were removed including division of the subscapular vessel. The wound was then primarily closed without drains.

Related references

(1) Meyer W. An improved method of the radical operation for carcinoma of the breast. *Medical Record* 1894; **46**:746.

(2) Banks WM. A plea for the more free removal of cancerous growths. *Liverpool and Manchester, Medical and Surgical Report* 1878; **5**:192.

(3) Winniwarter AV. *Beitrage zur Statistik der Carcinome.* Stuttgart: Breitkoff and Hartel, 1876.

Key message

Halsted proposed that breast cancer spreads in an orderly manner, firstly to regional lymph nodes and then systemically. By excising the breast and underlying muscles and the regional lymph nodes he argued that patients with breast cancer could be cured.

Why it's important

Until the middle of the 19th century women who developed breast carcinoma were doomed to an early death and many presented with local ulceration of disease. Halsted's publication demonstrated that radical surgical excision produced good long-term disease control. The strength of the paper was that for a publication at that time this was a large series of patients undergoing a standard operation which included follow-up data. The paper carefully reports details of each individual patient. It also presents the results of the same operation performed by Von Bergman, Bilroth, Czerny, Fisher, Gussenbauer, König, Küster, Lücke and Volkmann.

Strength

A consecutive series of patients were treated with a standard operation with follow-up data being available for the majority of patients.

Weaknesses

Data on local recurrence from Halsted's series and those of other series are not actuarial and no details of length of follow-up are provided. The Halstedian theory of breast cancer spread has now been shown to be incorrect, with many breast cancers having spread systemically at the time of diagnosis.

Relevance

This is one of the first papers to focus attention on the surgical aspects of the treatment of breast cancer. Although it subsequently became clear that radical mastectomy alone did not cure many patients, it demonstrated that mastectomy was a good operation for maintaining local control.

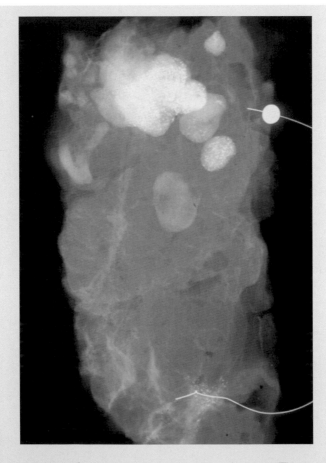

X-ray of a breast specimen after wide excision and axillary dissection. The tip of the hook wire is in a small area of microcalcifications (DCIS with microinvasion). Note however the extensive microcalcifications in the axillary lymphnodes. Histology revealed DCIS-like appearances in the lymphatic tissue suggesting the hypothesis that DCIS might not always be an in-situ lesion.

Paper 3

The prognosis of carcinoma of the breast in relation to the type of operation performed

Authors

Patey DH, Dyson WH

Reference

British Journal of Cancer 1948; **2**:7–13

Summary

This paper presents results of different combinations of surgery and radiotherapy treatment for carcinoma of the breast based on a personal series of 118 cases treated between 1930 and 1943 and followed up to the end of 1946. The authors concluded that a modified radical operation in which the pectoralis major was preserved produces results that are as good as a standard radical mastectomy. Patey and Dyson reported that partial mastectomy combined with axillary dissection was justifiable in occasional early cases with small cancers and that simple mastectomy combined with irradiation to the axilla gave as satisfactory results as a modified radical mastectomy, but they noted that irradiation was generally more upsetting to the patient than surgical dissection of the axilla.

Related references (1)   McWhirter R. Radiotherapy. *Lancet* 1947; **ii**:873.
(2)   Handley RS, Thackray AC. Invasion of the internal mammary lymph glands in carcinoma of the breast. *British Journal of Cancer* 1947; **1**:15.
(3)   Keynes G. Section of Surgery: summary of proceedings. *British Medical Journal* 1938; **ii**:302.

Key message

Removal of the pectoralis major muscle during mastectomy is not required to produce satisfactory rates of local control.

Why it's important

Until Patey's publication in 1948 it was routine practice in most units to perform a Halsted radical mastectomy for breast cancer. Patey was one of the first surgeons to suggest that removal of the pectoralis major was not necessary to perform an adequate dissection of the axilla. He reported that 'with elevation of the arm, retraction of the pectoralis major and removal of the pectoralis minor muscle it is easy to do a complete clearance of the axillary glands and fatty tissue right to the apex of the axilla and at the same time preserve the lateral pectoral nerve, the main nerve supply to the pectoralis major.' Furthermore he was one of the first surgeons to suggest that partial mastectomy combined with axillary dissection had a role in the treatment of at least some patients with breast cancer. Within this publication he also reported a series of patients treated by simple mastectomy and irradiation to the axilla. This publication represented a move away from the more radical surgery proposed by Halsted and Haagensen and the modified radical mastectomy described by Patey remains in common use today.

Strengths

1. Patey compared the results he obtained with his modified radical mastectomy with a series of patients treated by standard Halsted mastectomy.
2. Follow-up data was included in the publication although this did vary from 3 to 13 years.

Weakness

The series was small, with only 45 standard radical operations and 46 modified radical mastectomies. Data were only given on 3-year survival, which nowadays would be considered very short term follow-up. There was no statistical analysis.

Relevance

The Patey mastectomy remains in standard use today for patients with invasive breast cancer and it produces excellent long-term local control rates.

Paper 4

Radical mastectomy versus radical mastectomy plus internal mammary dissection: five year results of an international co-operative study

Authors

Lacour J, Bucalossi P, Cacers E, *et al.*

Reference

Cancer 1976; **37**:206–214

Summary

From 1963 to 1968 an international group collected 1580 cases of breast cancer, randomized into two therapeutic groups: radical mastectomy and extended mastectomy. No significant difference was observed between the two groups in the overall 5-year survival rate. However, a more detailed analysis, according to certain prognostic features, showed that extended mastectomy improved the results in one subgroup: cancers of inner or medial quadrants, axillary node-positive. Within this group the difference was highly significant for a smaller subgroup (190 patients) including only T1 and T2 tumours. It was concluded that there is no indication for extended mastectomy in any cancers of the outer quadrants or in those of the inner or medial quadrants without axillary involvement, although a limited indication for extended mastectomy may be provisionally retained for T1 and T2 cancers of the inner or medial quadrants with axillary involvement.

Related references (1)	Handley RS, Thackray AC. Invasion of internal mammary lymph nodes in carcinoma of the breast. *British Medical Journal* 1954; **i**:61–63.
(2)	Veronesi U, Valagussa P. Inefficacy of internal mammary nodes dissection in breast cancer surgery. *Cancer* 1981; **47**:1750–1753.
(3)	Urban JA, Marjani MA. Significance of internal mammary lymph node metastases in breast cancer. *American Journal of Roentgenology, Radium Therapy and Nuclear Medicine* 1971; **3**:130–136.

Key message

Extending breast surgery to include dissection of the internal mammary nodes does not improve overall survival.

Why it's important

The internal mammary nodes are involved in up to a quarter of patients with tumours in the medial and central part of the breast. These nodes are not traditionally removed during mastectomy. In the late 1950s and early 1960s there was a view that extending radical mastectomy to include internal mammary node dissection would improve survival and local disease control. This study showed that removing the internal mammary nodes in patients with breast cancer does not affect overall survival. It is one of the first papers demonstrating that supraradical breast cancer surgery does not improve survival.

Strength

This was a large international co-operative randomized study which included 737 patients with 15-year follow-up.

Weakness

In relation to the cancers seen today, the cancers were larger and more likely to be node-positive.

Relevance

This study showed that the initial optimistic results from small personal series which suggested an improvement in survival of patients undergoing extended radical mastectomy was misplaced and that extended radical mastectomy has no role in the management of patients with breast cancer.

Paper 5

Clinical classification of the stage of advancement of breast carcinoma

Author

Haagensen CD

Reference

In: *Diseases of the Breast* (Haagensen LD, ed.). Philadelphia: WB Saunders, 1981: 852–863

Summary

Haagensen describes a group of clinical characteristics associated with a high rate of local recurrence after radical mastectomy. This was the first study to identify a group of patients with what is now known as locally advanced breast cancer. The signs he identified were oedema of the skin overlying the breast, satellite nodules in the skin overlying the breast, inflammatory type of carcinoma, ulceration of the skin and direct involvement of the overlying skin or chest wall. In 75 patients with limited oedema of the skin the cure rate was only half that achieved in this overall series but for the 24 patients with oedema and satellite nodules or inflammatory skin changes none were cured. Similar poor outcomes were seen with the other signs of local advancement.

Related references (1) Fisher B, Montague E, Redmond C, *et al.* Comparison of radical mastectomy with alternative treatments for primary breast carcinoma. *Cancer* 1977; **39**:2827–2839.

(2) Handley RS, Thackray AC. Invasion of internal mammary lymph glands in carcinoma of the breast. *British Journal of Cancer* 1947; **1**:15.

(3) Warren JC. The operative treatment of cancer of the breast. *Annals of Surgery* 1904; **40**:805.

Key message

Patients with breast cancer having certain local signs had a high rate of local recurrence and poor overall survival rate if treated by mastectomy alone. Haagensen defined this group of local features (oedema of the skin, satellite nodules in the skin, inflammatory type carcinoma, ulceration of the skin and direct involvement of the skin or chest wall) as indicating inoperability.

Why it's important

This is the first paper to identify a group of patients whose initial treatment should not be surgical but who are best treated by radiotherapy or initial systemic therapy.

Strengths

1. Patients were carefully classified on the basis of clinical signs.
2. Five-year local recurrence and clinical cure data were provided.

Weakness

This was a personal series with data from only one institute.

Relevance

Haagensen's definition of locally advanced breast cancer remains in use today and the patients identified by Haagensen as inoperable are now managed by primary systemic therapy or radiotherapy.

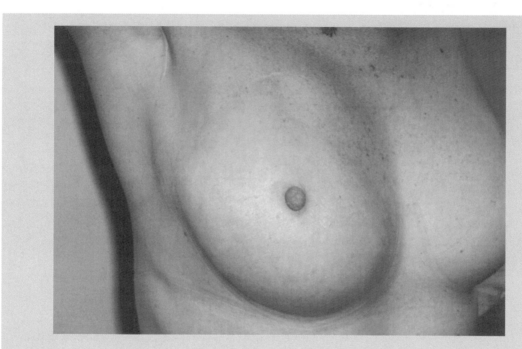

Good cosmetic appearances after modern conservative surgery and radiotherapy of the breast.

Paper 6

Comparison of radical mastectomy with alternative treatments for primary breast carcinoma

Authors

Fisher B, Montague E, Redmond C, *et al.*

Reference

Cancer 1977; **39**:2827–2839

Summary

This was a large randomized trial comparing different treatments for breast cancer and it showed no difference in survival between radical mastectomy and total mastectomy and postoperative irradiation in node-positive patients; in node-negative patients there was no difference in survival between radical mastectomy, total mastectomy with postoperative irradiation or total mastectomy followed by axillary dissection in those patients who developed clinically positive nodes. The fact that leaving nodes behind did not appear to have an adverse effect on overall survival indicates that lymph node metastases are a marker of the presence of distant metastases rather than a prerequisite and that there is not an orderly pattern of spread from primary tumour to regional nodes and then more widespread dissemination.

Related references (1)	Handley RS, The technic and results of conservative radical mastectomy (Patey's operation). *Progress in Clinical Cancer* 1965; **1**:462–470.
(2)	Fisher B, Slack NH, Cavanaugh PJ, Gardner B, Ravdin RG. Postoperative radiotherapy in the treatment of breast cancer: results of the NSABP clinical trial. *Annals of Surgery* 1970; **172**:711–732.
(3)	McWhirter R. Radiotherapy. *Lancet* 1947; **ii**:873.
(4)	Haybittle JL, Brinkley D, Houghton J *et al.*, Postoperative radiotherapy and late mortality: evidence from the Cancer Research Campaign trial for early breast cancer. *British Medical Journal* 1989; **298**: 1611–1614.

Key message

Local disease management does not appear to influence overall survival. A new theory of breast cancer spread emerged from this study which indicated that many patients already have metastatic disease at the time of initial presentation and that axillary nodal involvement is a marker of the presence of systemic disease but it is not a prerequisite for its development.

Why it's important

This was one of the first papers to show that local and regional treatments have little effect on overall survival. It started to question whether a complete axillary dissection is necessary for all patients with breast cancer.

Strengths

1. This was one of the first large randomized studies in breast cancer and involved 1665 women.
2. It was a multicentre study and presented 5-year follow-up data although the average follow-up at the time of publication was only 36 months.

Weakness

A number of the patients randomized in the clinically negative axillary node group randomized for treatment by mastectomy alone had some form of axillary dissection and these patients had a much lower rate of subsequent axillary recurrence than those patients who had no axillary nodes removed. This is not made very clear in this or subsequent publications.

Relevance

This was the first study to suggest involved axillary lymph nodes are a manifestation of tumour spread rather than a predecessor of systemic metastases. It showed that for many patients with breast cancer the Halstedian theory of the orderly spread of breast cancer is incorrect.

Paper 7

Comparing radical mastectomy with quadrantectomy, axillary dissection, and radiotherapy in patients with small cancers of the breast

Authors

Veronesi U, Saccozzi R, Del Vecchio M, *et al.*

Reference

New England Journal of Medicine 1981; **305**:6–11

Summary

From 1973 to 1980 a controlled study was carried out at the National Cancer Institute in Milan to consider the value of a conservative procedure in patients with breast cancer of small size. The authors randomized 701 patients with breast cancer measuring less than 2 cm in diameter and with no palpable axillary lymph nodes to Halsted radical mastectomy (349 patients) or to 'quadrantectomy' with axillary dissection and radiotherapy to the ipsilateral residual breast tissue (352 patients). The two groups were comparable in age distribution, size and site of primary tumour, menopausal status and frequency of axillary metastases. There were three local recurrences in the Halsted group and one in the quadrantectomy group. Actuarial curves showed no difference between the two groups in disease-free or overall survival. From these results, mastectomy appears to involve unnecessary mutilation in patients with breast cancer of less than 2 cm and no palpable axillary nodes.

Related references (1) Fisher B, Montague E, Redmond C, *et al.* Comparison of radical mastectomy with alternative treatments for primary breast carcinoma. *Cancer* 1977; **39**:2827–2839 (Paper 6 in this chapter).

(2) Fisher B, Bauer M, Margoleese R, *et al.* Five-year results of a randomized clinical trial comparing total mastectomy and segmental mastectomy with or without radiation in the treatment of breast cancer. *New England Journal of Medicine* 1985; **312**:665–673 (Paper 8 in this chapter).

(3) Keynes G. The treatment of primary carcinoma of the breast with radium. *Acta Radiologica* 1929; **10**:393–402.

(4) Atkins H, Hayward JL, Klyman DJ, Wayte AB. Treatment of early breast cancer: a report after ten years of a clinical trial. *British Medical Journal* 1972; **ii**:423–429.

Key message

The combination of a wide excision and radiotherapy produces the same disease-free and overall survival as mastectomy.

Why it's important

Until this paper, mastectomy was the only treatment available for patients with localized or operable breast cancer. Mastectomy is a mutilating procedure which results in significant psychological morbidity. This was the first study to demonstrate that excision of the tumour followed by radiotherapy gave equivalent results to mastectomy.

Strengths

1. This is a large study involving 701 patients.
2. Follow-up data were given to $7\frac{1}{2}$ years.

Weakness

Quadrantectomy removes a large volume of breast tissue. While it may be preferable to mastectomy, it produces a poor cosmetic result in at least 20% of patients. There was no assessment of cosmesis in this study, although a subsequent study from the same group did assess cosmetic outcomes.

Relevance

This was the first randomized study to show that breast conservation treatment (quadrantectomy and breast radiotherapy in this study) produced results equivalent to that of mastectomy.

Paper 8

Five-year results of a randomized clinical trial comparing total mastectomy and segmental mastectomy with or without radiation in the treatment of breast cancer

Authors

Fisher B, Bauer M, Margoleese R, *et al.*

Reference

New England Journal of Medicine 1985; **312**:665–673

Summary

In 1976, Fisher *et al.* began a randomized trial to evaluate breast conservation by a segmental mastectomy in the treatment of stage I and II breast tumours up to 4 cm in size. The operation removed only sufficient tissue to ensure that margins of resected specimens were free of tumour. Women were randomly assigned to total mastectomy, segmental mastectomy alone or segmental mastectomy followed by breast irradiation. All patients had axillary dissections, and patients with positive nodes received chemotherapy. Life-table estimates based on data from 1843 women indicated that treatment by segmental mastectomy, with or without breast irradiation, resulted in disease-free, distant disease-free and overall survival at 5 years that was no worse than after total breast removal. In fact, disease-free survival after segmental mastectomy plus radiation was better than disease-free survival after total mastectomy ($p = 0.04$) and overall survival after segmental mastectomy, with or without radiation, was better than overall survival after total mastectomy ($p = 0.07$ and 0.06, respectively). A total of 92.3% of women treated with radiation remained free of breast tumor at 5 years, as compared with 72.1% of those receiving no radiation ($p < 0.001$). Among patients with positive nodes, 97.9% of women treated with radiation and 63.8% of those receiving no radiation remained tumour-free ($p = 0.001$) although both groups received chemotherapy. Fisher *et al.* concluded that segmental mastectomy, followed by breast irradiation in all patients and adjuvant chemotherapy in women with positive nodes is appropriate therapy for stage I and II breast tumours up to 4 cm in size, provided that margins of resected specimens are free of tumour.

Related references **(1)** Veronesi U, Saccozzi R, Del Vecchio M, *et al.* Comparing radical mastectomy with quadrantectomy, axillary dissection, and radiotherapy in patients with small cancers of the breast. *New England Journal of Medicine* 1981; **305**:6–11 (Paper 7 in this chapter).

(2) Fisher B, Montague E, Redmond C, *et al.* Comparison of radical mastectomy with alternative treatments for primary breast carcinoma:. *Cancer* 1977; **39**:2827–2839 (Paper 6 in this chapter).

(3) Fisher B, Redmond C, Poisson R, *et al.* Eight-year results of a randomized clinical trial comparing total mastectomy and lumpectomy with or without irradiation in the treatment of breast cancer. *New England Journal of Medicine* 1989; **320**:822–828.

(4) Fisher B, Costantino J, Redmond C, *et al.* Lumpectomy compared with lumpectomy and radiation therapy for the treatment of intraductal breast cancer. *New England Journal of Medicine* 1993; **328**: 1581–1586.

Key message

Breast conserving treatment produces identical survival results to mastectomy.

Why it's important

This was the first large randomized trial (1843 women) to compare mastectomy with wide local excision with or without radiotherapy and it showed that survival following wide local excision was equivalent to that of mastectomy. It also showed the need for radiotherapy after breast conserving surgery to limit local recurrence.

Strengths

1. This was a large multicentre randomized study.
2. Five-year follow-up data were given on all patients.
3. Local disease-free, distant disease-free and overall survival were presented for all three groups of patients.
4. This was one of the first publications to discuss the importance of complete excision of both invasive and non-invasive disease.

Weakness

Although all patients undergoing wide local excision were supposed to have a complete excision to enter the study, a number of patients did have disease left at the margins which influenced the rate of local recurrence, particularly in the group having no radiotherapy.

Relevance

This was the first randomized study to show that wide local excision followed by radiotherapy produced local control and survival rates identical to mastectomy. Wide local excision has now become the treatment of choice for small localized breast cancers, largely as a consequence of this important trial.

Paper 9

Extent of metastatic axillary involvement in 1446 cases of breast cancer

Authors

Veronesi U, Luini A, Galimberti V, Marchini S, Sacchini V, Rilke F

Reference

European Journal of Surgical Oncology 1990; **16**:127–133

Summary

In this study, 1446 patients with carcinoma of the breast treated with Halsted mastectomy (167), Patey mastectomy (732) and conservative surgery with axillary dissection, either at the same time (340) or separately (207) were evaluated with regard to the number and distribution of axillary lymph nodes. A total of 29 378 were removed and examined: on average 20.3 per patient. The average number of nodes was 13.5 at the first level, 4.5 at the second and 2.3 at the third. The same number of nodes were removed in patients treated with extensive surgery such as Halsted mastectomy and limited surgery such as lumpectomy and in independent axillary dissection. In 839 cases metastases were found in the axilla. The average number of involved nodes was 6.4. Out of 839 patients, the first level was the site of metastases in 828, the second level in 364 and the third in 187. When a single lymph node was involved, it was nearly always at the first level. In only 11 cases were the second and/or third levels invaded without metastases at the first level. Therefore, the percentage of cases with skipping metastases was very low (1.3%). These results showed that the spread of breast cancer to the axilla follows a regular pattern: the first level is involved first, whilst in most cases, the second and third levels are involved only when the first is substantially affected.

Related references (1)	Berg JW. The significance of axillary node levels in the study of breast carcinoma. *Cancer* 1955; **8**:776–778.
(2)	Veronesi U, Rilke F, Luini A, *et al*. Distribution of axillary node metastases by level of invasion. An analysis of 539 cases. *Cancer* 1987; **59**:682–687.
(3)	Pigott J, Nichols R, Maddox WA, Balch CM. Metastases to the upper levels of the axillary nodes in carcinoma of the breast and its implications for nodal sampling procedures. *Surgical Gynecology and Obstetrics* 1984; **158**:255–259.

Key message

Breast cancer spreads in an orderly manner through the axillary lymph nodes, usually invading level I first with the second and third levels only being involved when the first is substantially affected.

Why it's important

This paper carefully demonstrates the pattern of axillary spread and showed that skip metastases, that is levels II and III of the axilla in the absence of level I, are very rare. It provided clear evidence that either sampling the axilla (usually the lower axilla) or level I dissection can theoretically be used to accurately stage the axilla. It also suggested that the majority of sentinel nodes in the axilla are at level I.

Strength

This is a very large series of patients carefully studied.

Weakness

These patients were collected over a long period of time. Nowadays extensive axillary lymph node involvement is the exception rather than the rule and many patients in this series had larger tumours and more extensive nodal disease than seen in current clinical practice.

Relevance

By demonstrating the orderly spread of disease within the axilla, this study provided a scientific basis for axillary staging procedures including sentinel node biopsy.

Paper 10

Lymphatic mapping and sentinel lymphadenectomy for breast cancer

Authors

Giuliano AE, Kirgan DM, Guenther JM, Morton DL

Reference

Annals of Surgery 1994; **220**:391–401

Summary

The sentinel lymph node is defined as the first node in the regional lymphatic basin which recovers lymph from the primary tumour. Using a supravital blue dye the authors were able to identify intra-operatively the sentinel lymph node draining a breast cancer and were able to show that this reflected axillary node status in the majority of patients.

Related references (1)	Morton D, Wen D, Cochran A. Management of the early-stage melanoma by intra-operative lymphatic mapping and selective lymphadenectomy: an alternative to routine elective lymphadenectomy or 'watch and wait'. *Surgical Oncology Clinics of North America* 1992; **1**:247–259.
(2)	Cabanas RM. Lymph node metastases: indicators, not governors of survival. *Archives of Surgery* 1977; **119**:1067–1072.
(3)	Krag DN, Asikaga T, Harlow SP, Weaver DL. Development of sentinel node targeting technique in breast cancer patients. *Breast* 1998; **4**:67–74.

Key message

It is possible to identify intra-operatively sentinel nodes in patients with breast cancer and these sentinel nodes accurately predict whether other nodes in the axilla are involved by cancer.

Why it's important

This study showed that the sentinel node concept was clinically relevant in breast cancer. It demonstrated that intraoperative lymphatic mapping can identify accurately the sentinel node in a high percentage of patients and that the sentinel node is the node most likely to contain breast cancer metastases.

Strengths

1. This is a consecutive series of 174 patients.
2. All patients studied by this technique were included, even those who had disease which would now not be considered suitable for sentinel lymph node mapping because of lymphatic obstruction by metastatic tumour.

Weakness

Patients were included in the study with large tumours and clinically involved axillary lymph nodes which are known to be associated with a lower rate of sentinel lymph node detection and from first principles it could have been deduced that the technique would not work in these patients. Only axillary nodes can be identified with blue dye, which is a problem as in up to 8% of patients the sentinel node is in the internal mammary chain.

Relevance

Sentinel lymph node biopsy for breast cancer using supravital dye and radioactive tracer is currently being evaluated in clinical trials and is likely to become the method of choice for staging the axilla of patients with small breast cancers.

Paper 11

Mammillary fistula

Author

Atkins HJB

Reference

British Medical Journal 1955; **ii**:1473–1474

Summary

Atkins describes a series of 28 patients with what was termed 'mammillary fistula' (now known as mammary duct fistula). Their treatment was on the lines of that practised for fistula *in ano*, by laying open of the fistula, with excellent results. The procedure described involves placing a probe along the line of the fistula tract and opening down on to the probe. After using this technique, Atkins reported no recurrences.

Related references (1)   Zuska JJ, Crile G Jr, Ayres WW. Fistulas of lactiferous ducts. *American Journal of Surgery* 1951; **81**:312.

(2)   Kilgore AR, Fleming R. *California Medicine* 1952; **77**:190.

(3)   Dixon JM, Thompson AM. Effective surgical treatment for mammillary fistula. *British Journal of Surgery* 1991; **78**:1185–1186.

Key message

These fistulae which are responsible for recurrent periareolar sepsis can be cured by appropriate surgery.

Why it's important

Until the description by Atkins of laying open of fistulae, patients developed frequent recurrent infections, with a number of patients requiring mastectomy.

Strengths

1. Mammary duct fistula is rare and 28 cases is a reasonably large number.
2. The operation is well described and easy to perform.

Weaknesses

1. Credit for recognizing the true nature of these fistulae must go to Zuska, Crile and Ayres (related reference 1). It is not clear from the paper whether this was Atkins own method of treatment or whether Kilgore and Fleming (related reference 2) gave him the initial idea of how to treat mammary duct fistula.

2. The operation produces an ugly scar across the nipple. Excision of the fistula through a more cosmetically placed incision is now standard practice.

Relevance

Until recently, laying open of the fistula was the treatment of choice for mammary duct fistula secondary to periductual mastitis. As mammary duct fistula can cause recurrent episodes of infection, the procedure described by Atkins has cured many women over many years and significantly improved their quality of life.

Paper 12

Are the lesions of duct ectasia sterile?

Authors

Bundred NJ, Dixon JMJ, Lumsden AB, *et al.*

Reference

British Journal of Surgery 1985; **2**:844–845

Summary

This paper demonstrated the presence of bacteria in periareolar inflammatory conditions. Using special transport media, *Staphylococcus aureus* and a variety of anaerobic organisms were isolated from the majority of the lesions which we now refer to as periductal mastitis (for more up-to-date discussion of terminology, see related reference 4).

Related references (1)   Walker JC, Sandison AT. Mammary duct ectasia. *British Journal of Surgery* 1964; **51**:350–355.

(2)   Sandison AT, Walker JC. Inflammatory mastitis, mammary duct ectasia and mammillary fistula. *British Journal of Surgery* 1963; **50**:57–64.

(3)   Pearson HE. Bacteroides in areolar breast abscesses. *Surgery Gynecology and Obstetrics* 1967; **125**:800–802.

(4)   Dixon JM. In: *Breast Infection. ABC of Breast Diseases*, 2nd edn. London: BMJ Publishing Group, 2000: 21–25.

Key message

The lesions of what we now call periductal mastitis – it was called at the time of this publication duct ectasia – are not sterile but contain both aerobic and anaerobic organisms.

Why it's important

Prior to this study the lesions of recurrent periareolar infection secondary to what is now known as periductal mastitis were thought to be sterile. Using special transport media both aerobic and anaerobic bacteria were identified from a high proportion of patients. Antibiotics covering both the aerobic and anaerobic bacteria identified in this study are now used as a routine part of the treatment of this condition.

Strength

This was a large series of patients with a relatively rare condition.

Weakness

There were problems with terminology and there was until recently confusion as to what constituted periductal mastitis and what constituted duct ectasia.

Relevance

By identifying the range of organisms present in periductal mastitis, it is possible to identify which antibiotics are likely to be effective in this condition. Patients with periductal mastitis can now be effectively treated with antibiotics which cover the range of organisms first identified in these lesions by Bundred *et al.*

CHAPTER 11

Radiotherapy

JAY R HARRIS

Introduction

The use of radiotherapy has evolved slowly but substantially over the last 100 years. In November 1895, Roentgen developed a cathode tube capable of producing ionizing radiation and discovered 'X-rays'. It is remarkable that Emil Grubbe treated the first person for breast cancer using X-rays in January 1896. In 1898, the Curies discovered radium, a radioactive substance, thus establishing the other major source of ionizing radiation. The use of radiotherapy has evolved in an intertwined manner along technical and conceptual lines over the last 100 years.

Low-energy treatment machines (100–250 kV) with high skin doses and poor penetration into tissues limited the initial uses of radiotherapy. Over time:

- the energy of machines has been improved (4–10 mV), providing 'skin-sparing' and more homogeneous dosage;
- the dosage of irradiation has become standardized, initially measured in 'erythema doses', then the rad, and now the gray (Gy or cGy);
- methods of precise simulation and treatment planning have been developed, and, more recently, computed tomography (CT)-based three-dimensional treatment planning and intensity-modulated radiotherapy have been introduced.

Radiotherapy has been used as primary local treatment after breast conserving surgery in an effort to improve quality of life and as primary local-regional treatment after mastectomy in an effort to improve survival. It was only with improved techniques that these primary treatment approaches would prove practical both in efficacy and in minimizing toxicity.

The use of breast conserving treatment for invasive breast cancer is now well established. However, it took many randomized trials and long follow-up for this approach to be widely accepted. Even as recently as 2001, only about half of the patients with early-stage breast cancer in the USA were treated. The strategy in this treatment approach is to remove the bulk of the tumor in the breast surgically and to use moderate doses of radiation to eradicate any residual cancer. Multiple randomized clinical trials, now with large numbers of patients and long follow-up, show equivalent survival following total mastectomy and breast conserving treatment. The effective use of breast conserving treatment requires close cooperation between the surgeon and radiation oncologist, working with pathologists and breast imagers, to achieve appropriately low rates of local-regional recurrence with acceptable cosmetic results.

Current evidence suggests that breast irradiation should be routine following breast-conserving surgery. (It is remarkable that wide resection alone, even with very clear margins, is associated with a high rate of local recurrence.) There are six randomized clinical trials with published results comparing breast conserving surgery with and without radiotherapy in patients with early-stage breast cancer. These trials vary with regard to patient selection, the details of the surgery and radiotherapy, the use of adjuvant systemic therapy, and the length of follow-up. These trials all show a large reduction in the rate of local recurrence, with a crude reduction averaging about 75%. The effect of radiotherapy on survival is considerably more modest. None of the five trials shows a survival benefit for radiotherapy; however, in the 2000 Overview date from Oxford, a small mortality improvement has been seen (unpublished data).

There is recent evidence that post-mastectomy local-regional radiotherapy improves long-term survival. The reports of the Danish trials testing post-mastectomy radiotherapy in breast cancer patients treated with adjuvant systemic therapy are a major contribution to the oncology literature. In these trials, large numbers of patients were randomized, and premenopausal patients received adjuvant chemotherapy and postmenopausal patients adjuvant tamoxifen for 1 year. These reports, corroborated by the report of the smaller British Columbia trial, establish an important principle about the value of establishing local-regional control in the presence of effective systemic therapy. It is important to note that the mortality improvement seen with post-mastectomy radiotherapy is similar in magnitude to that seen with adjuvant systemic therapy.

Without detracting from the importance or validity of the principle, it is legitimate to question the clinical implications of these results for practice in the USA. Of note in all three trials, patients had a higher rate of local and regional recurrences than seen in series from the USA, where a more complete axillary dissection is typically employed. Also, the systemic therapy used in these trials might not have been adequate.

Studies on radiotherapy inevitably deal with the basic understanding of the disease as either a strictly local process (as originally espoused by William Halsted) or a strictly systemic process (as originally espoused by Bernard Fisher). While the former is certainly not true, the latter appears also to be not completely true based on recent results of randomized trials showing a small survival advantage with improved local control. Moreover, the advent of effective systemic therapy mandates a new evaluation of the importance of local-regional therapy. To date, systemic therapy by itself has had a modest ability to improve local tumor control. One can anticipate that the importance of local therapy will be 'parabolic' with increasing effectiveness of systemic therapy. As we see incremental improvements in systemic therapy, it is likely that local therapy will increase in importance. In the long run, however, systemic therapy will become effective locally and systemically, and the role of surgery and radiotherapy will decline.

Paper 1

Statistical study of radiation therapy in eight hundred and one cases of carcinoma of the breast

Authors

Pfahler GE, Widmann BP

Reference

American Journal of Roentgenology 1925; **14**:550–562

Summary

This paper presents a summary of personal experience using orthovoltage radiotherapy from 1900 to 1925 in treating 801 various cases of breast cancer in Philadelphia, USA.

Related references (1)   Finzi NS. X-rays and radium in the treatment of carcinoma of the breast. *British Medical Journal* 1927; **ii**:728–733.

(2)   Lee B. Results of the treatment by radiation of primary inoperable carcinoma of the breast. *Annals of Surgery* 1922; **76**:359–385.

(3)   Soiland A. Cancer problem of the female breast: an analysis based upon 25 years personal experience with radiation therapy. *Acta Radiologica* 1925; **4**:391–396.

Key message

Radiotherapy appeared effective at improving local control after mastectomy.

Why it's important

These early results using primitive equipment inspired further exploration of the approach.

Strength

This was a large experience, carefully documented with regard to survival.

Weakness

It was a retrospective review with incomplete documentation of local control and complications.

Relevance

This was an early demonstration of the ability of radiotherapy to improve local tumor control following surgery, leading to more systemic evaluations of its use and improved methods of irradiation.

Paper 2

Conservative treatment of cancer of the breast

Author

Keynes G

Reference

British Medical Journal 1937; **ii**:643–647

Summary

Radium needle implantation of the breast and axilla was used as an alternative to radical surgery. In this study 250 patents were reported with 3 years of follow-up and 201 with 5 years. In the 85 patients with disease apparently restricted to the breast, the 5-year survival rate was 86%, comparable to that seen with radical surgery. The technique evolved over time, and later in the series, patents first underwent local removal of the tumor. The cosmetic results appeared good, but some patients developed excessive fibrosis and many developed 'neuralgia' in the treated area. (Of historical interest, the procedure was discontinued at the start of World War II because of the danger of bombing in relation to the radium needles and because Professor Keynes became heavily involved in the war effort.)

Key message

Breast conserving therapy (optimally using limited breast surgery) is possible using irradiation.

Why it's important

This article is the first description of the use of irradiation to avoid radical surgery. Since high-energy external beam irradiation was not available, Keynes used radium needles to deliver sufficient doses. The results that he achieved were comparable to those achieved by radical surgery, thus establishing a proof of principle. Keynes intuitively realized the benefit of limited breast surgery prior to irradiation.

Strength

The paper provides a meticulous record of the treatment method in consecutive patients.

Weakness

The follow-up is too short to assess long-term results. Implantation of the entire breast and axilla is technically challenging and could not be instituted as a public health method of treating breast cancer. The comparison with radical mastectomy is retrospective.

Relevance

The techniques and results are not directly relevant to today's treatment, but are of historical significance.

Paper 3

The value of simple mastectomy and radiotherapy in the treatment of cancer of the breast

Author

McWhirter R

Reference

British Journal of Radiology 1948; **21**:599

Summary

A total of 757 patients with operable breast cancer and 389 patients with locally advanced disease were treated with total (or 'simple') mastectomy and radiotherapy to the chest wall and draining lymph node areas. The 5-year actuarial survival rate was 62% for operable cases and 29% for advanced cases. In contrast, radical surgery and postoperative radiotherapy during the preceding time period at the same institution yielded a 50% 5-year survival rate.

Related reference (1)   Kaae S, Johansen H. Does simple mastectomy followed by irradiation offer survival comparable to radical procedures? *International Journal of Radiation Oncology, Biology, Physics* 1977; **2**:1163–1166.

Key message

This article is the first description of combining less than radical surgery with external beam radiotherapy. Previously, radiotherapy was primarily used following radical surgery but in this new approach the axilla was left undissected. There was still uncertainty about the ability of external beam radiotherapy to eradicate disease in the breast, so a simple mastectomy was performed. The survival results achieved using this approach appeared comparable to (or better than) those achieved with radical mastectomy. Of related interest is a Danish study conducted between 1951 and 1957 which compared simple mastectomy followed by irradiation with extended radical mastectomy. No differences in efficacy of either treatment was observed (see related reference 1).

Why it's important

This study extended the use of radiotherapy to treatment of the axilla.

Strength

The paper provides a meticulous follow-up of this treatment method in systematically staged consecutive patients.

Weakness

This is not a randomized comparison with radical surgery and the follow-up was relatively short.

Relevance

The ability of radiotherapy to assure local tumor control with less than radical surgery helped to decrease the use of radical surgery.

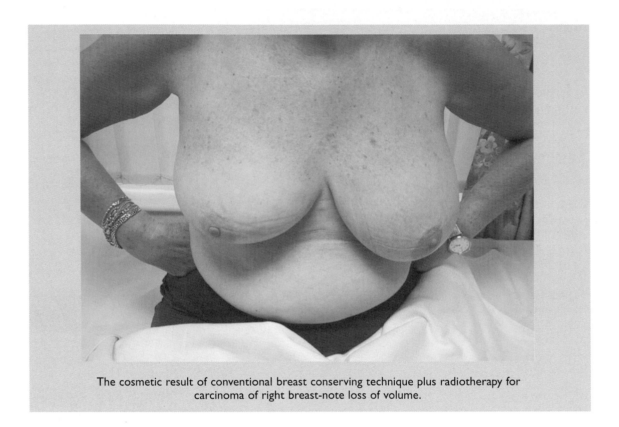

The cosmetic result of conventional breast conserving technique plus radiotherapy for carcinoma of right breast-note loss of volume.

Paper 4

Roentgentherapy alone in the cancer of the breast

Author

Baclesse F

Reference

Acta Universitatis International Cancer 1959; **15**:1023–1026.

Summary

Stage II, III and IV breast cancer patients were treated with 'Roentgenrays' only. In 310 patients radiation was directed systematically to the breast and draining lymph node regions. The crude 5-year relapse-free survival rate was 32% and the 10-year rate was 15%. Treatment failure was primarily due to distant metastasis. Of the 54 patients free of relapse at 5 years, 12 developed distant metastasis and only 5 developed a local recurrence between 5 and 10 years.

Related references (1) Calle R, Pilleron JP, Schlienger P, Vilcoq JR. Conservative management of operable breast cancer: ten years experience at the Foundation Curie. *Cancer* 1978; **42**:2045–2053. [This is a follow-up report from the same institution describing the use of breast conserving therapy in 514 patients with operable cancer treated with magavoltage radiotherapy between 1960 and 1970. In this study 120 patients had lumpectomy and 394 were treated with 'exclusive radiotherapy'.]

(2) Pierquin B. Peut-on traiter les cancers de sein de petite taille par la seule radiotherapie? [Is it possible to treat small size breast cancer with radiotherapy alone?] *Annales de Medicine Interne* 1971; **122**:575–579. [Peirquin popularized the use of interstitial radioactive implantation as part of breast-conserving therapy, primarily with exclusive radiotherapy.]

(3) Amalric R, Santamaria F, Robert F, *et al*. Radiation therapy with or without primary limited surgery for operable breast cancer. A 20-year experience at the Marseilles Cancer Institute. *Cancer* 1982; **49**, 30–34.

Key message

External beam radiotherapy can provide long-term control of cancer in the breast.

Why it's important

Prior to this report, there was uncertainty about the ability of external beam radiotherapy to permanently eradicate cancer in the breast. It was also among the first to describe an effective radiotherapy technique for treating the breast and nodal areas.

Strength

There was meticulous follow-up of this treatment method in consecutive patients.

Weakness

This was a retrospective analysis. Local recurrence may have been underestimated because of the larger competing risk of distant failure in these patients.

Relevance

The experience provided assurance that radiotherapy was effective in treating cancer in the breast and led the ways to its use in breast conserving therapy.

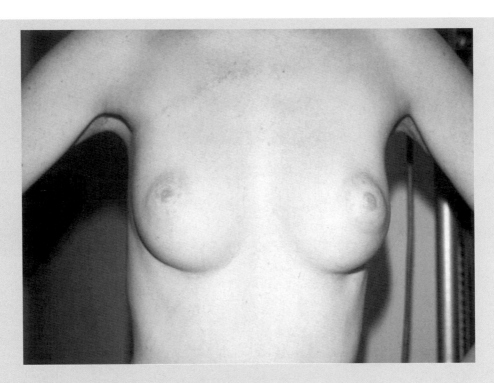

The cosmetic result of breast conserving surgery plus radiotherapy for carcinoma of the right breast- note line of teliangectasia where there has been a slight overlap of radiation fields.

Paper 5

Wedge resection and irradiation: An effective treatment in early breast cancer

Author

Peters MK

Reference

Journal of the American Medical Association 1967; **199**:18–19.

Summary

From 1935 to 1960, 124 clinical stage I and II patients were treated with excisional biopsy and radiotherapy at the Princess Margaret Hospital in Toronto and compared retrospectively to similar patients treated with mastectomy. The results at 5–10 years were similar for the two groups.

Related references **(1)** Nelson AJ, Montague ED. Resectable localized breast cancer: the rationale for combined surgery and irradiation. *Journal of the American Medical Association* 1975; **231**:189–191.

(2) Levene MB, Harris JR, Hellman S. Treatment of carcinoma of the breast by radiation therapy. *Cancer* 1977; **39**:2840–2845.

(3) Mustakallio S. Conservative teatment of breast carcinoma: review of 25 years follow-up. *Clinical Radiology* 1972; **23**:110–116.

Key message

Lumpectomy and radiotherapy is a feasible local treatment of early-stage breast cancer.

Why it's important

This article was among the first to articulate the basis of breast conserving therapy employing limited breast surgery and breast irradiation. This approach became feasible with the development of megavoltage irradiation. In 1967, Peters argued that the outcome in breast cancer patients is determined primarily by 'host influences' and not by the type of local treatment. Also, as a woman, Peters articulated the concept that 'the woman who discovers a lump in her breast would seek medical advice earlier … if she were fortified by the knowledge that she did not need to face an extensive and mutilating operation.' (A historical note is that I first met Dr Peters in the late 1970s and she strongly advocated breast conserving therapy but warned me about its use in young patients with prominent intraductal involvement.)

Strength

This was among the first papers to articulate the concept of combining 'lumpectomy' and moderate-dose radiotherapy and to demonstrate long-term results in selected patients.

Weakness

This was a retrospective study of selected patients. In subsequent papers, Peters attempted to correct for biases by use of a matched pair analysis.

Relevance

The concept of 'lumpectomy' or excisional biopsy is still used today.

Paper 6

Local results of irradiation in the primary management of localized breast cancer

Author

Fletcher G

Reference

Cancer 1972; **29**:545–551

Summary

In this study, 89 pathologically node-positive patients received 4000 rad in 4 weeks with 250 kV irradiation to the supraclavicular fossa and 6 (7%) developed a supraclavicular failure. A further 273 pathologically node-positive patients received 5000 rad in 4 weeks with cesium, cobalt or electron beam irradiation to the supraclavicular fossa and 4 (1.3%) developed a supraclavicular failure. In the absence of irradiation, supraclavicular failure was seen in 20–25% of cases. Similar findings were seen for control in the axilla.

Related references		
(1)	Lenze M. Tissue dosage in roentgentherapy of mammary cancer. *Acta Radiologica* 1947; **18**:583–592.
(2)	Cohen L. Theoretical iso-survival formulae for fractionated radiation therapy. *British Journal of Radiology* 1968; **41**:522–528.
(3)	Fletcher GH. Clinical dose–response curves of human epithelial tumors. *British Journal of Radiology* 1973; **46**:1–12.

Key message

This article established the dose required to eradicate breast cancer in the draining lymph node areas. Fletcher established the concept of 'subclinical disease'. For treatment of 'subclinical disease' in a clinically negative nodal area, 4500–5000 cGy in 4–5 weeks was necessary to provide greater than 90% control. For treatment of palpable nodal disease, much higher doses of irradiation were necessary.

Why it's important

This study provided a basis for nodal treatment in breast cancer using radiotherapy.

Strength

This experience provided a useful guideline for radiation dosage of nodal areas.

Weakness

This was a retrospective analysis of the data. The concept of subclinical disease was initially applied to irradiation of the cancer in the breast, and this turned out to be inappropriate.

Relevance

These guidelines for radiation dose to nodal areas are still in use today.

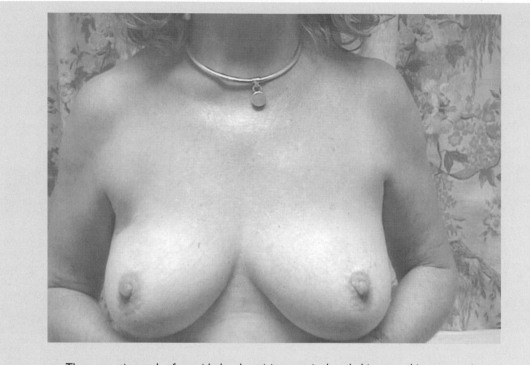

The cosmetic result after wide local excision, sentinel node biopsy and intraoperative radiotherapy for carcinoma of the upper outer quadrant of the right breast.

Paper 7

Ten-year results of a randomized clinical trial comparing radical mastectomy and total mastectomy with or without radiation

Authors

Fisher B, Redmond C, Fisher ER, *et al.*

Reference

New England Journal of Medicine 1985; **312**:674–681

Summary

A total of 1089 eligible patients with clinically node-negative breast cancer were randomized to radical mastectomy or total mastectomy with or without radiotherapy. 17.8% of patients treated with total mastectomy developed an axillary recurrence and underwent delayed axillary dissection. Despite this, the 10-year results showed no statistically significant differences in freedom from distant failure or overall survival among the treatment arms. Local control was similar for radical mastectomy and total mastectomy and radiotherapy. An additional 586 patients with clinically-postive axillary nodes were randomized to radical mastectomy or total mastectomy and radiotherapy and there were no differences in 10-year results between these arms.

Related reference (I)

Fisher B, Redmond C, Fisher ER, *et al.* Findings from NSABP Protocol No. B-04 – comparison of radical mastectomy with alternative treatments for primary breast cancer: a first report of results from a prospective randomized clinical trial. *Cancer* 1977; **39**:2827–2839.

Key message

Variations in local treatment do not result in large differences in long-term survival from breast cancer.

Why it's important

This article demonstrated the limited importance of local therapy and led to the conclusive demise of the radical mastectomy.

Strength

A formal randomized clinical trial simultaneously not only tested different local treatments, but also established an important biological principle.

Weaknesses

1. The trial size was relatively small and slight but clinically significant survival could not be eliminated.
2. Many patients assigned to total mastectomy alone underwent some removal of axillary nodes.

Relevance

This trial conclusively demonstrated that the main site of treatment failure was systemic and not local and that improvements in outcome would require effective systemic therapy.

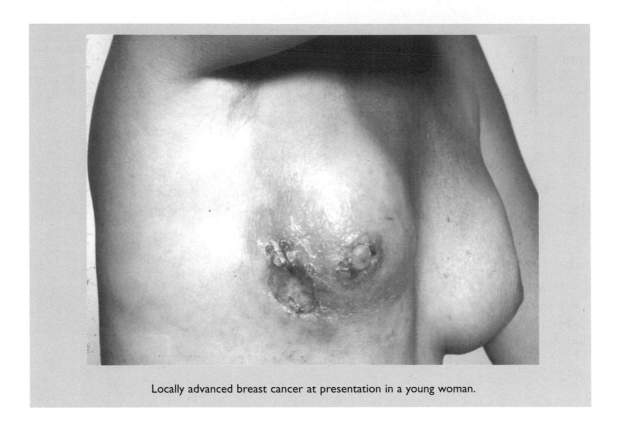

Locally advanced breast cancer at presentation in a young woman.

Papers 8 and 9

8: *Comparing radical mastectomy with quadrantectomy, axillary dissection, and radiotherapy in patients with small cancers of the breast.*

9: *Five-year results of a randomized clinical trial comparing total mastectomy and segmental mastectomy with or without radiation in the treatment of breast cancer*

Authors

8: Veronesi U, Saccozzi R, Del Vecchio M, *et al.*
9: Fisher B, Bauer M, Margolese R, *et al.*

References

8: *New England Journal of Medicine* 1981; **305**:305–306
9: *New England Journal of Medicine* 1985; **312**:665–673

Summary

In the Veronesi study, 701 patients were randomized to a wide resection of the tumor in the breast ('quandrantectomy'), axillary dissection, and radiotherapy or to radical mastectomy. In the Fisher study, 1843 patients were randomized to total mastectomy or a limited resection of the tumor ('lumpectomy') with or without radiotherapy. The 5-year results from both studies showed equivalent survival for patients treated with breast conserving therapy and with mastectomy. In the Fisher study, breast cancer recurrence was seen in 28% of patients without radiotherapy and 8% with radiotherapy.

Related references (1) Veronesi U, Salvadori B, Luini A, *et al.* Breast conservation is a safe method in patients with small cancer of the breast. Long-term results of three randomised trials on 1973 patients. *European Journal of Cancer* 1995; **31A**:1574–1579.

(2) Fisher B, Anderson S, Redmond CK, *et al.* Reanalysis and results after 12 years of follow-up in a randomized clinical trial comparing total mastectomy with lumpectomy with or without irradiation in the treatment of breast cancer. *New England Journal of Medicine* 1995; **333**:1456–1461.

(3) NIH Consensus Development Panel. Consensus Statement: treatment of early-stage breast cancer. *Journal of the National Cancer Institute Monographs* 1992; No. **11**:1–6. [Based on the Milan, NSABP B-06 and other trials, it was concluded that 'breast-conservation treatment is an appropriate method of primary therapy for the majority of women with stage I and II breast cancer and is preferable because it provides survival equivalent to total mastectomy and axillary while preserving the breast'.]

(4) Schnitt SJ, Hayman J, Gelman R, *et al*. A prospective study of conservative surgery alone in the treatment of selected patients with stage I breast cancer. *Cancer* 1996; **77**:1094–1100. [This prospective study demonstrated a substantial rate of breast recurrence, even in a very highly selected group of patients.]

Key message

Breast conserving therapy is equivalent to mastectomy, and breast conserving surgery alone is associated with a high risk of local recurrence.

Why they're important

These studies provided firm evidence supporting breast conserving therapy using radiotherapy.

Strength

These were randomized trials with large numbers of patients.

Weakness

Even these large trials cannot rule out a small survival difference.

Relevance

They led to the widespread use of breast conserving therapy in North America and Europe.

Paper 10

The presence of an extensive intraductal component following a limited excision correlates with prominent residual disease in the remainder of the breast

Authors

Holland R, Connolly J, Gelman R, *et al.*

Reference

Journal of Clinical Oncology 1990; **8**:113–118

Summary

Previous studies of patients with infiltrating ductal breast cancer treated with limited excision and radiotherapy have indicated that the presence of an extensive intraductal component (EIC) in the excision specimen is highly associated with subsequent breast recurrence. The presence or absence of an EIC in the primary tumors of 214 women who underwent mastectomy was related to the likelihood of finding additional foci of cancer in their mastectomy specimens using a correlated pathologic–radiologic mapping technique. Patients with primary tumors that were EIC-positive were significantly more likely to have carcinoma in the remainder of the breast than those with tumours that were EIC-negative. This difference was primarily due to the presence of residual intraductal carcinoma. In particular, 44% of EIC-positive patients had 'prominent' residual intraductal carcinoma compared with only 3% of EIC-negative patients, ($p < 0.00001$). It was concluded that patients whose tumors contain an EIC more frequently have a large subclinical tumor burden in the remainder of the breast compared with patients whose tumors do not contain an EIC.

Related references (1) Holland R, Veling SH, Mravunac M, *et al.* Histologic multifocality of Tis, T1–2 breast carcinomas: implications for clinical trials of breast-conserving treatment. *Cancer* 1985; **56**:979–990. [This prior study detailed the distribution of cancer in the breast in relation to the primary lesions.]

(2) Schnitt SJ, Connolly JL, Khettry U, *et al.* Pathologic findings on re-excision of the primary site in breast cancer patients considered for treatment by primary radiation therapy. *Cancer* 1987; **59**:675–681. [This was a similar pathologic study using re-excision instead of mastectomy specimens.]

(3) Gage I, Schnitt SJ, Nixon AJ, *et al.* Pathologic margin involvement and the risk of recurrence in patients treated with breast-conserving therapy. *Cancer* 1996; **78**:1921–1928. [This clinical study of patients treated with lumpectomy and radiotherapy demonstrated that an EIC is not predictive of breast recurrence when margin status is known.]

Key message

This article demonstrated that the concept of 'subclinical disease' (established for nodal disease by Fletcher) did not apply to the breast. Many patients whose tumors show an EIC will have prominent amounts of residual intraductal involvement in the breast and moderate dose irradiation is unlikely to eradicate it.

Why it's important

This study demonstrated the importance of an EIC in the context of breast conserving therapy and the reason for its importance.

Strength

This was a fastidious and detailed pathologic study by dedicated breast pathologists at separate institutions.

Weakness

The study did not provide a clear-cut and reproducible definition of EIC or identify subgroups of EIC most often associated with extensive involvement.

Relevance

Surgeons are now conscious of the need to achieve clear margins in patients whose tumors show an EIC.

Paper 11

Mortality patterns over 34 years of breast cancer patients in a clinical trial of postoperative radiotherapy

Authors

Jones JM, Ribeiro GG

Reference

Clincal Radiology 1989; **40**:204–208

Summary

Very long-term follow-up was obtained on 1461 patients with operable breast cancer who were treated with radical mastectomy and then randomized between postoperative radiotherapy or to no further treatment between January 1949 and June 1955 in Manchester, UK. Orthovoltage radiotherapy was used and the technique resulted in irradiation of substantial portions of the heart. During the first 15 years of follow-up, there was no difference in survival between the treatment arms. However, after 15 years, there was increased mortality (relative risk = 1.43) for the irradiated group, which was attributable to deaths from cardiovascular disease.

Related references **(1)** Haybittle JL, Brinkley D, Houghton J, *et al.* Postoperative radiotherapy and late mortality: evidence from the Cancer Research Campaign trial for early breast cancer *British Medical Journal* 1989; **298**:1611–1614. [Similar findings were seen in this CRC trial using orthovoltage radiotherapy.]

(2) Rutqvist LE, Lax I, Fornander T, Johansson H. Cardiovascular mortality in a randomized trial of adjuvant radiation therapy versus surgery alone in primary breast cancer. *International Journal of Radiation Oncology, Biology, Physics* 1992: **22**:887–896. [Similar findings were seen in this Stockholm trial and related to the volume and dose of irradiation to the heart.]

(3) Nixon AJ, Manola J, Gelman R, *et al.* No long-term increase in cardiac-related mortality after breast-conserving surgery and radiation therapy using modern techniques. *Journal of Clinical Oncology* 1998; **16**:1374–1379. [In contrast, no increase in cardiovascular deaths were seen in this series using current techniques and megavoltage radiotherapy.]

Key message

There is long-term potential for late cardiac mortality with radiotherapy for breast cancer that inadvertently irradiates the heart.

Why it's important

The potential for late cardiac mortality from breast cancer radiotherapy can offset its benefits in local and systemic control of the breast cancer.

Strength

This article provided very long-term (up to 34 years) follow-up from a carefully performed randomized clinical trial with very few patients lost to follow-up.

Weakness

The technique of radiotherapy used in the trial is no longer used today and its relevance to current practice is uncertain.

Relevance

Techniques of radiotherapy used to treat breast cancer should minimize or exclude cardiac irradiation.

Papers 12 and 13

12: *Postoperative radiotherapy in high-risk premenopausal women with breast cancer who received adjuvant chemotherapy.*

13: *Postoperative radiotherapy in high-risk postmenopausal breast cancer patients given tamoxifen: Danish Breast Cancer Cooperative Group DBCG 82c randomized trial*

Authors

12: Overgaard M, Hansen PS, Overgaard J, *et al.*
13: Overgaard M, Jensen M-B, Overgaard J, *et al.*

References

12: *New England Journal of Medicine* 1997; **337**:949–955
13: *Lancet* 1999; **353**:1641–1648

Summary

In companion trials, 1708 premenopausal patients with stage II or III breast cancer were treated with modified radical mastectomy and eight cycles of CMF chemotherapy and randomized to post-mastectomy radiotherapy or no further treatment (Paper 12) and 1375 postmenopausal patients with stage II or III breast cancer were treated with modified radical mastectomy and 1 year of tamoxifen and randomized to postmastectomy radiotherapy or no further treament (Paper 13). With a median follow-up of about 10 years, both trials showed about a 70% reduction in local recurrence and about a 30% reduction in overall mortality with radiotherapy.

Related reference (1)   Early Breast Cancer Trialists' Collaborative Group. Favourable and unfavourable effects on long-term survival of radiotherapy for early breast cancer: an overview of the randomised trials. *Lancet* 2000; **355**:1757–1770 (Paper 16 in this chapter).

Key message

Postmastectomy radiotherapy when used in conjunction with adjuvant systemic therapy and using techniques that spare the heart not only improves local control, but also impacts on breast cancer and overall mortality.

Why it's important

This study provided firm evidence that improvements in local control can impact on survival.

Strength

Both trials are large and well conducted and have long follow-up.

Weakness

The rate of local recurrence in the absence of radiotherapy was over 30%, considerably higher than seen in most centers in the USA and in other countries in Europe. As a result, the generalizability of the results has been questioned. In addition, the specific systemic therapies used have been criticized for not being ideal.

Relevance

These studies increased the routine use of postmastectomy radiotherapy, particularly in patients with four or more nodes.

features

t year to early a

gout

Paper 14

Five versus more than five years of tamoxifen therapy for breast cancer patients with negative lymph nodes and estrogen receptor-positive tumors

Authors

Fisher B, Dignam J, Bryant J, *et al.*

Reference

Journal of the National Cancer Institute 1996; **88**:1529–1542

Summary

In this trial, node-negative estrogen receptor-positive patients were randomized to 20 mg of tamoxifen per day for 5 years or to a placebo. (There was a secondary randomization to continue or not continue tamoxifen after 5 years.) Overall, the results showed a benefit for tamoxifen that persisted through 10 years of follow-up. In particular, among the 1062 patients treated with conservative surgery and radiotherapy, the 10-year rate of recurrence in the ipsilateral breast was 10.3% for placebo and only 3.4% with tamoxifen.

Related references **(1)** Fisher B, Dignam J, Mamounas HP, *et al.* Sequential methotrexate and fluorouracil for the treatment of node-negative breast cancer patients with estrogen-receptor negative tumors: eight year results from NSAPB B-13 and first report of findings from NSABP B-10 comparing methotrexate and fluorouracil with conventional cyclophosphamide, methotrexate and fluorouracil. *Journal of Clinical Oncology* 1996; **14**:1982–1992. [In the NSABP B-13 trial, node-negative ER-negative patients were randomized to chemotherapy or to a no-treatment control group. Among the 235 patients treated with breast conserving sugery and radiotherapy, the 8-year rate of recurrence in the ipsilateral breast was 13.4% without chemotherapy and 2.6% with chemotherapy.]

(2) Dalberg K, Johansson H, Johansson U, Rutqvist L, for the Stockholm Breast Cancer Study Group. A randomized trial of long term adjuvant tamoxifen plus postoperative radiation therapy versus radiation therapy for patients with early stage breast carcinoma treated with breast-conserving surgery. *Cancer* 1998; **82**:2204–2211. [A similar result was seen in the Stockholm Breast Cancer Study Group among node-negative patients randomized to tamoxifen or to a placebo. Among the 432 patients treated with breast conserving surgery and radiotherapy, the 10-year rate of recurrence in the ipsilateral breast was 12% without tamoxifen and only 3% with tamoxifen.]

Key message

The use of adjuvant tamoxifen (and also adjuvant chemotherapy) results in a large improvement in local tumor control in the breast when combined with radiotherapy.

Why it's important

This trial demonstrated a substantial (albeit fortuitous) radiosensitization with adjuvant tamoxifen. A similar effect is seen with adjuvant chemotherapy. Prior efforts to develop radiation sensitizers had been largely unsuccessful.

Strength

Firm evidence was presented, based on large randomized clinical trials.

Weakness

The article did not clarify whether the timing of systemic therapy and radiotherapy is important in achieving this result.

Relevance

Since adjuvant systemic therapy is now commonly recommended, breast recurrence rates are much lower than during the prior time period when adjuvant systemic therapy was not routinely used.

Paper 15

Lumpectomy and radiation therapy for the treatment of intraductal breast cancer: Findings from the National Surgical Adjuvant Breast and Bowel Project B-17

Authors

Fisher B, Dignam J, Wolmark N, *et al.*

Reference

Journal of Clinical Oncology 1998; **16**:441–452

Summary

A total of 818 patients with localized ductal carcinoma *in situ* (DCIS) were randomized to lumpectomy (with negative margins) or lumpectomy plus breast radiotherapy. With a median follow-up time of 90 months, radiotherapy resulted in a persistent reduction in non-invasive breast recurrences (13.4% to 8.2%) and in invasive breast recurrences (13.4% to 3.9%), with a similar benefit observed in all subsets.

Related references (1) Julien J-P, Bijker N, Fentiman IS, *et al.* Radiotherapy in breast-conserving treatment for ductal carcinoma *in situ*: first results of the EORTC randomized phase III trial 10853. *Lancet* 2000; **355**:528–533.

(2) Fisher B, Dignam J, Wolmark N, *et al.* Tamoxifen in treatment of intraductal breast cancer: National Surgical Adjuvant Breast and Bowel Project B-24 randomized controlled trial. *Lancet* 2000; **353**:1993–1999.

Key message

Radiotherapy is effective following lumpectomy in reducing local recurrence, although the magnitude of the benefit is not as great as seen with radiotherapy for invasive breast cancer.

Why it's important

This study established the benefit of radiotherapy for DCIS.

Strength

This was a large well-conducted randomized clinical trial.

Weaknesses

The mammographic and pathologic evaluation of patients and their specimens was variable and local recurrence rates for lumpectomy were higher than seen in other series. It did not clarify whether some subsets of patients are adequately treated with lumpectomy alone and which require mastectomy.

Relevance

Radiotherapy is generally used following lumpectomy for DCIS, except for small, low-grade lesions that have been widely excised.

Paper 16

Favourable and unfavourable effects on long-term survival of radiotherapy for early breast cancer: An overview of the randomized trials

Authors

Early Breast Cancer Trialists' Collaborative Group

Reference

Lancet 2000; **355**:1757–1770

Summary

A meta-analysis was done of 10-year and 20-year results from 40 unconfounded randomized trials of radiotherapy for early breast cancer with central review of 20 000 individual patients' data on recurrence and cause-specific mortality. Radiotherapy followed various types of surgery (total mastectomy, mastectomy with axillary surgery, and breast conserving surgery), but overall reduced local recurrence by two-thirds (27% vs. 9% at 10 years). In aggregate, radiotherapy was associated with improved breast cancer mortality and increased non-breast cancer mortality (chiefly due to 'vascular' causes). The overall 20-year survival rate slightly favoured radiotherapy (37% vs. 36%). There was improved breast cancer mortality and less non-breast mortality in more recent trials, in larger trials and in trials using systemic therapy compared respectively to older trials, smaller trials and trials not using systemic therapy.

Related references

(1) Whelan TJ, Julian J, Wright J, *et al.* Does locoregional radiation therapy improve survival in breast cancer? A meta-analysis. *Journal of Clinical Oncology* 2000; **18**:1220–1229. [This was a meta-analysis restricted to 63 000 patients receiving adjuvant systemic therapy demonstrating that local recurrence was reduced by 75%, any recurrrence by 31%, and mortality by 17% (confidence interval 6–26%).]

(2) Early Breast Cancer Trialists' Collaborative Group. Updated results presented in Oxford in September 2000. Personal communication. [In a preliminary analysis, the use of radiotherapy was now associated with a small but statistically significant improvement in survival; however, this result needs confirmation.]

Key message

Radiotherapy for breast cancer is highly effective at improving local control and can decrease breast cancer mortality, but it can also increase non-breast cancer mortality.

Why it's important

This article helped to establish that local therapy can have a systemic effect and that breast cancer is not strictly a systemic disease.

Strength

The overview combines the results of all trials involving radiotherapy, both published and unpublished.

Weaknesses

1. This article has the weaknesses attributable to meta-analysis in general: it gives equivalent weight to all studies. Since radiotherapy is a complex procedure, the heterogeneity associated with the various trials is greater than for trials of systemic therapy. This is shown in the large variation in non-breast cancer mortality among the individual trials in the overview.
2. This article can, furthermore, be criticized in analyzing cause-specific mortality, since this endpoint is less reliable than overall mortality and creates problems in analysis because of competing risks.

Relevance

This study resulted in greater use of radiotherapy and encouraged creative technological advances to insure minimal irradiation to the heart.

Paper 17

The role of radiotherapy and tamoxifen in the management of node negative invasive breast cancer < 1.0 cm treated with lumpectomy

Authors

Wolmark N, Dignam J, Margolese R, *et al.*

Reference

Proceedings of the American Society of Clinical Oncology 2000; **19**:70a

Summary

A total of 1009 pathologic node-negative breast cancer patients with tumors measuring 1 cm or less were randomized to radiotherapy, tamoxifen or both combined. With a median follow-up time of 73 months, the annual rate of ipsilateral breast recurrence was 1.17% per year for radiotherapy, 2.44% per year for tamoxifen, and 0.36% for the combination. (Assuming a constant hazard over the first 8 years, this would result in 8-year rates of 9%, 20% and 3% for the arms, respectively.)

Related reference (1)

Fyles A, Mccready D, Manchul L, *et al.* Prelimary results of a randomized study of tamoxifen ± breast radiation in T1/2 N0 disease in women over 50 years of age. *Proceedings of the American Society of Clinical Oncology* 2001; **20**:24a. [This study was designed to determine whether tamoxifen resulted in similar disease-free survival as tamoxifen plus breast irradiation in women over 50 with T1 and T2 node-negative breast cancer.]

Key message

Tamoxifen is not as effective as radiotherapy in preventing local recurrence in the breast and, as noted above, the combination is considerably more effective than the use of radiotherapy alone.

Why it's important

This trial, in patients with very early-stage breast cancer, demonstrated a substantial local recurrence rate following lumpectomy and adjuvant tamoxifen in the absence of radiotherapy. It demonstrated the inability of tamoxifen to substitute for radiotherapy following lumpectomy. Prior related articles had demonstrated a substantial rate of local recurrence in the most highly selected patients following wide resection alone. It had been hoped – even assumed by some – that tamoxifen could substitute for radiotherapy locally, and this trial failed to show this.

Strength

Firm evidence was presented, based on a large randomized clinical trial.

Weakness

Not all patients had estrogen receptor-positive tumors.

Relevance

Based on the results of this trial, all patients with invasive breast cancer are recommeded to receive breast radiotherapy, even if tamoxifen is being used.

CHAPTER 12

Endocrinology

MITCHELL DOWSETT

WILLIAM R MILLER

Introduction

The hormonal dependence of a large proportion of breast cancer has been recognized for over 100 years due to the classic observations of Beatson (see Chapter 13, Paper 1). During the intervening period, hormonal therapy has become a mainstay of the treatment of women at all stages of breast cancer. In the advanced disease setting it has been considered to be primarily palliative, but over the last decade it has become clear that survival gains can be made using modern hormonal therapy, even at that late stage. In the adjuvant treatment of early breast cancer the use of tamoxifen is now known to have saved many thousands of lives. The excellent tolerability of this approach has resulted in the active consideration of these agent for breast cancer prevention. Hormonal therapy and the biological understanding of the underlying mechanism of hormonal dependence have developed hand in hand, particularly over the last 30 years since the discovery of the oestrogen receptor.

The discovery by Beatson that the removal of the ovaries from women with advanced disease could result in a substantial regression in the disease in some patients laid the foundation for the advances in hormonal therapy that we have seen over the last 50 years. During the first part of the 20th century, surgical manoeuvres (oophorectomy in premenopausal women and adrenalectomy and/or hypophysectomy in postmenopausal women) were widely used in the treatment of breast cancer patients. During the latter half of that century those surgical procedures were largely replaced by medical manoeuvres that resulted in the same hormonal change. Thus oophorectomy has been replaced by the use of gonadotrophin-releasing hormone agonists and the treatment of postmenopausal women involves the use of anti-oestrogens or aromatase inhibitors.

Jensen and his colleagues in the 1960s (Paper 1), found a protein that bound oestrogen at high affinity in the cytosol of organs which were responsive to this hormone; this led to the discovery that this same protein existed in a large proportion of breast carcinomas. This oestrogen receptor (ER) has become the single most important biochemical measurement to be made in breast carcinomas, since it predicts the likely benefit to patients from hormonal manoeuvres. The group of McGuire promoted the use of ER extensively during the 1970s with their exploitation of a ligand binding assay. In more recent years, the application of specific antibodies to the ER has allowed specific, inexpensive and rapid analysis to be conducted on very small amounts of tissue, including those which have been formalin-fixed. Thus in the 21st century, all patients with primary breast cancer should have ER status measured as part of their standard work-up. The recent discovery of the *ERβ* gene has yet to be shown to be important for breast cancer management.

While much of the understanding of the interaction of hormones with breast cancer has been made by clinical observations, enormous advances have also taken place as a result of numerous studies of the MCF-7 human breast cancer cell line (over 2000 published over the last four years). The importance of this cell line is particularly great given that the establishment of breast cancer cell lines has been enormously difficult. Thus, having one that is both oestrogen-dependent and tamoxifen-sensitive has been of great value. The work by Lippman's group (Paper 2) on these cells led to the development of concepts of autocrine and paracrine growth factor pathways. The exploitation of the MCF-7 line by Jordan's group (see Paper 2 and related references) has been particularly extensive and has paralleled much of the clinical development of tamoxifen, allowing the testing of hypotheses relating to resistance to anti-oestrogens.

A role for oestrogens in the aetiology of breast cancer has been clear for many years: early menarche, late menopause, late first childbirth, and postmenopausal obesity are all aspects which impact on the exposure of the normal breast to oestrogen and are risk factors for breast cancer. Thus a large number of studies have assessed the relationship between breast cancer incidence and the prevailing level of oestrogen in the plasma of the patients. However, these studies were of little value until the establishment of prospective collections of blood were constructed from normal women prior to the occurrence of breast cancer. The first of these was the Guernsey study by Bulbrook and his colleagues at the Imperial Cancer Research Fund at Guy's Hospital, London. Moore *et al.* (Paper 4) demonstrated that the binding of oestradiol could be important in establishing breast cancer risks, and many papers since have confirmed the positive relationship between plasma oestrogens and breast cancer risk.

The use of hormone replacement therapy (HRT) in millions of women after the menopause has been of concern in relation to breast cancer risk and has elicited very large numbers of epidemiological studies. The overview analysis by Beral and colleagues (Paper 7) brought together data from a large number of studies on many tens of thousands of women who had taken HRT. This revealed a small increase in the relative risk of breast cancer of 2.3% for every year of HRT taken. This is, however, a relatively modest increased risk compared with the benefits of HRT.

Over the last 30 years, by far the most important agent for the treatment of breast cancer has been tamoxifen. About one-third of patients with advanced disease not selected on the basis of ER show an objective clinical response to first-line tamoxifen. The most important advances in the use of tamoxifen, however, have taken place in the adjuvant setting as a result of a series of studies starting in the mid 1970s. The first of the overview analyses of adjuvant therapy for breast cancer established that tamoxifen enhanced the survival of breast cancer patients when given in early disease (Paper 5); the widespread use of tamoxifen in this setting has probably contributed to the marked reduction in mortality from breast cancer that has occurred in Western countries over recent years.

Observations of the excellent tolerability of tamoxifen and its effect on reducing contralateral breast cancer incidence led to its investigative use as a prophylactic agent in the Royal Marsden Hospital (London) feasibility study which started in 1986. The National Surgical Adjuvant Breast and Bowel Project (NSABP) P-1 study started in the early 1990s and was the first one to establish that tamoxifen can reduce the incidence of breast cancer in a high-risk population by approximately 50% over the first four years of follow-up (Paper 8). Much controversy surrounds the early publication of these data, but this publication will undoubtedly have a marked influence on the conduct of further prevention studies during the early part of the current century.

These observations on the early prophylactic effect of tamoxifen were nearly concurrent with results from the MORE (Multiple Outcomes of Raloxifene Evaluation) study (Paper 9) which revealed that another selective oestrogen receptor modulator, raloxifene, reduced the incidence of breast cancer – in this case in a low-risk breast cancer group. Importantly, this compound has been licensed for the treatment of osteoporosis in postmenopausal women. This has led to concepts being developed that women may be able to take agents for HRT which, far from having a detrimental effect on breast cancer risk, might in fact reduce this risk. The applicability of these observations in a high-risk breast cancer population is currently being assessed in the STAR (Study of Tamoxifen Against Raloxifene) study.

While the mixed agonist activity of compounds like tamoxifen and raloxifene may be advantageous in reducing the complications of anti-oestrogenic therapy in breast cancer patients, it has been considered for many years that this agonist activity may be disadvantageous so far as efficacy is concerned. Thus a series of pure anti-oestrogens has been developed which are now under in-depth study in the advanced breast cancer setting (Paper 6). In addition, compounds such as fulvestrant (ICI 182,780, Faslodex) have been instrumental in increasing our understanding of hormonal dependence in models such as the MCF-7 human breast cancer cell line (Paper 6).

During the last 30 years another series of hormonal agents has become increasingly important – the aromatase inhibitors. The prototype for these compounds was aminoglutethimide, which Santen's group (Paper 3) showed to be an aromatase inhibitor during the late 1970s. The newer compounds such as letrozole, anastrozole and exemestane are highly potent and specific, well-tolerated compounds, and most excitingly recent data indicate that some of these compounds have greater efficacy than tamoxifen in patients with advanced or early disease. For over 25 years, the ultimate goal has been to displace tamoxifen as the most efficacious compound. At last we seem to be making a significant stride forward.

Paper 1

Estrogen receptors in hormone-dependent breast cancers

Author

Jensen EV

Reference

Cancer Research 1975; **35**: 3362–3364

Summary

Assays of oestrogen receptors in either primary or metastatic disease provide useful information on the likelihood of response to endocrine therapy in patients with advanced breast cancer. Thus, response to therapy is largely restricted to patients who have tumours with substantial levels of oestrogen receptors; conversely, women having tumours without receptors have little chance of responding to endocrine manipulations and should be treated with other therapeutic modalities.

Related references (1)   De Sombre ER, Carbone PP, Jensen EV, *et al.* Special Report. Steroid receptors in breast cancer. *New England Journal of Medicine* 1979; **301**: 1011–1012.

(2)   King WJ, Greene GL. Monoclonal antibodies localize estrogen receptor in the nuclei of target cells. *Nature* 1984; **307**; 745–747.

Key message

The response of breast cancer to hormone therapy is confined to tumours possessing oestrogen receptors.

Why it's important

The publication of this paper marked the transition from the indiscriminate use of hormone therapy, with a success rate of only 1 in 3, to a rational approach in which patients were selected on the basis of tumour phenotype.

Strengths

1. The observations are based on substantial numbers of patients with breast cancer treated with a variety of endocrine treatments.
2. Most results are derived from a relatively simple *in vitro* assay.
3. The data are presented clearly, are easy to interpret and provide clear conclusions.

Weaknesses

1. The assay, although simpler and less invasive than previous *in vitro* techniques, is nevertheless laborious, requiring access to substantial amounts of fresh tissue and sophisticated equipment and technology. (It has therefore been superseded by immunohistochemical techniques which can be used on archival material: see related reference (2).)

2. There is a mention of an erroneous concept that receptor protein is mostly localized in the cytoplasm and only moves to the nucleus after combination with hormone.

3. No details are provided on assessment of response.

Relevance

The paper illustrates how understanding the mechanisms of hormone action can help distinguish between breast cancers that are hormone-sensitive and those that are not. In practice, a relatively simple assay on a tumour biopsy could identify a cohort of patients who were unlikely to derive benefit from a major treatment modality and therefore be spared the unnecessary side effects of ineffective therapy. Assessment of oestrogen receptors is the only biochemical measurement universally accepted as being important in early breast cancer management

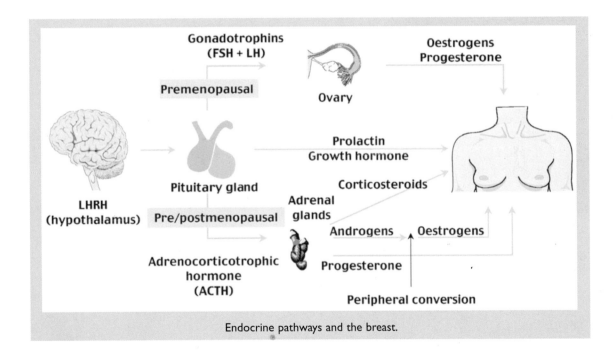

Endocrine pathways and the breast.

Paper 2

The effects of estrogens and antiestrogens on hormone-responsive human breast cancer in long-term tissue culture

Authors

Lippman M, Bolan G, Hulf K

Reference

Cancer Research 1976; **36**: 4595–4601

Summary

The paper describes the characterization of six cell lines derived from breast cancers and maintained in long-term culture with regard to their responsiveness to oestrogens and anti-oestrogens. The authors focus on one of the cell lines (MCF-7) which is markedly stimulated by physiological concentrations of oestradiol as determined by effects of cell numbers and macromolecular synthesis. Higher concentrations of oestrogen are inhibitory and very high levels kill the cells. These latter effects appeared to be non-specific since they could also be observed with other steroids and in other cell lines which neither were sensitive to oestrogen nor contained specific oestrogen receptors. By contrast, the responsive cell lines contained receptors which bound oestradiol with high affinity; anti-oestrogens competed with oestradiol but had a lower affinity for the receptor. Anti-oestrogens also inhibited the growth of cells and blocked the stimulatory effects of oestrogen. At very high concentrations, anti-oestrogens could be cytotoxic. The authors suggest that the cell lines would prove to be valuable models by which to study hormone sensitivity in target tissues, most notably the effects of endocrine therapy in patients with breast cancer.

Related references **(1)** Soule HD, Vazquez J, Long A, Albert S, Brennan M. A human cell line from a pleural effusion derived from a breast carcinoma. *Journal of the National Cancer Institute* 1973; **51**: 1409–1413.

(2) Lippman M, Bolan G, Huff K. The effects of glucocorticoids and progesterone on hormone-responsive human breast cancer in long term tissue culture. *Cancer Research* 1976; **36**: 4602–4609.

(3) Lippman M, Bolan G, Huff K. The effects of androgens and anti-androgens on hormone responsive human breast cancer in long term tissue culture. *Cancer Research* 1976; **36**: 4610–4618.

Key message

Using a well-defined model system, it is possible to characterize the effects of oestrogens and antioestrogens on cell division and macromolecule synthesis in breast cancer cells, in terms of (i) effective concentrations, (ii) specificity of oestrogens and sensitive cell lines, and (iii) antagonistic properties of antioestrogen and their potential for cell kill.

Why it's important

These cell lines, most particlarly the MCF-7 cell line, have proven to be invaluable models by which to study cellular processes. MCF-7 cells are universally used and are the yardstick by which to monitor oestrogen-mediated events and by which to screen anti-oestrogenic agents.

Strengths

1. The study used viable monoclonal cell populations which grow in defined media.
2. These were well-designed experiments producing definitive results.
3. It was possible to appreciate the relevance of the observations and translate them into what may be clinically meaningful.

Weaknesses

1. The monoclonal nature of the cell lines and their culture on plastic means that paracrine and endocrine effects are not truly assessed.
2. The MCF-7 cell line was derived from a pleural effusion, i.e. an advanced stage of disease, and its relevance to other early cellular components can be questioned.
3. Although it was claimed that the cells are grown in completely hormonally defined media, it was not appreciated that the phenol red marker in DMEM (Dulbecco's minimal essential medium) is oestrogenic. The effects of tamoxifen in this system therefore could be competitive of oestrogen rather than an inherent cytostatic property.
4. Subsequently other workers have found it difficult to reproduce some of the more dramatic effects.

Relevance

These observations are a good example of what can be achieved with appropriate model systems and well-designed experiments. MCF-7 cells remain the major cell line to be used to characterize mechanisms of endocrine sensitivity and against which to screen anti oestrogenic agents *in vitro*.

Paper 3

Aminoglutethimide inhibits extraglandular estrogen production in postmenopausal women with breast cancer

Authors

Santen RJ, Santner S, Davis B, Veldhuis J, Samojlik E, Ruby E

Reference

Journal of Clinical Endocrinology and Metabolism 1978; **47**: 1257–1265.

Summary

Results were presented on the measurement of peripheral aromatization of androgen to oestrogens and levels of circulating oestrogens in postmenopausal women before and after treatment with aminoglutethimide. The drug was shown to be a potent inhibitor of aromatization, treatment reducing values by 95–98%. As a consequence, circulating oestrogens were also reduced to levels comparable to those in adrenalectomized postmenopausal patients. The authors concluded that aminoglutethimide's effects on aromatase inhibition in peripheral tissues, including breast cancers themselves, might be at least as important as previously noted effects on adrenal steroidogenesis. They also suggested that drugs such as aminoglutethimide might provide a unique agent for treatment of patients with oestrogen-dependent metastatic breast cancer, and recommended comparative trials with other endocrine therapies.

Related references   **(1)**   Hughes SWM, Durling DM. Aminoglutethimide, a side effect turned to therapeutic advantage. *Postgraduate Medical Journal* 1970; **46**: 409–416.

       (2)   Samojlik E, Santen RJ, Wells SA. Adrenal suppression with amino-glutethimide. II. Differential effect on plasma androstenedione and estrogen levels. *Journal of Clinical Endocrinology and Metabolism* 1977; **45**: 480–487.

       (3)   Brodie AMH, Schwarzel WC, Shaikh AA, Brodie HJ. The effect of an aromatase inhibitor, 4-hydroxy-4-androstene-3,17-dione, on estrogen-dependent processes in reproduction and breast cancer. *Endocrinology* 1977; **100**: 1684–1695.

       (4)   Geisler J, Haynes B, Anker G, Dowsett M, Loming PE. Influence of letrozole and anastrozole on total body aromatization and plasma estrogen levels in postmenopausal breast cancer patients evaluated in a randomized, cross-over study. *Journal of Clinical Oncology* 2002; **20**; 751–757.

Key message

The paper presents unequivocal evidence that drugs such as aminoglutethimide which were first introduced as a form of medical adrenalectomy inhibiting steroidogenesis in the adrenal could have profound effects on peripheral tissues, most notably inhibiting the aromatization of androgens to oestrogens. The further implications of this are that effects on oestrogen biosynthesis are biologically important and have clinical utility in the treatment of hormone-dependent breast cancers in postmenopausal women.

Why it's important

The demonstration that aminoglutethimide could inhibit oestrogen biosynthesis peripherally provided the impetus to develop drugs which could block the aromatase enzyme with greater potency and specificity. Subsequent studies have shown that the inhibition of aromatase is a practical and attractive option by which to treat hormone-sensitive breast cancer. New generations of drugs have recently been developed which can reduce circulating levels of oestrogens in postmenopausal women to values undetectable by current assay whilst not affecting other classes of steroid hormones. These drugs now represent major treatment options for postmenopausal patients with breast cancer.

Strengths

1. This study employed a definitive and well validated methodology by which to monitor peripheral aromatase activity in postmenopausal women before and after treatment with an aromatase inhibitor
2. It was possible to correlate effects on peripheral aromatase with those on circulating oestrogen
3. It was realized that aminoglutethimide's effects on peripheral aromatase (including that in breast tissue) represents an important mechanism of action which could be exploited in the treatment of breast cancer.

Weaknesses

1. The studies were performed with a regime of aminoglutethimide plus corticosteroids such that the effects could not be definitively or totally attributed to aminoglutethimide
2. The number of subjects (5) was small
3. The assays for circulating oestrogens were relatively insensitive.

Relevance

This is one of the pioneering papers to elucidate the mechanism of action of a class of drugs that are now routinely used to treat hormone-sensitive breast cancer. The methodology used has (in a modified form) become established as the gold standard for comparing the pharmacological effectiveness of different aromatase inhibitors.

Paper 4

Binding of oestradiol to blood proteins and aetiology of breast cancer

Authors

Moore JW, Clark GMG, Hoare SA, *et al.*

Reference

International Journal of Cancer 1986; **38**: 625–630

Summary

Five thousand blood samples were collected from healthy women on the island of Guernsey and stored frozen for several years until a group of these had developed breast cancer. Samples taken earlier from this subgroup of precancer cases were matched with controls from unaffected women and analysed for non-protein-bound oestradiol and sex hormone-binding globulin (SHBG). Precancer cases had a significantly higher proportion of protein-free oestradiol and significantly lower level of SHBG. The data indicate that women who are exposed to higher levels of biologically active oestradiol are at greater risk of breast cancer. It is not possible, however, to conclude that this exposure is directly causative.

Related references   **(1)**   Bulbrook RD, Hayward JL. Abnormal urinary steroid excretion and subsequent breast cancer. *Lancet* 1971; **ii**: 395–398.

(2)   Thomas HV, Reeves GK, Key TJ. Endogenous estrogen and postmenopausal breast cancer: a quantitative review. *Cancer Causes Control* 1997; **8**: 922–928.

(3)   Cuzick J, Wang DY, Bulbrook RD. The prevention of breast cancer. *Lancet* 1986; **i**: 83–86.

(4)   Endogenous Hormones and Breast Cancer Collaborative Group. Endogenous hormones and breast cancer in postmenopausal women. *Journal of the National Cancer Institute* 2002; **94**: 606–616.

Key message

This prospective collection of samples was the first to demonstrate convincingly that oestrogenic exposure was greater in women who eventually develop breast cancer as a result of differences in protein binding.

Why it's important

This paper was one of a series published by the same group on studies emanating from a prospective collection of blood and urine from normal women who were subsequently followed-up for their development of breast cancer. This prospective collection was the first of its kind but it has since been followed by many others of similar design. The first papers from the ICRF group using this study design were on urinary analyses and were published 15 years earlier, but the findings are of less contemporary importance (related reference 1).

The conduct of such studies is a formidable task, requiring collection of many thousands of samples (in this case 5000) from normal subjects with follow-up for several years. It has become clear that for hormonal–epidemiological studies, prospective designs are needed to avoid the confounders of case–control studies: the positive and important data resulting from prospective studies contrasts with the variable data of doubtful significance from numerous earlier and later case–control studies.

This paper was particularly novel since it examined the small proportion of oestradiol in blood not bound to plasma proteins and reflected the contemporary interest in this being the biologically active fraction. The proportion of protein-free oestradiol and the concentration of SHBG, the predominant binding protein for oestradiol, were measured in 24 women who developed breast cancer and 212 controls matched individually for patient age and storage time. The samples were collected on the island of Guernsey as the population was geographically stable and the local health authority had an excellent cancer registry, both factors allowing comprehensive follow-up. The proportion of protein-free oestradiol was significantly higher in the precancer cases for both pre- and postmenopausal subjects ($p = 0.0032$ and 0.0002, respectively). Less substantial differences in the same direction were found in the proportion of oestradiol bound to albumin. In contrast SHBG levels were significantly lower in the precancer cases. The lower SHBG levels partially accounted for the increase in the proportion of free oestradiol.

The date were compelling and the ICRF group as a result made a proposal that SHBG levels might be used to identify patients at a higher risk of breast cancer for inclusion in a breast cancer prevention trial with tamoxifen (related reference 3). Subsequent findings from the group that women from the cohort who developed breast cancer later did not have decreased SHGB have detracted from the importance of the result reported but not from the study design.

There has recently been a series of papers, including one using the Guernsey cohort, reporting that the total concentration of oestradiol in postmenopausal women is higher in precancer cases than controls (related reference 2) Thus a body of evidence has developed which directly supports a higher oestrogenic stimulus being related to increased breast cancer incidence.

Strength

This study had a prospective design and novel analytical approaches.

Weakness

The number of cases at the time of analysis was small. The analysis of protein-free oestradiol is complicated and was not suitable for widespread application.

Relevance

Larger studies are presently attempting to refine the relationships first demonstrated in the Guernsey studies, and a recent overview confirmed and extended these original results. These relationships are being extended further to the study of genetic polymorphisms which might identify low penetrance or modifier genes of breast cancer risk amongst the controlling factors for the hormone levels.

Paper 5*

Effects of adjuvant tamoxifen and of cytotoxic therapy on mortality in early breast cancer: An overview of 61 randomized trials among 28 896 women

Authors

Early Breast Cancer Trialists' Collaborative Group (EBCTG)

Reference

New England Journal of Medicine 1988; **319**: 1681–1692

Summary

Data were collected from all identified randomized clinical trials of adjuvant tamoxifen (or cytotoxic) therapy for early breast cancer that began before 1985. Randomization required tamoxifen to be compared with no treatment, or tamoxifen plus treatment A versus treatment A. In 28 trials of adjuvant tamoxifen, nearly 4000 of 16 513 women had died. Twenty-five of the trials involved tamoxifen use for 2 years or less. The data on individual patients were subjected to novel overview statistical analysis. There was a clear reduction in mortality by about one-fifth with tamoxifen ($p < 0.0001$) at 5 years: 68.2% of women on no tamoxifen survived compared with 73.0% on tamoxifen. This difference was accounted for by the difference in women aged 50 years or more. For younger women there was no demonstrable difference, but there were relatively few women in this comparison ($n = 1062$). It was notable that for those younger women receiving tamoxifen alone there was a strong trend to a benefit, but those receiving chemotherapy as well obtained no benefit, possibly because of the ovarian effects of cytotoxics.

Related references **(1)** Early Breast Cancer Trialists' Collaborative Group. Systemic treatment of early breast cancer by hormonal, cytotoxic, or immune therapy: 133 randomised trials involving 31 000 recurrences and 24 000 deaths among 75 000 women. *Lancet* 1992; **339**: 1–15; 71–85.

(2) Early Breast Cancer Trialists' Collaborative Group. Tamoxifen for early breast cancer: an overview of the randomised trials. *Lancet* 1998; **351**: 1451–1467.

Key message

Tamoxifen reduces the 5-year mortality of women with early breast cancer.

---

* See also Paper 7 in Chapter 13.

Why it's important

This was the first report of the overview approach to assessing the benefits of therapy by combining data from many different trials for hormonal (and cytotoxic) treatment of early breast cancer. There had already been a number of reports of individual clinical trials showing survival benefits with tamoxifen, but also of others showing no benefits, such that until the publication the position was unclear. The data from this overview were sufficiently persuasive for it to have a profound effect on the treatment of early breast cancer. The results, combined with the good tolerability and relative inexpensiveness of tamoxifen, led to wide usage of tamoxifen in postmenopausal patients. World-wide, hundreds of thousands of patients' lives have been extended as a result. In the UK the dramatic downturn in the mortality statistics with breast cancer through the 1990s has recently been ascribed largely to this change in practice during the late 1980s.

The overview approach required the collaboration of large numbers of trials organizations to pool their results – in many cases prior to the publication of data from their own studies. This collaborative overview approach has been built upon in subsequent years by updates of the data at approximately 5-yearly intervals.

It is notable that in this paper the comment was made that: 'there is no reason to suppose that either the tamoxifen or chemotherapy regimens tested represent the best that these treatments can offer'. Subsequent overviews (related references 1 and 2) have indeed refined the initial observation by confirming that the survival benefit:

- persisted beyond 10 years
- occurred also in premenopausal women
- was greatest in those tumours containing high concentrations of ER
- was greater in those patients receiving a least 5 years of tamoxifen.

Thus, 5 years of tamoxifen is currently the norm for early treatment of ER-positive breast cancer.

These subsequent overviews have extended the analyses to relapse-free survival – a step which was initially controversial but is now accepted as an important intermediate end-point for overall survival.

Overview analyses have thus become the most powerful analytical tool for establishing or modifying medical practice in early breast cancer, and each new 5-year analysis is keenly anticipated. It has, however, become increasingly clear that a level of sophistication is required to ensure that interactive confounding factors do not obscure or minimize real significant effects. The individual randomized clinical trial retains an important role in itself as well as in contributing to the next overview.

Strengths

Overview analysis brought together large data sets to give otherwise unavailable statistical power. Contacting individual trial groups minimized publication bias.

Weakness

There was no analysis of subgroups that might or might not derive benefit. To a limited extent such analyses would occur in the later overviews.

Relevance

The data indicating reduced mortality with tamoxifen are as relevant today as 15 years ago. Adjuvant treatment with tamoxifen remains the gold-standard for hormone-dependent disease.

Paper 6

A potent specific pure antiestrogen with clinical potential

Authors

Wakeling AE, Dukes M, Bowler J

Reference

Cancer Research 1991; **51**: 3867–3873

Summary

A new anti-oestrogen devoid of agonist activity was described for the first time: ICI 182,780 (now known as fulvestrant (Faslodex)). The compound was 10 times more potent than the prototype pure anti-oestrogen ICI 164,384. The structure of these compounds was a departure from all earlier anti-oestrogens, in that they were steroids and identical to oestradiol, save for a long aliphatic, poly-fluorinated side-chain at carbon 7 of the chemical structure. The compound had similar binding affinity for the oestrogen receptor as oestradiol.

The pure antagonism was well illustrated by the lack of any uterotrophic effect when fulvestrant was administered to immature rats and by its ability to antagonize the uterotrophic effects of tamoxifen in immature animals. The compound blocked the oestrogen-stimulated growth of MCF-7 human breast cancer cells *in vitro* to a greater degree than 4-hydroxytamoxifen. Similar antitumour effects to tamoxifen were shown on two hormone-dependent animal tumours.

Related references   **(1)**   Howell A, De Friend D, Robertson J, Blamey R, Walton P. Response to a specific antioestrogen (ICI 182,780) in tamoxifen resistant breast cancer. *Lancet* 1995; **345**: 29–30.

         (2)   De Friend DJ, Howell A, Nicholson RI, *et al.* Investigation of a new pure antiestrogen (ICI 182,780) in women with primary cancer. *Cancer Research* 1994; **54**: 408–414.

         (3)   Wakeling AE, Bowler J. Novel antioestrogens without partial agonist activity. *Journal of Steroid Biochemistry* 1988; **31**: 645–653.

Key message

A steroidal anti-oestrogen which lacked any agonist activity had antitumour effects in a series of model systems. The 10-fold higher potency than the prototype anti-oestrogen ICI 164,384 indicated a compound with the potential for clinical usage.

Why it's important

During the 1980s, the complex pharmacology of tamoxifen and like compounds was increasingly recognized as being characterized by mixed agonist and antagonist action (related reference 3). The hypothesis was developed that the clinical anti-breast cancer effects of tamoxifen were limited by this agonist component of its pharmacology. It was clear that breast cancer cells could be stimulated to grow *in vitro* by some doses of tamoxifen. This was paralleled by the observation of clinical tumour flare at the start of tamoxifen treatment in some patients and others in whom responses could be seen on tamoxifen withdrawal. Thus an anti-oestrogen which lacked this agonist activity was a highly attractive concept.

Pharmacological characterization of the prototype compound ICI 164,384 had established the principle that such pure anti-oestrogens could be derived but the greater potency of fulvestrant was needed for the drug to have potential for clinical usage.

Early phase II clinical trials were highly encouraging, with excellent response rates after previous tamoxifen failure and particularly impressive response duration (related reference 1). The ongoing clinical trials of fulvestrant in first- and second-line therapy will establish if this promise is confirmed and will determine the future assessment of this agent in the adjuvant setting.

Flvestrant has also become a favoured tool of molecular and cell biologists, and their work with it has revealed an interesting and potentially valuable aspect to its mode of action, namely that ER levels are markedly reduced, apparently due to destabilization of the receptor protein (mRNA levels are unaffected). The marked reduction in ER levels was confirmed in breast tumours in a short-term presurgical clinical trial with fulvestrant (related reference 2). This effect on ER may have additional benefits by decreasing any ligand-independent effects of ER. The potential for such agents to be effective in disease resistant to conventional endocrine disease is particularly important.

Strengths

1. The paper has a comprehensive set of data on female reproductive and breast tissues (as xenografts) in rodents.
2. This was the first report of an agent from this new class of hormonal drugs.

Weakness

The paper lacks information on other oestrogen-dependent tissues such as bone. The compound itself has the weakness of poor effectiveness when given orally.

Relevance

The paper remains relevant to those interested in hormonal therapy and treatment of disease that is resistant to other hormonal agents. It is yet more relevant to biologists using fulvestrant as an investigational tool. The compound is so widely used in that setting that it is generally referred to merely as 'ICI'!

Paper 7

Breast cancer and hormone replacement therapy: Collaborative re-analysis of data from 51 epidemiological studies of 52 705 women with breast cancer and 108 411 women without breast cancer

Authors

Collaborative Group on Hormone Factors in Breast Cancer

Reference

Lancet 1997; **350**: 1047–1059

Summary

The Collaborative Group assembled and analysed 90% of the worldwide epidemiological data on the relation between risks of breast cancer and the use of hormone replacement therapy (HRT). This represents results on more than 160 000 women world-wide derived from 51 different epidemiological investigations spanning a 25-year period. The main findings are that the risk of breast cancer: (i) is significantly increased in women using HRT (by a factor of 1.023) and (ii) increases with increasing duration of use, but (iii) the excess risk is reduced after discontinuation of use (and has largely disappeared after 5 years); (iv) the relative risk among current/recent users is greater for women with low weight; (v) the breast cancers diagnosed in women who had used HRT were less advanced clinically than those diagnosed in newer users. The authors discuss confounding factors and potential biases within their analyses, the consistency of effect within individual studies, the explanation for the finding and the need to balance the increased risk to breast cancer with other risks/benefits of HRT.

Related references **(1)** Colditz GA, Egan KM, Stampfer MJ. Hormone replacement therapy and risk of breast cancer: Results from epidemiologic studies. *American Journal of Obstetrics and Gynecology* 1993; **168**: 1473–1480.

(2) Ross RK, Kraito M, Pike MC, Henderson BE. Breast cancer in mothers given diethylstilbestrol in pregnancy. *New England Journal of Medicine* 1985; **312**: 1059.

Key message

1. HRT use is associated with a small but significant increase in breast cancer risk amongst women currently or recently using HRT for more than 5 years.
2. Risk is associated with duration of use.
3. The effect is equivalent to delaying the menopause.
4. Cancers diagnosed in women who had used HRT tended to be less advanced clinically.

Why it's important

HRT is increasingly being used at the menopause to treat symptoms associated with loss of ovarian function. Given the evidence that steroid hormones may stimulate the growth of breast cancer and epidemiological evidence that delayed menopause may increase risk of the disease, it is essential to know the impact of HRT on the natural history of breast cancer. Prior to the publication of the Collaborative Group paper there had been many reports on the subject, some of which had come to conflicting conclusions and none of which individually had the power in terms of numbers and follow-up to provide a definitive analysis of the cost–benefit of HRT. This paper, which provides a meta-analysis of most of the available data, crosses geographical boundaries and has sufficient power to detect even small differences in hazards and to permit subgroup analysis. As such it provides the most reliable evidence that current or recent HRT is associated with a small but definitive increased risk of breast cancer. This is important knowledge for women contemplating HRT use and those likely to advise or prescribe its use.

Strengths

1. There was a comprehensive search for all relevant studies addressing HRT and breast cancer risk.
2. There was meticulous scrutiny of source data for each study.
3. The paper used the power of meta-analysis in employing a huge database of women and encompassing diverse sources and extended study period (such that smaller studies would be unable to detect any association).
4. There was careful consideration of confounding factors and biases.
5. Conservative 99% confidence intervals were used for all but the main comparison.
6. There was internal consistency between individual studies.
7. It was possible to ascertain whether other aetiological factors might increase risk either alone or in combination with HRT.

Weaknesses

1. Information on hormonal constitution or the therapy was known in only the minority of women (39%).
2. The majority of women were likely to be taking hormone preparations (oestrogen only) which may not be relevant to future HRT.
3. The possibility still exists that the meta-analysis might either underestimate or overestimate the true magnitude of breast cancer risk associated with HRT.
4. No data are presented on mortality to breast cancer.

Relevance

HRT is relatively common and increasingly used to treat menopausal symptoms. It is therefore essential to be able to assess accurately the increased risk to breast cancer (if any) and identify those who might be particularly susceptible.

Paper 8

Tamoxifen for prevention of breast cancer: report of the National Surgical Adjuvant Breast and Bowel Project P-1 study

Authors

Fisher B, Constantino JP, Wickerham DL, *et al.*

Reference

Journal of the National Cancer Institute 1998; **90**: 1371–1388

Summary

Women ($n = 13\,388$) at increased risk of breast cancer according to Gail's algorithm were randomly assigned to receive placebo or tamoxifen 20 mg/day for 5 years to assess the possible role of tamoxifen in breast cancer prevention. After a mean follow-up time of 47.7 months, tamoxifen reduced the risk of invasive breast cancer by 49% ($p < 0.000\,01$). Risk was reduced in women aged less than 50 years (44%), 50–59 years (51%) and 60 years or older (55%). The risk of non-invasive breast cancer was also reduced by 50%. The effect of tamoxifen on invasive breast cancer was confined to ER-positive tumours (69% reduction). There was no reduction in the rate of ischaemic heart disease, but a reduction in hip, radius and spine fractures was observed. Endometrial cancer incidence was higher (RR, 2.53; CI, 1.35–4.97), predominantly in women older than 50 years. Rates of stroke, pulmonary embolism and deep vein thrombosis were also increased with tamoxifen. The results unequivocally demonstrate that tamoxifen decreased the early incidence of invasive and non-invasive breast cancer in this population.

Related references **(1)** Powles TJ, Eeles R, Ashley S, *et al.* Interim analysis of the incidence of breast cancer in the Royal Marsden Hospital tamoxifen chemoprevention trial. *Lancet* 1998; **352**: 98–101.

(2) Veronesi U, Maisonneuve P, Costa A, *et al.* Prevention of breast cancer with tamoxifen: preliminary findings from the Italian randomized trial among hysterectomized women. Italian Tamoxifen Prevention Study. *Lancet* 1998; **352**: 93–97.

(3) Cuzick J, Wang DY, Bulbrook RD. The prevention of breast cancer. *Lancet* 1986; **i**: 83–86.

(4) Cuzick J, Powles TJ, Veronesi U, *et al.* Overview of the main outcomes in breast cancer-prevention trials. *Lancet* 2003; **361**: 296–300.

Key message

Tamoxifen can reduce the incidence of invasive and non-invasive breast cancer in a population of women at increased risk of breast cancer based on the Gail model. Increased risk of several other health concerns diminishes the value of the decreased risk.

Why it's important

This paper presents the outcome of one of the most widely discussed studies on any aspect of breast cancer in recent years. While it demonstrated very clearly that breast cancer incidence could be reduced by tamoxifen, at least over the first few years of treatment, the early stopping of the trial has meant that the balance of long-term beneficial effects to deleterious side-effects remains to be established. Many commentators reasonably contend that it was already known through the study of reduced contralateral breast cancer incidence in adjuvant studies that tamoxifen 'prevented' breast cancer and that the role of the trial was to elicit the long-term data which this early stopping negated.

The controversy around the study was heightened by the near simultaneous publication of data from the Royal Marsden trial (related reference 1) and the Italian trial (related reference 2), neither of which confirmed the NSABP result. Attention has focused on trying to rationalize the different result in the Marsden trial, which despite randomizing far fewer subjects (2500) had much longer follow-up, having started 6 years prior to the NSABP study. Lower statistical power and use of HRT by some of the Marsden patients have been cited as possible confounds, but the most likely explanation seems to be different characteristics of the study populations with much stronger family history determining the increased risk in the Marsden study. Nonetheless, the fourth tamoxifen prevention trial (IBISI) has recently confirmed a reduced incidence of breast cancer in women receiving tamoxifen, and an overview of the four trials reveals a 38% reduction in breast cancer incidence.

The NSABP P-1 trial resulted in a license being granted by the American Food and Drug Administration (FDA) for tamoxifen's use to reduce breast cancer risk in women with a risk similar to the P-1 population and it established tamoxifen as the gold-standard comparator for future prevention studies, at least in the USA. For example, the STAR (Study of Tamoxifen Against Raloxifene) trial will compare raloxifene with tamoxifen in a similar (postmenopausal) population to that of the P-1 trial.

Although not powered to establish a decrease in heart disease by tamoxifen, data was collected and disappointingly found no reduced incidence. This contrasts with data from some adjuvant trials. The reduction in the incidence of fractures of the spine was not trivial and can be considered as a real benefit to taking tamoxifen. Comparative efficacy on this end-point with that achieved by raloxifene will be assessed in STAR. The increase in thromboembolic events remains a worrying feature.

Strengths

1. These included the size of the study, its placebo-controlled design, and the systematic collection of side-effect data.
2. This was the first substantive chemoprevention trial in breast cancer to report.

Weakness

The short follow-up and early termination of the trial leave the important questions on long-term benefit unanswered.

Relevance

The paper is likely to remain relevant for many decades. The reasons for the trial's early termination set challenges for future prevention studies. Tamoxifen is considered the comparator for new studies in the USA as a result of this trial.

Paper 9

The effect of raloxifene on risk of breast cancer in postmenopausal women. Results from the MORE randomized trial

Authors

Cummings SR, Eckert S, Krueger KA, *et al.*

Reference

Journal of the American Medical Association, 1999; **281**: 2189–2197

Summary

This study aimed to determine whether osteoporotic women taking raloxifene (a selective oestrogen receptor modulator, SERM) have lower risk of invasive breast cancer. The Multiple Outcomes of Raloxifene Evaluation (MORE) was a multicentre, randomized double-blind trial in which 7705 osteoporotic postmenopausal women (mean age 66.5 years) received raloxifene or placebo for a median of 40 months. Randomization was 2:1, respectively. There were 13 cases of breast cancer among 5129 women assigned raloxifene and 27 among 2576 women assigned placebo (relative risk (RR), 0.24; 95% confidence interval (CI), 0.13–0.44; $p < 0.01$). The relative risk of oestrogen receptor-positive breast cancer on raloxifene was reduced by 90% (RR, 0.10; 95% CI, 0.04–0.24). Raloxifene was associated with a 3.1-fold increase risk of thromboembolism. There was no increase in the risk of endometrial cancer, but the confidence intervals were wide.

Related references   **(1)**   Jordan VC, Phelps E, Lindgren JU. Effects of antiestrogens on bone in castrated and intact female rate. *Breast Cancer Research and Treatment* 1987; **10**: 31–35.

(2)   Jordan VC. Designer oestrogens. *Scientific American* 1998; October: 36–43.

(3)   Delmas PD, Bjarnason NH, Mitlak BH, *et al.* Effects of raloxifene on bone mineral density, serum cholesterol concentration and uterine endometrium in postmenopausal women. *New England Journal of Medicine* 1997; **337**: 1641–1647.

Key message

Raloxifene, a drug with reduced endometrial stimulatory effects compared with tamoxifen, decreased the risk of invasive breast cancer in postmenopausal women with osteoporosis by 76%.

Why it's important

The concept of agents like tamoxifen, which were previously described as anti-oestrogens, having differential agonist and antagonist effects between tissues was developed during the early 1990s and the term 'selective estrogen receptor modulator' (or SERM) was coined to describe such compounds. During the 1980s, it was already known that the balance of agonist and antagonist effects of tamoxifen and like compounds within a tissue was affected by prevailing levels of oestrogen. Jordan and colleagues showed that tamoxifen could inhibit the growth of mammary tumours but enhance the growth of endometrial tumours in the same animal. Importantly, agonist effects on bone could also be demonstrated in ovariectomized rats with not only tamoxifen but also keoxifene, which later became known as raloxifene.

Confirmation of bone preservation by tamoxifen in postmenopausal patients heightened interest in the use of such compounds for treatment/prevention of osteoporosis in postmenopausal women, a condition for which hormone replacement therapy (HRT) was normally used (with its associated concerns related to breast cancer). The increase in endometrial cancer risk with tamoxifen precluded its use for this indication; instead the era of so-called designer oestrogens (i.e. SERMs) was initiated with the aim of producing the perfect HRT – a compound with anti-breast cancer and anti-endometrial cancer properties, but with the beneficial effects of oestrogens on bone, lipids, vasculature and brain. Raloxifene has been the predominant compound in this group over the last few years, as a result of it already being 'on the shelf'. Many more have since been synthesized and will enter trials over the coming years.

The MORE study confirmed the expectation from preclinical studies that raloxifene enhanced bone density in postmenopausal women through its interaction with the oestrogen receptor, and also reduced breast cancer risk (rather than enhancing it like HRT). The study revealed, however, that like tamoxifen, raloxifene enhanced the risk of thromboembolism. Concerns remain about whether these compounds will have positive or negative effects on cognitive function and Alzheimer's disease. Like other non-steroidal SERMs, raloxifene is not effective against hot flushes. It is important to recognize that the apparent breast cancer preventive effects of raloxifene in this trial were in osteoporotic patients, a group at reduced risk of breast cancer. The effectiveness in a higher-risk study will be tested in the STAR (Study of Tamoxifen Against Raloxifene) prevention trial, which was initiated in 1999.

Strengths

1. This was a placebo-controlled, large double-blind trial.
2. Multiple end-points were assessed.
3. All breast cancer cases were carefully reviewed.

Weaknesses

1. The follow-up period was short.
2. There were relatively small numbers of breast cancer cases.
3. The trial population was at low risk of breast cancer before treatment.

Relevance

For women needing treatment for osteoporosis, raloxifene is a drug without associated breast cancer worries. The relevance of the breast cancer protective effects is reduced by this being a low-risk population.

CHAPTER 13

Endocrine therapy

MICHAEL BAUM

Introduction

Breast cancer and prostate cancer are especially sensitive to endocrine manipulation. As a result, the endocrine therapy of breast cancer has been a remarkable success story. Over the last 15 years there has been a dramatic fall in mortality from the disease in both the UK and the USA. Most commentators attribute this to the direct or indirect effect of adjuvant hormonal manipulation. A large component of this has been the cross-talk between clinical scientists and endocrinologists. The clinicians tend to make the original observations that then provoke the laboratory research. This may then suggest further clinical interventions with further 'biological fall-out'. And so the cycle continues from Beatson in 1896 (Paper 1) to the ATAC trial starting in 1996 (Paper 10).

The original observations by Beatson over 100 years ago (Paper 1) started a quest that is a model of scientific endeavour. This chapter needs to be read alongside Chapter 12 to trace the history of the discovery of the endocrine system, the metabolic pathways of steroidogenesis, the understanding of endocrine response in target tissues and the subclassification of breast cancers into hormone-responsive and non-responsive phenotypes. Many of the clinical studies referred to were to some extent ahead of their time, with some quite heroic surgery undertaken without a full understanding of the endocrinological consequences. About 50 years after Beatson's landmark series of surgical castration, Huggins and his colleagues first described surgical adrenalectomy as second-line endocrine therapy (Paper 2). Following these two seminal accounts the scene was set to learn how best to exploit these clinical observations in an attempt to either palliate or prolong the life of women with early breast cancer.

Some readers might think there is a notable absence of reports of trials of endocrine therapy in advanced disease in this chapter. That is for two reasons. First, there have been so many trials of endocrine therapy in the advanced setting that it would be invidious to choose 'a classic' within the limited space available. Second, although such trials always report differences in objective response rates, little is written on quality of life, and at its best variations in endocrine therapy (or for that matter chemotherapy) have achieved little more than, say, 6 months' prolongation of median survival. For those reasons I have concentrated on those studies with the first description of a new mode of therapy or the first trials in the adjuvant setting to demonstrate reduction in mortality. Thus, in addition to the two papers cited above, I have chosen the first description of tamoxifen (Paper 4), the first description of a medical adrenalectomy (Paper 5) and the first description of a medical castration (Paper 8). To accompany these in chronological order I have selected the first trial of adjuvant ovarian ablation (Paper 3), the first trial of adjuvant tamoxifen (Paper 6), the overview of adjuvant tamoxifen studies (Paper 7) and the first trial of medical adrenalectomy using a specific oral aromatase inhibitor (Paper 10). Finally, to complete the picture and to understand a continuing controversy I have chosen the first trial comparing ovarian ablation with chemotherapy for node-positive premenopausal patients (Paper 9).

A thread that runs through these studies is the search for the mechanism of response and the identification of the role of the oestrogen receptor (ER) in selecting the most appropriate patients for treatment. Of course the ER status of the primary tumour might be considered an inevitable limitation to endocrine therapy, but such is the success of endocrine approach, I predict that the next challenge endocrinologists will face up to is the mechanism leading to the loss of the ER mechanism. If this turns out to be an epigenetic phenomenon then within a generation it might be possible to convert ER− tumours to an ER+ phenotype, and that I hope would be the beginning of the end of non-specific chemotherapy.

Finally, I hope the inclusion of the ATAC trial (Paper 10) as a 'classic' will not be considered too self-indulgent, but the justification is described below. No one could argue against the fact, that whatever the longer-term outcomes, this trial marks a culmination of 100 years' work involving surgeons, biochemists, endocrinologists, medical and clinical oncologists, statisticians and, of course, the pharmaceutical industry.

Paper 1*

On the treatment of inoperable cases of carcinoma of the mamma: Suggestions for a new method of treatment, with illustrative cases

Author

Beatson GT

Reference

Lancet 1896; **ii**:104–107

Summary

The history of the science and therapeutic relevance of endocrinology starts with these extraordinary observations of George Beatson in 1896.

Long before the endocrine system was described, Beatson deduced by simple observation of the lactation of farm animals that there must be a link between the physiology of the breast and the activity of the ovaries. The anecdotal spectacular responses of three young women with locally advanced or locally recurrent breast cancer to surgical oophorectomy set the scene for the future. Beatson describes a young woman with rapidly recurrent breast cancer on the chest wall not long after radical surgery, who is sent to see him for a second opinion. He then digresses on the current theories about the nature and aetiology of breast cancer before going on to describe his MD research on the physiology of lactation in farm animals, starting with sheep.

At that time it had been assumed that lactation was controlled by nervous stimuli, yet dissections failed to demonstrate the nerves of lactation. He then made the observation that lactation terminates when menses restart after a calf has been weaned and that in Australia cows are spayed to prolong lactation. He also describes his animal experiments on rabbits that confirm these natural observations. He concludes his theoretical development by suggesting that cancer results from a failure of the natural involution of the lining of the breast ducts. With this in mind he embarks on his clinical experiments in an attempt to normalize the breast cancer cells by removing the as yet unknown stimulus of ovarian activity.

His description of seeking informed consent from the first case is very moving and incidentally demonstrates a degree of compassion and ethical probity which would be in keeping with modern attitudes.

The three anecdotes of unequivocal objective remissions leave little doubt that he had discovered a new class of therapeutic intervention. Curiously enough, the first patient was also treated with high doses of thyroid extract for reasons he fails to explain.

---

* See also Paper 1 in Chapter 16.

Key message

This paper is a model of how the prepared mind of an inquisitive and brilliant man can help to build a biological theory of disease and its therapeutic consequences. Beatson then has the courage to carry out animal and clinical experiments to test this hypothesis. I wonder, however, if it would have got past a multicentre research ethics committee of the day if such institutions had existed. Nevertheless he describes the informed consent procedure for the experimental therapy, and history is his judge.

Why it's important

For the first time Beatson demonstrates that the function of one organ can have profound physiological effects on another remote organ independent of the nervous system, thus giving birth to the science of endocrinology.

Strength

Objective remissions were induced in previously untreatable advanced breast cancer.

Weakness

We have the numerator but not the denominator. Recent work by David Smith of Glasgow, Beatson's home, using the original operative records of Beatson's operating theatre, has shown that he had completed nine cases of oophorectomy before his report in *The Lancet* (personal communication). Three out of nine successes would be the anticipated 30% response rate for unselected cases of advanced breast cancer to endocrine manipulation!

Paper 2

Inhibition of human mammary and prostatic cancers by adrenalectomy

Authors

Huggins C, Bergenstal DM

Reference

Cancer Research 1952; **12**:134–141

Summary

For over 50 years since Beatson's original work on castration for metastatic breast cancer little had changed. The discovery of the sex steroid hormones of course provided a rational explanation for the therapeutic benefit of sugical ovarian ablation and led Haddow and his colleagues to experiment with synthetic oestrogens and Adair and Herrman to use androgens for advanced breast cancer in the early 1940s (see related references 1 and 2).

Huggins and Bergenstal took the next courageous leap forward with the description of bilateral adrenalectomy for metastatic breast and prostate cancer. The scientific rationale they describe is bizarre in retrospect – with justification being based on animal experiments with a variety of tumours, only some of which might be considered hormone-sensitive. Because the role of the adrenal gland in the synthesis of oestrogen precursors had not yet been described, they thought that any responses seen in the experimental setting were related to a non-specific effect of the corticosteroid hormones.

They describe 18 cases of bilateral adrenalectomy: 7 breast cancers, 7 prostate cancers and 4 'miscellaneous'. There were two postoperative deaths. (Unlike Beatson's paper there is no description of informed consent for this dangerous experimental therapy!) Six of the breast cancer cases were premenopausal and had undergone prior oophorectomy. There were 2 partial responses and 1 stable disease, and 3 cases progressed (this can only be deduced, since criteria for measuring objective responses had not been defined). This response rate is what might be expected for second-line endocrine therapy of advanced disease.

Related references

(1)   Haddow A, Watkinson JM, Patterson E, Koller PC. Influence of synthetic oestrogens upon advanced malignant disease. *British Medical Journal* 1944; **ii**:393–398.

(2)   Adair FE, Herrman JB. The use of testosterone propionate in the treatment of advanced carcinoma of the breast. *Annals of Surgery* 1946; **123**:1023–1035.

Key message

This was the first paper in 50 years to demonstrate another biological pathway that might influence the natural history of what we have now come to describe as hormone-sensitive cancers. Although published after the description of the steroidal sex hormones, the mechanism of action was not well understood.

Why it's important

The supreme surgical skills of the authors together with the medical support with adrenocortical hormones allowed 16 out of 18 patients to survive the procedure. The observation that at least two of the premenopausal patients who had previously undergone surgical castration subsequently experienced a further response was the first suggestion of the notion of second-line endocrine therapy.

Strength

The strength of this paper lies with the courage of the authors (not to mention the patients) to undertake such heroic surgery among patients with incurable disease, many of whom were far from fit. The procedure followed on from animal experiments and appeared logical at the time. Objective and subjective benefits are described clearly, setting the scene for further medical and surgical approaches to the management of advanced breast cancer.

Weakness

The theoretical underpinning for the procedures was very weak and one could argue that they were lucky rather than clever. Furthermore, there is no evidence or description of informed consent for what was a highly hazardous experimental operation. Finally the description of 'responses' is hard to follow and would not be accepted by modern criteria.

Relevance

This paper was an adumbration of the future work on the extra-ovarian source of oestrogen synthesis and the search for a safe and efficient way of downregulating peripheral aromatase activity that ultimately led to the ATAC trial (Paper 10). The perfecting of the technique was also of value for the treatment of adrenal tumours.

Paper 3

Suppression of ovarian function in primary breast cancer

Author

Nissen-Meyer R

Reference

Acta Radiologica 1965; **259**(Suppl):

Summary

Between 22 November 1957 and 31 December 1963 a total of 932 women under the age of 70 years were admitted as in-patients for their first treatment of operable breast cancer (stage I and II). They were all registered for a prospective study of 'prophylactic' versus 'therapeutic' castration. Oophorectomy was performed as part of the primary treatment of 74 cases, ovarian irradiation in 590 cases. In the remaining 268 cases, castration was planned to be performed as soon as recurrences were diagnosed. In 448 of the cases a controlled clinical trial with random allocation was found to be ethically justified. All other treatment was kept as standardized as possible. In the primarily castrated groups, the time free of symptoms as well as total survival time was increased. This was found also in the postmenopausal groups. Oophorectomy was not found to be superior to ovarian irradiation as a method of primary castration.

Related references **(1)** Nissen-Meyer R. The role of prophylactic castration in the therapy of human mammary cancer. *European Journal of Cancer* 1967; **3**:395–403.

(2) Cole MP. The place of radiotherapy in the management of early breast cancer. *British Journal of Surgery* 1964; **51**:216–220.

(3) Nevinny HB, Nevinny D, Rossof CB, Hall TC, Muench H. Prophylactic oophorectomy in breast cancer therapy. *American Journal of Surgery* 1969; **117**:531–536.

(4) Ravdin RG, Lewison EF, Slack NH, *et al*. Results of a clinical trial concerning the worth of prophylactic oophorectomy for breast carcinoma. *Surgery, Gynecology and Obstetrics* 1970; **130**:1055–1064.

(5) Meakin JW, Allt WEC, Beale FA, *et al*. Ovarian irradiation and prednisone therapy following surgery and radiotherapy for carcinoma of the breast. *Canadian Medical Association Journal* 1979; **120**:1221–1238.

(6) Early Breast Cancer Trialists' Collaborative Group. Ovarian ablation in early breast cancer: overview of the randomized trials. *Lancet* 1996; **348**:1189–1196.

Key message

Prophylactic, now described as adjuvant, oophorectomy can prolong the disease-free and overall survival in patients with early breast cancer.

Why it's important

Although not the first 'randomized controlled trial' of adjuvant ovarian suppression in early breast cancer, some of which were 'quasi-randomized', this study was the first one to show a significant improvement in 'symptom-free' and actual survival for early breast cancer. It took 30 years and a world overview before this practice was accepted by the profession.

Strength

Nissen-Meyer, almost single-handed and without the help of computers (in fact he used punched cards), held together a multicentre Nordic group for what was at the time a large clinical trial. He stated his experimental method clearly and the predetermined endpoints. Curiously enough, he considered withholding prophylactic ovarian suppression in stage II premenopausal women to be unethical (30 years ahead of his time!). He also attempted to stratify by menopausal status and method of ovarian suppression for subgroup analysis. He justified the use of the procedure in post-menopausal women by his studies of oestrogen metabolites in the urine as evidence of continuing ovarian function in the days before the extra-ovarian source of oestrogens was discovered. The fact that he found a significant advantage in *postmenopausal* women is bizarre and difficult to explain.

Although not widely recognized, later analyses of this trial demonstrated an 80% reduction in the incidence of contralateral disease in the premenopausal group.

Weaknesses

1. These studies were for unselected women in the days before the discovery of the oestrogen receptor (ER). The attempts at subgroup analyses without any discussion of statistical power and the statistical methods used would be considered naive today.
2. He makes no mention of the permanent loss of fertility or the later risk of development of osteoporosis.
3. He was misled by the urinary excretion of oestrogen metabolites as evidence of continued ovarian function in women up to the age of 70.

Relevance

This and related trials were the first to demonstrate the benefits of adjuvant systemic therapy for early breast cancer even before Fisher's classical papers (see Chapter 14) had fully worked up their rationale. In selected ER+ cases adjuvant ovarian ablation is still in use, although these days gonadotrophin-releasing hormone (GnRH) agonists are more likely to be favoured.

Paper 4

A new anti-oestrogenic agent in late breast cancer: An early appraisal of ICI 46,474

Authors

Cole MP, Jones CIA, Todd IDH

Reference

British Journal of Cancer 1971; **25**:270–275

Summary

An introductory trial of the anti-oestrogenic agent ICI 46,474 (now known as tamoxifen) in late or recurrent breast cancer was described. Forty-six patients have been treated, of whom 10 showed a good response. This is of the same order as that seen with oestrogens and androgens. The particular advantage of this drug was the low incidence of troublesome side effects.

Related reference (1)   Harper MJK, Walpole AL. *Nature* 1967; **212**:000–000.

Key message

This was the first description of tamoxifen, and the first novel approach to the medical treatment of advanced breast cancer since the use of stilboestrol, androgens and the alkylating agents.

Why it's important

Until this point the only treatments for advanced breast cancer were castration in premenopausal women, and stilboestrol, androgens and the alkylating agents for postmenopausal women. The last three meant that treatments for the older woman were associated with considerable toxicity, whereas taxoxifen, a molecule synthesized by Arthur Walpole, could produce similar results with minimal toxicity.

Strength

This was truly original work based on some brilliant biochemistry and biological research of ICI scientists. There was also an informal comparison with historical controls in a randomized clinical trial of stilboestrol versus an androgen. Also this paper may have been the first to suggest that hormonal agents act via a specific binding mechanism at the cancer cell target.

Weakness

The criteria of response were not very rigorous and of course the cases were not selected by ER status or meaningful clinical criteria. Nevertheless this might be accepted as a phase II trial.

Relevance

These modest observations ultimately led to an explosion of interest in the drug which until today has been considered to be the gold standard in the treatment of both early and advanced disease for ER+ tumours. Tamoxifen is the cancer drug with the largest sales in history, and has also been a valuable agent to explore mechanisms of endocrine response in experimental systems.

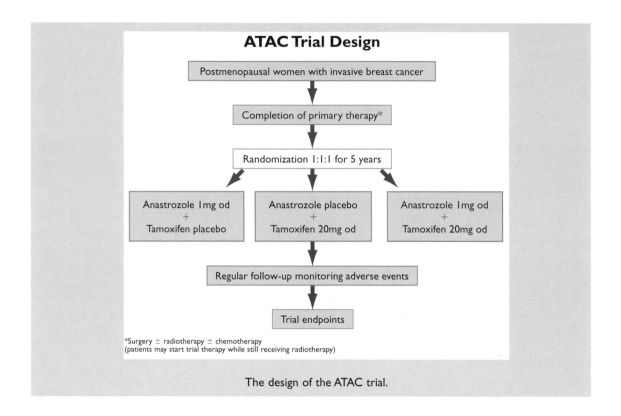

The design of the ATAC trial.

Paper 5

Preliminary trial of aminoglutethimide in breast cancer

Authors

Griffiths CT, Hall TC, Saba Z, *et al.*

Reference

Cancer 1973; **32**:31–37

Summary

Adrenalectomy had been effective in the management of breast cancer, but many patients were poor operative risks. A medical ablation of adrenal function would have wider application. Aminogluthimide blocks adrenal steroidogenesis high in the biosynthetic pathway. Nine patients with absent ovarian function and enlarging metastases received the drug in daily oral doses of 1.0–2.5 g. Corticosteroid replacement consisted of dexamethasone 0.75 mg daily and fludrocortisone acetate 0.1 mg every other day. Regression of osseous disease and disappearance of skin metastases were observed in three patients for 7, 9 and 2 months, respectively. Tumour growth ceased for 4 and 7 months in two patients. Suppression of urinary 17-ketosteroids and 17-hydroxycorticosteroids was only transient in 8 patients, presumably because of compensatory increase in ACTH secretion. Oestrogen secretion rates were similarly affected. The patient with a 9-month remission on 2.5 g daily demonstrated permanent hypoadrenocorticism. Dose-related CNS toxicity ranging from drowsiness to semicoma predominated, but relative hypoadrenocorticism may have contributed. The authors suggested that anticancer action may result from a peripheral effect of the drug or from suppression of an unidentified steroid. Concurrent pharmacological doses of glucocorticoids may reduce toxicity and inhibit compensatory ACTH secretion.

Related references **(1)** Santen RJ, Lipton A, Kendall J. Successful medical adrenalectomy with amino-gluthimide. Role of altered drug metabolism. *Journal of the American Medical Association* 1974; **23**:1661–1665.
(2) Smith IE, Fitzharris BM, McKinna JA, *et al.* Aminogluthimide in treatment of metastatic breast cancer. *Lancet* 1978; **2(8091)**:646–649.
(3) Santen RJ, Worgul TJ, Samojlik E, *et al.* A randomized trial comparing surgical adrenalectomy with aminogluthimide plus hydrocortisone in women with advanced breast cancer. *New England Journal of Medicine* 1981; **305**:545–551.

Key message

'Medical adrenalectomy' induced by the interruption of steroidogenesis at the level of the conversion of cholesterol to pregnenolone can achieve objective responses in metastatic breast cancer among women without ovarian function to a similar extent as a surgical adrenalectomy, and thus can be more widely applicable to women who are a poor operative risk.

Why it's important

This paper was the first of its kind to demonstrate that a medical interference with steroidal biosynthetic pathways can influence the behaviour of advanced breast cancer. Furthermore, it opened the door to less aggressive approaches for women who were either postmenopausal or who had already undergone oophorectomy. Although the mechanisms for the conversion of cholesterol to mineralocorticoids, glucocorticoids and sex steroids were understood at this time, the authors concluded that another mechanism of action was required and postulated the suppression of an as yet unidentified steroid. In fact they were wrong, but these early observations set in train the work that eventually led to the discovery of peripheral aromatization of androgens into oestrogens and later the synthesis of the specific third generation of aromatase inhibitors that look likely to replace tamoxifen in the metastatic and adjuvant settings for postmenopausal women.

Strength

This paper was a truly innovative piece of work based on a fundamental understanding of the endocrine function of the adrenal gland. The rationale for the phase II trial was therefore secure. The authors also took the opportunity of studying serum and urinary metabolites of patients on therapy to gain further insights into the mechanisms of action. Unlike earlier papers described above, they clearly defined their criteria of response.

Weaknesses

1. This was a small phase II study with no recommendations of how to carry it forward into a phase III setting.
2. The toxicity of the treatment was so severe that some might consider it no better than a surgical adrenalectomy.
3. There were no selection criteria for entry and none suggested for the future, although there was a hint that the treatment might be of specific value for bone pain and skeletal metastases.

Relevance

Following this paper and other studies (see related references 1–3), a search for more specific and less toxic methods of palliation achieved by adrenalectomy began. Ultimately, the biosynthetic pathways of the extra-adrenal origins of oestrogens in the postmenopausal women were described, leading to the synthesis of the oral specific aromatase inhibitors that are likely to replace tamoxifen in early and advanced disease for ER+ cases.

Paper 6

Controlled trial of tamoxifen as adjuvant agent in management of early breast cancer: Interim analysis at four years by the Nolvadex Adjuvant Trial Organization

Authors

Baum M, Brinkley DM, Dossett JA, *et al.*

Reference

Lancet 1983; 5th Feb:257–261

Summary

Tamoxifen (Nolvadex), an anti-oestrogen, was evaluated as an adjunct to the local treatment of early breast cancer in a prospective randomized trial in which 1285 women (with pathological stage II premenopausal and pathological stage I and II postmenopausal disease) were treated by total mastectomy with either axillary node clearance or axillary node sampling and then randomized to receive either tamoxifen 10 mg twice daily for 2 years or no further treatment. Treatment failure (recurrent disease or death) at 21 months was reduced in patients receiving tamoxifen (14.2%) compared with controls (20.5%) ($p = 0.01$). This was equivalent to prolongation of the disease-free interval from 21 months to 30 months at a mean follow-up time of 21 months. Subgroup analyses by menopausal, axillary node and oestrogen receptor status did not reveal a significantly different treatment effect in any of these subgroups. There was no significant effect on mortality at this point in the study. This endocrine adjuvant therapy was well tolerated and treatment was discontinued in only 14 (2.2%) patients as a direct result of side effects. Thus, it was shown that tamoxifen significantly delayed recurrence in early breast cancer. The magnitude of the effect was comparable with that associated with adjuvant cytotoxic chemotherapy at a similar follow-up time, but with minimal toxicity and excellent compliance.

Related references **(1)** Scottish Breast Cancer Trials Committee. Adjuvant tamoxifen in the management of operable breast cancer: the Scottish trial. *Lancet* 1987; **i**:171–175.

(2) Fisher B, Redmond C, Brown A, *et al.* Adjuvant chemotherapy with and without tamoxifen in the treatment of primary breast cancer: 5-year results from the National Surgical Adjuvant Breast and Bowel Project Trial. *Journal of Clinical Oncology* 1986; **4**:459–471.

(3) Fornander T, Rutqvist LE, Cedermark B, *et al.* Adjuvant tamoxifen in early breast cancer: occurrence of new primary cancers. *Lancet* 1989; **ii**:117–120.

Key message

Two years of tamoxifen reduced the chance of recurrence by about 30% at a mean follow-up of approximately 2 years. The treatment was well tolerated.

Why it's important

This was the first report of a randomized controlled trial to show that adjuvant tamoxifen had a significant effect on disease-free survival. The study was also one of the first to include premenopausal women and was not diluted in its effect by the inclusion of concurrent or prior adjuvant cytotoxic chemotherapy.

Strength

This was a pragmatic and large trial for its day. The inclusion of both pre- and postmenopausal women and both ER+ and ER− cases could be looked upon as one of its strengths, by not pre-judging the outcome. The same group were later to be the first to demonstrate the impact of tamoxifen on the contralateral breast. The choice of an acronym (NATO) drew attention to the study and established a vogue.

Weaknesses

1. The trial was underpowered to investigate interaction between treatment and predetermined patient subgroups.
2. The method of determining ER status by a modification of the ligand binding assay was flawed in retrospect, leading to the erroneous conclusion that tamoxifen was equally likely to demonstrate a benefit in ER− as well as ER+ cases.
3. The choice of duration of therapy was arbitrary at 2 years, and as chance would have it the benefit was exaggerated when ultimately compared with 5 years of treatment.

Relevance

As is often the case in the history of science, other groups unknown to each other were studying adjuvant tamoxifen at the same time. So, although this was the first study to report a benefit, it must not be considered in isolation. The NATO trial together with others (some of which are cited in the related references) paved the way for the first overview in 1985 that revolutionized the treatment of breast cancer for the next 15 years. The Scottish trial (related reference 1) suggested a greater benefit of 5 years therapy, the NSABP study (related reference 2) showed the benefit of adding tamoxifen to chemotherapy and the Swedish trial (related reference 3) was the first to point out the important long-term side-effect of endometrial cancer.

Paper 7*

Effects of adjuvant tamoxifen and of cytotoxic therapy on mortality in early breast cancer. An overview of 61 randomized trials among 28 896 women

Authors

Early Breast Cancer Trialists' Collaborative Group (EBCTG)

Reference

New England Journal of Medicine 1988; **319**:1681–1692

Summary

Information was sought worldwide on mortality according to assigned treatment in all randomized trials that began before 1985 of adjuvant tamoxifen or cytotoxic therapy for early breast cancer (with or without regional lymph-node involvement). Coverage was reasonably complete for most countries. In 28 trials of tamoxifen nearly 4000 of 16 513 women had died, and in 40 chemotherapy trials slightly more than 4000 of 13 442 women had died. The 8106 deaths were approximately evenly distributed over 1,2,3,4 and 5+ years of follow-up, with little useful information beyond 5 years.

A systematic overview of the results of these trials demonstrated reductions in mortality due to treatment that were significant when tamoxifen was compared to no tamoxifen ($p < 0.0001$), and any chemotherapy with no chemotherapy ($p = 0.003$). In tamoxifen trials, there was a clear reduction in mortality only among women aged 50 or older, for whom assignment of tamoxifen reduced the annual odds of death during the first 5 years by about one-fifth. In the chemotherapy trials there was a clear reduction only among women under 50, for whom assignment of chemotherapy reduced the annual odds of death during the first 5 years by about a quarter. Direct comparisons showed that combination chemotherapy was significantly more effective than single-agent therapy, but suggested that the administration for chemotherapy for 8–24 months may offer no survival advantage over administration of the same chemotherapy for 4–6 months. Because it involved several thousand women, this overview was able to demonstrate particularly clearly that both tamoxifen and cytotoxic chemotherapy can reduce 5-year mortality.

Related references (1)   Early Breast Cancer Trialists' Group. Tamoxifen for early breast cancer: an overview of the randomized trials. *Lancet* 1998; **351**:1451–1467.

Key message

Ignoring the data for the chemotherapy trials which are covered elsewhere in this book, this paper confirms unequivocally that two or more years of adjuvant tamoxifen will reduce mortality following surgery for early breast cancer in women aged over 50 years.

---

* See also Paper 5 in Chapter 12.

Why it's important

Until this overview, conducted in 1985 and published three years later, there was a lot of uncertainty: some trials pointed one way and others showed no advantage. Many of the smaller trials were under-powered to detect a 20% risk reduction in mortality. By bringing all the studies together and using the new statistical tools available (see Chapter 2) it was possible to see the 'signal against the background noise'.

Strength

To bring together all the trials groups from around the world and persuade them to share their data was a *tour de force* in itself. The statistical methodology was so robust that no one could argue with the headline result. Therefore, almost overnight, tamoxifen became standard therapy for most post-menopausal women, leading ultimately to a sizeable proportion of the fall in mortality seen in the UK and the USA since 1988.

Weakness

Because of the large numbers and hence statistical power, small benefits in absolute reduction in mortality reached high levels of statistical significance, leading clinicians to treat according to '*p*-value' rather than a mature harm/benefit analysis. It took nearly another 10 years to appreciate that tamoxifen was also of benefit in premenopausal patients, even though this was apparent in some of the European trials that retained an untreated control arm. Unfortunately, the large American trials that kept chemotherapy as a control arm against which to judge the benefit of adding tamoxifen appeared to dilute the effect in the under-50s. On the other hand, the lack of quality control of the measurement of ER in the UK trials delayed the recognition of the interaction between tamoxifen and ER status for a similar period.

Relevance

Having established the methodology and the collaboration of the EBCTG, the process will continue to be repeated every 5 years under the leadership of Professor Sir Richard Peto. The next overview planned for 2005 should clear up the matter of the optimum duration of tamoxifen. In the meantime, other groups are working on user-friendly methods of translating the results for planning treatment of the individual woman.

Paper 8

Medical castration produced by the GnRH analogue leuprolide to treat metastatic breast cancer

Authors

Harvey HA, Lipton A, Max DT, *et al.*

Reference

Journal of Clinical Oncology 1985; **3**:1068–1072

Summary

Leuprolide, a gonadotrophin-releasing hormone (GnRH) analogue, was administered to 26 pre-menopausal women with metastatic breast cancer. Of 25 evaluable patients, 11 (44%) had a partial response with a median duration 39 weeks and 5 (20%) remained stable. Six patients showed early rapid progression of their disease. Toxicity was mild and included hot flushes, nausea, vomiting and headache. Leuprolide induced amenorrhoea in all cases who received treatment for 10 weeks or longer. The authors concluded that this GnRH analogue provided a safe and effective means of producing medical castration in premenopausal patients with metastatic breast cancer.

Related references **(1)** Hayward JL, Atkins HJB, Falconer MA *et al.* Clinical trials comparing transfrontal hypohysectomy with adrenalectomy and with transethmoidal hypohysectomy. In: *Clinical Management in Advanced Breast Cancer. Second Tenovus Workshop* (Joslin CAF, Gleave EN, eds). Cardiff: Alpha Omega Alpha Publishing, 1970: 50–53.

(2) Scally AV. Aspects of hypothalamic regulation of the pituitary gland. Its implication for the control of reproductive processes. *Science* 1978; **202**:18–28.

(3) Nicholson RJ, Finney EJ, Maynard PV. Activity of a new analogue of luteinising releasing hormone, ICI 118,630, on the growth of rat mammary tumours. *Journal of Endocrinology* 1976; **79**:51–52.

Key message

Medical castration by indirectly inhibiting ovarian function at the hypothalamic–pituitary level can achieve similar results in advanced breast cancer to those achieved by surgical oophorectomy.

Why it's important

Once it was established that the reduction of circulating oestradiol levels was associated with an objective response in a proportion of 'hormone-responsive' cases of metastatic breast cancer, and that these levels were controlled at the hypothalamic–pituitary level, a search went on to discover a treatment that inhibited this control mechanism. There was a short inglorious period, best forgotten, when surgeons undertook hypophysectomy, either as an open procedure or stereotactically, with insertion of radioactive sources. The morbidity of this procedure was awful, with diabetes insipidus being added to adrenocortical insufficiency and occasionally blindness from damage to the optic chiasma. The relatively non-toxic class of drugs, GnRH analogues, achieved all this safely and provided a simple reversible alternative to permanent ovarian ablation.

Strength

The authors describe evaluable patients and provide clear descriptions of criteria of response. They also demonstrate the impact of the drug on circulating oestradiol levels. In addition, patients are classified according to ER status and an attempt is made to correlate responses to pattern of disease and ER status.

Weakness

This was a small study of only 25 patients of whom 14 were ER+ and 10 ER− with a cut-off of >5 fmol/mg cytosol protein. It is not surprising that they failed to find a correlation of response with ER status.

Relevance

This description of a medical castration followed rapidly on the heels of a medical adrenalectomy. However, the morbidity of a surgical castration is nothing like that of an adrenalectomy. The relevance, therefore, is subtly different. First of all, to add castration to a woman who may already have been subjected to a mastectomy is psychologically damaging, adding insult to injury. Furthermore, as the ovarian suppression is reversible for some women, it leaves open the possibility of starting or completing their families, once treatment of their breast cancer is completed.

A whole raft of randomized trials of GnRH analogues has recently been completed, presented at meetings and awaiting publication, that addresses these issues (see the review by the author – Breast Cancer On-Line, October 2001). These have to be seen in conjunction with Paper 9, which begins to explore the possibility that at least part of the benefit of adjuvant chemotherapy in premenopausal women is achieved via a chemical castration.

Paper 9

Adjuvant ovarian ablation versus CMF chemotherapy in premenopausal women with pathological stage II breast cancer: The Scottish trial

Authors

Scottish Cancer Trials Breast Group and ICRF Breast Unit, Guy's Hospital London

Reference

Lancet 1993; **341**:1293–1298

Summary

During 10 years, 332 premenopausal women with node-positive breast cancer were randomized, after mastectomy or conservative therapy, to receive either ovarian ablation or CMF chemotherapy, each with or without prednisolone 7.5 mg daily for 5 years. After a maximum follow-up of 12 years, no significant overall differences were detected in relapse rates or in event-free or overall survival for ovarian ablation compared with chemotherapy or for prednisolone versus no prednisolone, nor was there any suggestion of interaction between these factors. Actuarial survival at 8 years was 60% overall, irrespective of treatment, with hazard ratio and confidence interval of 1.12 (0.76–1.63) for the comparison of CMF with ovarian ablation and 1.26 (0.86–1.84) for prednisolone versus no prednisolone. Oestrogen receptor (ER) assays were done in 270 (81%) primary tumours, but these results played no part in the randomization procedure. When patient outcome was analysed in relation to the concentration of ER in the tumour, there was a statistically significant interaction between ER content and treatment, such that ovarian ablation was associated with improved survival in patients with ER concentrations 20 fmol/mg protein or more, and CMF was more beneficial for patients with values less than 20 fmol/mg protein. No such interaction was seen for prednisolone therapy. The authors pointed out that ER content has a role to play in decisions about treatment for primary breast cancer.

Related references

(1) Rose DP, Davis TE. Ovarian function in women receiving chemotherapy for breast cancer. *Lancet* 1977; **ii**:1174–1176.

(2) Bianco AR, Del Mastro L, Gallo C, *et al.* Prognostic role of amenorrhoea induced by adjuvant chemotherapy in premenopausal women with early breast cancer. *British Journal of Cancer* 1991; **63**:799–803.

(3) Kaufman M, Jonat W, Blamey, J, *et al.* Survival analysis from the ZEBRA study: goserelin (Zoladex) versus CMF in premenopausal women with node-positive breast cancer. *European Journal of Cancer* 2003; **39**:1711–1717.

Key message

In unselected premenopausal patients with stage II breast cancer the outcome of ovarian ablation is similar to that of CMF chemotherapy. However, those with tumours that are ER+ fare better with the endocrine approach, while those with ER− tumours fare better on chemotherapy.

Why it's important

Adjuvant chemotherapy became 'default' therapy for node-positive premenopausal women shortly after the 1985 overview. At that time dissenting voices pointed to a number of facts suggesting that a component of this response could be mediated via a chemical castration. First, the benefit of chemotherapy appeared confined to the group under 50 years of age; second, chemotherapy lowers oestradiol and raises luteinizing hormone (LH)/follicle-stimulating hormone (FSH), and finally chemotherapy-induced amenorrhoea itself was a prognostic factor. This trial was the first of its kind to test this hypothesis. More recent trials have substituted a GnRH analogue for ovarian ablation.

Strength

This trial took a lot of courage to challenge the new dogma of adjuvant chemotherapy for node-positive premenopausal women. At the same time the authors tried to relate the outcome to ER status. They also attempted to answer a further question concerning the role of corticosteroids in the treatment of early breast cancer.

Weakness

The researchers were too ambitious and the trial was seriously underpowered and took so long to recruit that interest waned. In effect this was a 2×2 factorial trial with 85 or less patients in each of the possible treatment allocations. ER status was missing in 20% patients. Although 'equivalence' was claimed for the unselected patients, the confidence intervals were wide (0.76–1.63) for survival at 8 years. Although tests for interaction based on ER status were significant, these were not based on an *a priori* agreement on the cut-off level for ER content of the tumour and therefore have to be considered hypothesis generation.

Relevance

The subject of this trial is extremely topical at this time, although considering GnRH analogues instead of permanent ovarian ablation. Several trials have been reported, although at the time of writing none was published in full, comparing CMF-like regimens with a GnRH analogue alone or together with tamoxifen. Other trials have looked at the addition of a chemical castration to patients who have completed chemotherapy. The subject is in flux at the moment but two consensus conferences (one in the USA and one in Europe) have acknowledged that reversible chemical ovarian suppression should at least be offered as an alternative to chemotherapy for young women with good-prognosis ER+ tumours and might be added to chemotherapy for poor-prognosis ER+ cases who fail to achieve amenorrhoea.

Paper 10

Anastrozole alone or in combination with tamoxifen versus tamoxifen alone for adjuvant treatment of postmenopausal women with early breast cancer: First results of the ATAC randomised trial

Authors

The ATAC Trialist's Group

Reference

Lancet 2002; **359**:2131–2139

Summary

In the adjuvant setting, tamoxifen is the established treatment for postmenopausal women with hormone-sensitive breast cancer. However, it is associated with several side-effects, including endometrial cancer and thromboembolic disorders. The ATAC (Arimidex, Tamoxifen, Alone or in Combination) trial aimed to compare the safety and efficacy outcomes of tamoxifen with those of anastrozole (Arimidex) alone and the combination of anastrozole plus tamoxifen for 5 years.

Participants were postmenopausal patients with invasive operable breast cancer who had completed primary therapy and were eligible to receive adjuvant hormonal therapy. The primary endpoints were disease-free survival and occurence of adverse events. Analysis for efficacy was by intention to treat.

The study recruited 9366 patients, of whom 3125 were randomly assigned anastrozole, 3116 tamoxifen, and 3125 the combination. The median follow-up was 33.3 months. Of the patients, 7839 (84%) were known to be hormone receptor-positive. The disease-free survival rate at 3 years was 89.4% on anastrozole and 87.4% on tamoxifen (hazard ratio 0.83 [95% confidence interval (CI) 0.71–0.96], $p = 0.013$). Results with the combination were not significantly different from those with tamoxifen alone (87.2%, 1.02 [0.89–1.18], $p = 0.8$). The improvement in disease-free survival with anastrozole was seen in the subgroup of hormone receptor-positive patients. but not the receptor-negative patients. The incidence of contralateral breast cancer was significantly lower with anastrozole than with tamoxifen (odds ratio 0.42 [0.22–0.79], $p = 0.007$). Anastrozole was significantly better tolerated than tamoxifen with respect to endometrial cancer ($p = 0.02$), vaginal bleeding and discharge ($p = 0.0001$ for both), cerebrovascular events ($p = 0.0006$), venous thromboembolic events ($p = 0.0006$), and hot flushes ($p = 0.0001$). Tamoxifen was significantly better tolerated than anastrozole with respect to musculoskeletal disorders and fractures ($p < 0.0001$ for both).

The authors concluded that anastrozole is an effective and well-tolerated endocrine option for the treatment of postmenopausal patients with hormone-sensitive early breast cancer. They pointed out that longer follow-up is required before a final benefit–risk assessment can be made.

Related references **(1)**   Miller WR, O'Neill J. The importance of local synthesis of estrogen within the breast. Steroids 1987; **50**:4–6.

Key message

After only 2½ years' median period of treatment, anastrozole shows superior efficacy and tolerability to tamoxifen. In addition, anastrozole shows an approximate 60% reduction in the incidence of contralateral breast cancers compared with tamoxifen. The addition of anastrozole does not appear to add any advantage to tamoxifen on its own.

Why it's important

This paper has only recently appeared, yet is likely to become a classic in its time. Recruitment started 100 years after Beatson's description of surgical castration for advanced breast cancer. With over 9000 patients recruited, it is the largest trial of its kind to date and represents a remarkable collaboration of groups from around the world and between Industry (Astra-Zeneca) and academia. Anastrozole is one of the third-generation oral specific aromatase inhibitors that represents a culmination of the biochemical and endocrinological studies provoked by Huggins' work of 50 years ago (Paper 2). The size of the study bypasses the need for meta-analysis of several small studies and the result suggests that for the first time in nearly 20 years there may be an agent that is better than tamoxifen for the adjuvant treatment of early breast cancer and the prevention of cancer in high-risk populations.

Strengths

The very size of the trial is one of its strengths, allowing for a three-way analysis as well as the study of predefined subgroups based on ER status and presence or absence of prior chemotherapy. In addition prospective sub-protocols looking at the pathology of the primary tumour, pharmacokinetics of the drug interactions, endometrial pathology, lipid and bone mineral metabolism and quality of life, will allow a full harm/benefit analysis to be calculated after more mature follow-up. Furthermore, the counter-intuitive result for the combination arm is likely to keep another generation of endocrinologists in gainful employment!

Weakness

Like the overview, the large scale of this trial means that very small absolute differences in disease-free survival reach high levels of statistical significance and may provoke an over-reaction of the lay and medical populations. Only about 80% of the patients are of known ER+ status, the relevant group. Although an early side effect of anastrozole-induced oestrogen deprivation, namely fractures, is reported, there is a lingering concern about the long-term effects on cognitive function.

Relevance

Watch this space!

CHAPTER 14

Chemotherapy

CAROLINE LOHRISCH

MARTINE PICCART

Introduction

Chemotherapy is fairly new on the menu of therapies for breast cancer compared with local surgery, castration and radiotherapy. Initial randomized trials which showed a benefit of chemotherapy in early breast cancer did not emerge until the late 1960s. These early reports, demonstrating a survival advantage for single-agent melphalan and cyclophosphamide, stimulated a profusion of randomized trials which established many of the chemotherapy regimens which are still in regular use today, including cyclophosphamide–methotrexate–5 fluorouracil (CMF) and doxorubicin (Adriamycin)–cyclophosphamide (AC). Various combinations and strategies have been employed to try to improve upon these regimens in the ensuing years.

Adjuvant chemotherapy was initially targeted to women with node-positive disease, recognizing that node-negative breast cancer was associated with a lower recurrence risk, and appreciating the potential short and long term sequelae associated with chemotherapy. However, as experience and understanding of these side-effects increased, supportive care measures have been developed to minimize them. More recent studies established a survival benefit for chemotherapy in node-negative disease, particularly tumors associated with adverse prognostic features, and in young women. Studies have convincingly demonstrated a lower dose intensity threshold, below which results are compromised; however, dose intensification beyond that threshold have yet to further enhance survival.

The comprehensive Oxford meta-analyses, which reviewed all randomized comparisons of chemotherapy (among other topics), confirmed the survival advantage of both CMF and anthracycline-based chemotherapy, in both node-positive and negative disease, in young and older women, regardless of the added use of tamoxifen. As a result of this mammoth undertaking, we feel confident today that the majority of women with early breast cancer derive benefit from adjuvant polychemotherapy.

New cytotoxic drugs have emerged for the treatment of metastatic disease over the last two decades, the most promising of which are the taxanes and vinorelbine. Biologic agents which target molecules that may enhance tumor cell survival are available (trastuzumab (Herceptin)) or in various stages of clinical investigation (such as inhibitors of angiogenesis, of cell cycle regulators, and of multi-drug resistance protein pumps). The arsenal of therapeutic agents for metastatic disease has thus increased substantially. The high activity of taxanes in metastatic disease has led to randomized trials in the adjuvant setting to determine whether or not they are beneficial in early disease. With one trial showing a disease-free survival advantage for the addition of paclitaxel to AC, results of other ongoing adjuvant taxane trials are eagerly awaited.

The new paradigm in chemotherapy research for breast cancer involves targeted therapy by maximizing the use of markers predictive of response to various treatments. Recent advances in this area include the recognition that tumors that overexpress c-*erb*B-2 (HER2/neu) may be particularly sensitive to trastuzumab (Herceptin, an anti-HER2 monoclonal antibody) and to anthracycline dose intensity, that estrogen receptor-negative tumors may benefit preferentially from prolonged non-cross resistant chemotherapy (such as with AC followed by paclitaxel), and that tumors with *p53* mutations may be particularly succeptible to taxanes.

Despite the great strides that have been made in breast cancer chemotherapy, there are numerous outstanding questions being actively investigated. In the adjuvant setting, these include the additive role of chemotherapy and ovarian ablation in premenopausal women, the best regimen for specific tumor and patient profiles, and the role of taxanes and biologic agents. In the metastatic setting, herceptin has been one of the few new drugs to improve survival, and intense research combining classic cytotoxic therapies with new biologic agents is ongoing with the hope of finding other highly active combinations. The following chapter outlines the major representative trials which have contributed to the field of chemotherapy for early and advanced breast cancer to date, with emphasis on the points outlined above. Despite clear advantages of chemotherapy, it is ultimately a coordinated approach of individualized local therapy, hormonal and chemotherapy, and biologic therapy directed by the use of predictive and prognostic markers, that offers the best chance of continued survival gains in patients with breast cancer.

Paper 1

Combination chemotherapy as an adjuvant treatment in operable breast cancer

Authors

Bonadonna G, Brusamolino E, Valagussa P, *et al.*

Reference

New England Journal of Medicine 1976; **294**:405–410

Summary

This single-center trial compared relapse in women up to 75 years of age with operable node-positive breast cancer who were randomized to either CMF (cyclophosphamide 100 mg/m^2/d d1–14; methotrexate 40 mg/m^2 i.v. d1,8; 5-fluorouracil (5-Fu) 600 mg/m^2 i.v. d1,8 q28d for 12 cycles) or observation following surgery. Stratification was according to age ($\leq$49 vs. 50–75), number of positive nodes (1–3 vs. >3), and type of mastectomy (radical vs. extended radical), and 5 of 391 enrolled patients were not evaluable. With a follow-up of 27 months, the relapse rate for CMF-treated patients ($n = 207$) was 5.3%, while for control patients ($n = 179$) it was 24%, representing a highly significant difference, $p < 10^{-6}$. The improvement in relapse-free survival observed with CMF was evident in all stratification groups, as well as pre- and postmenopausal women, and tumor T^m stages 1–3. Nausea during cyclophosphamide treatment was experienced in the majority of patients, and mucositis, alopecia, cystitis, and amenorrhea occurred in 18%, 55%, 28%, and 54%, respectively. Hematologic toxicity was modest, with grade 2 leucopenia and thrombocytopenia (both of which required treatment delay according to the protocol rules) occurring in 4% and 14%, respectively; only 10 patients (4.8%) received < 6 cycles. The average dose intensities of the three drugs were cyclophosphamide 76%, methotrexate 80%, and 5-FU 81%.

Related references (1)   Bonadonna G, Valagussa P, Moliterni A, *et al.* Adjuvant cyclophosphamide, methotrexate, and fluorouracil in node-positive breast cancer. The results of 20 years of follow-up. *New England Journal of Medicine* 1995; **332**:901–926.

(2)   Howell A, Bush H, George WD, *et al.* Controlled trial of adjuvant chemotherapy with cyclophosphamide, methotrexate, and fluorouracil for breast cancer. *Lancet* 1984; **ii**:307–311.

Key message

The natural history of node-positive early breast cancer can be influenced by the use of systemic adjuvant CMF chemotherapy (CT), resulting in superior relapse-free survival compared with that observed with only local therapy (surgery with or without radiation).

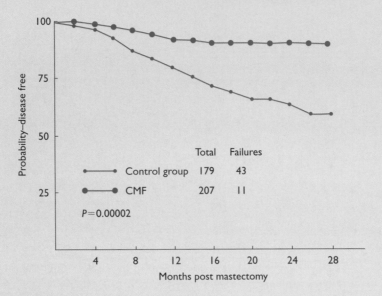

Figure 14.1 Recurrence-free survival with CMF compared with observation in node-positive breast cancer.

Why it's important

This trial was among the first, along with the Scandinavian Adjuvant chemotherapy Study Group trial of cyclophosphamide vs observation [1] and the National Surgical Adjuvant Breast and Bowel Project (NSABP) comparison of melphalan vs. placebo in a similar patient populations [2], to demonstrate an advantage of adjuvant CT in node-positive operable breast cancer in terms of relapse, and with longer follow-up, of survival [3]. These results were subsequently confirmed by numerous trials and by the Oxford overviews [4,5]. Adjuvant CT, and in particular CMF, became the standard of care throughout Europe and America almost universally as a result. It also inspired investigators to examine the ability of systemic therapies to alter the natural history of node-negative breast cancer, leading to a generation of randomized trials in this population.

Strengths

1. The accrual period was short (just over 2 years), with no patients lost to follow-up and only a minor percentage of protocol violations (4.8%).
2. There was stratification for prognostic factors known at that time (age, number of positive nodes).
3. There was a reasonable work-up to exclude metastatic disease prior to enrolment, and during the follow-up period.

Weakness

There is no description of the statistical design and/or the method used to determine the number of patients to be enrolled.

Relevance

This same chemotherapy combination, developed over 30 years ago, is still widely used in adjuvant therapy of breast cancer, although anthracyclines are now generally preferred in node-positive disease. The recognition that adjuvant CT is warranted in the majority of women with early breast cancer remains unchallenged today.

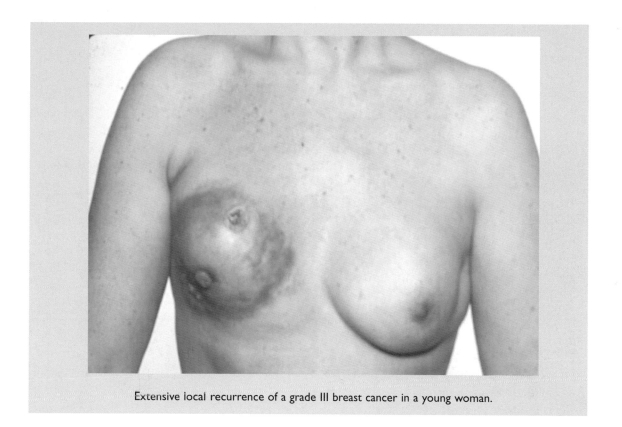

Extensive local recurrence of a grade III breast cancer in a young woman.

Paper 2

Adjuvant CMF in breast cancer: comparative 5-year results of 12 versus 6 cycles

Authors

Tancini G, Bonadonna G, Valagussa P, Marchini S, Veronesi U

Reference

Journal of Clinical Oncology 1983; **1**:2–10

Summary

This randomized trial examined whether a reduction in the duration of adjuvant CMF CT could be safely achieved in node-positive breast cancer without compromising its efficacy. Four hundred and fifty-nine eligible patients were randomized to 12 or 6 monthly cycles of CMF (Bonadonna regimen [6]) after primary surgery and exclusion of metastatic disease. Based on early results from the CMF vs. observation trial by the same group, which suggested that CMF did not benefit postmenopausal women [6], randomization of postmenopausal women was discontinued after the first year, instead allocating them all to 12 CMF for the following 12 months, and thereafter excluding them from the trial (last 14 months of accrual). At 59 months of follow-up, relapse-free survival which was the primary endpoint of the trial, was not significantly different in the 12- and 6-month CMF groups (59% vs. 65.6%, $p = 0.17$, respectively), and no significant differences were observed when treatment assignment was examined in subgroups of 1–3 or >3 nodes for both the population as a whole and divided by menopausal status. Treatment at the time of relapse was uniform according to menopausal and estrogen receptor status, and overall survival was not significantly different in the two arms. Toxicity was similar in the two groups, although a description of any added toxicity with the longer CT course is not provided.

Key message

Adjuvant CMF chemotherapy can be safely reduced from 12 to 6 months without compromising efficacy (in terms of relapse-free and overall survival) in node-positive early breast cancer.

Why it's important

After demonstrating that adjuvant CT could improve the natural history of early breast cancer [6], it became important to identify the minimum amount of effective therapy, both in terms of duration, the focus of this trial, and dose intensity, which was the focus of subsequent trials. The advantage of equally effective shorter therapy is in being able to minimize toxicity, thus enhancing patient acceptance and physician recommendation of adjuvant therapy, which although relatively routine now, was at that time still a novel concept.

Strength

This was a randomized controlled trial with short accrual period, uniform follow-up and few protocol violations.

Weaknesses

1. There is no description of statistical design, so it is impossible to determine if there was truly no difference between the two treatment arms, or if the study was not adequately powered to detect a clinically important difference. However, the fact that both relapse-free and overall survival figures were higher in the 6-month CMF group suggests that this latter possibility is unlikely.

2. The way in which treatment randomization and allocation for postmenopausal women was altered during the trial is unclear. When the decision was made to act on the observation from another trial that they did not benefit from CMF, exclusion of all postmenopausal women from further enrolment would have been the cleanest modification to the protocol. Since postmenopausal women were allocated to 12 months of CMF for 12 of the 32-month accrual period, the proportion of postmenopausal women was higher in the 12- than 6-month CMF group. If their hypothesis that postmenopausal women did not benefit from CMF was correct, this could have reduced the observed efficacy in the 12-month CMF arm, thus resulting in a non-significant difference between the two arms. However, we know from more mature data of the first trial [7] and from the Oxford overview [5], that postmenopausal NP breast cancer patients do benefit from adjuvant CT, both in the presence and absence (such as these patients) of hormonal therapy.

Relevance

This trial demonstrated that 6 months of adjuvant CT for early breast cancer was equivalent to 12 months, a finding later confirmed by the Oxford overview [3]. This resulted in a change in practise, with many oncology centers worldwide currently giving less than 12 months of adjuvant CMF.

Paper 3

A randomized clinical trial evaluating sequential methotrexate and fluorouracil in the treatment of patients with node-negative breast cancer who have estrogen-receptor-negative tumors

Authors

Fisher B, Redmond C, Dimitrov NV, *et al.*

Reference

New England Journal of Medicine 1989; **320**:473–478

Summary

This trial randomized women ≤70 years old, with node-negative breast cancer thought to be at high risk of recurrence by virtue of having estrogen receptor-negative (< 10 fmol) disease, to observation or 12 monthly cycles of methotrexate (100 mg/m^2 d1,8 i.v.) and 5-fluorouracil (600 mg/m^2 d1,8 i.v.) (MF). Patients were stratified by age (≤49, ≥50 years old), T^m size, type of operation, and estrogen receptor level (0–2, 3–9 fmol). With four years of follow-up, disease-free survival was significantly better in the MF arm: 80% vs. 71%, $p = 0.003$. This was true for both older and younger women. There were fewer local and distant recurrences in the MF group; however, overall survival for all ages was similar (87% MF, 86% observation, $p = 0.8$). Compliance was relatively high: 66% of the 235 patients eligible to receive 12 cycles of MF received 100% of the cycles, and a minimal number of dose reductions were required due to hematological toxicity.

Related references **(1)**   Systemic therapy in patients with node-negative breast cancer. A commentary based on two National Surgical Adjuvant Breast and Bowel Project (NSABP) clinical trials. *Annals of Internal Medicine* 1989; **111**:703–712.

        (2)   Fisher B, Dignam J, Mamounas EP, *et al.* Sequential methotrexate and fluorouracil for the treatment of node-negative breast cancer patients with estrogen receptor-negative tumors: eight-year results from National Surgical Adjuvant Breast and Bowel Project (NSABP) B-13 and first report of findings from NSABP B-19 comparing methotrexate and fluorouracil with conventional cyclophosphamide, methotrexate, and fluorouracil. *Journal of Clinical Oncology* 1996; **14**:1982–1992.

Key message

The risk of recurrence following high-risk node-negative breast cancer can be reduced with the addition of adjuvant chemotherapy.

Why it's important

This trial provided clear evidence that superior outcome was achievable in high-risk node-negative breast cancer with systemic adjuvant CT. Prior to this study, physicians were reluctant to give adjuvant CT for this type of breast cancer, because the relapse risk was felt to be low and did not justify the CT-associated morbidity. However, based on the NSABP B-06 trial [8], in which 25% of node-negative patients with no systemic therapy relapsed and 15% died within 5 years, an exploration of whether CT might be of benefit in this high-risk disease was undertaken. A superior disease-free survival with MF was observed for both younger and older women with estrogen receptor-negative disease, which was maintained through 8 years of follow-up [9]. Overall survival was also shown to be prolonged in older women at 8 years follow-up (89% MF, 80% observation, $p = 0.03$) but not in younger women (although subset analyses limit the power of these observations). Building on these results, subsequent trials demonstrated superior disease-free and borderline overall survival improvement in node-negative, estrogen receptor-positive disease with CMF versus MF (NSABP B-19) [9], and in node-negative, estrogen receptor-positive disease with CMF + tamoxifen versus tamoxifen (disease-free survival 90% vs. 84%, $p < 0.01$; overall survival 97% and 94%, respectively) (NSABP B20) [10]. Additionally, this trial suggested that young age might be an adverse prognostic factor, which has since been incorporated in the St Gallen risk stratification guidelines [11]. More recent trials explored the value of anthracycline-containing CT over CMF [12], and are attempting to better define the population of node-negative breast cancers with high recurrence risk [13].

Strengths

1. This was a large randomized trial in a relatively narrow risk population (those who are both node and estrogen receptor-negative), allowing a specific question to be answered.
2. The protocol was modified to allow lumpectomy with radiation therapy when it became clear that this approach was equivalent to mastectomy [8]. Radiotherapy was given concurrently with MF, so systemic treatment delivery timing was preserved.

Weaknesses

1. No power calculation is provided to describe how the number of enrolled patients was selected.
2. It is not clear whether the follow-up schedule for the two groups was similar.

Relevance

This pivotal trial demonstrated both the need to establish markers of high risk in node-negative breast cancer, and the benefit of chemotherapy in such high-risk patients. Estrogen receptor-negative status and young age are now accepted as adverse prognostic factors, and women with these characteristics are routinely offered adjuvant CT in the majority of centers. Refinement of systemic therapy, in terms of both the optimal regimen and the optimal target population, has been the focus of numerous subsequent trials.

Paper 4

Adjuvant chemotherapy with doxorubicin plus cyclophosphamide, methotrexate, and fluorouracil in the treatment of resectable breast cancer with more than three positive axillary nodes

Authors

Buzzoni R, Bonadonna G, Valagussa P, Zambetti M

Reference

Journal of Clinical Oncology 1991; **9**:2134–2140

Summary

This randomized trial demonstrated that in early breast cancer patients with >3 positive nodes, giving 4 cycles of doxorubicin followed by 8 cycles of CMF (sequential regimen) produced superior 5-year relapse-free and overall survival than giving the same drugs at the same total doses, given as 2 cycles of CMF alternating with 1 cycle of doxorubicin (alternating regimen). Delivered dose intensity and toxicities were similar in both arms. The superior relapse-free survival for the sequential regimen has been maintained at 10 years of follow-up [13], at which time superior overall survival was also demonstrated for this group.

Related reference   **(1)**   Bonadonna G, Zambetti M, Valagussa P. Sequential or alternating doxorubicin and CMF regimens in breast cancer with more than three positive nodes. Ten-year results. *Journal of the American Medical Association* 1995; **273**:542–547.

                           (2)   Citron M, Berry D, Cirrincione C, *et al.* Superiority of dose-dense (DD) over conventional scheduling (CS) and equivalence of sequential (SC) vs. combination adjuvant chemotherapy (CC) for node-positive breast cancer (CALGB 9741, INT C9741). *Breast Cancer Research and Treatment* 2002; **76** (Supp 1): S32, abstract 15.

Key message

Alternating cytotoxic drugs leads to longer inter-treatment intervals between exposure of malignant cells to drugs to which they are potentially sensitive, and thus drug resistance may develop, resulting in inferior survival compared to the same total drug doses given sequentially (i.e. the same drug at shorter inter-treatment intervals).

Why it's important

These results support the Gompertzian growth theory [15], in which a tumor doubling time increases as the tumor size increases. Although small tumors grow faster, they are also more susceptible to CT. The corollary is that as the number of cells decreases and the proportion killed increases with each cycle, the rate of regrowth also increases. Increasing CT dose increases cell kill but does not influence the regrowth kinetics, which may be more effectively targeted by shortening the inter-treatment interval. Thus longer intervals between the same cytotoxic drugs in the alternating regimen may enable some previously sensitive cells to develop multidrug resistance.

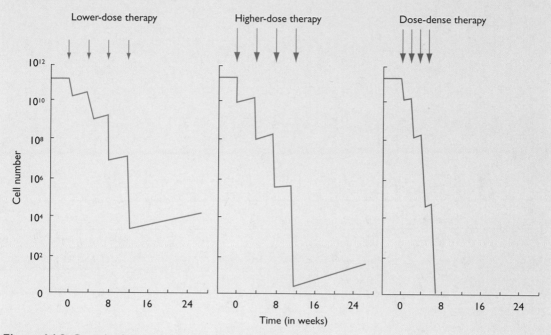

Figure 14.2 Growth of tumors between chemotherapy cycles.

Strengths

1. The same drugs and total drug doses were given in both arms, making this a pure sequence comparison.

2. The delivered dose intensity was high in both arms (92% sequential, 94% alternating).

3. There was stratification for menopausal status and complimentary local therapy as well as a similar follow-up schedule in both arms.

Weaknesses

1. There was a long accrual period, 8.4 years.

2. A higher proportion of women with >10 nodes positive were randomized to the alternating regimen, so this group had an overall worse baseline risk, which may in part account for their inferior outcome.

3. Dose reductions for hematologic toxicity were substantially higher than what would be recommended currently.

4. The CMF schedule used (d1 every 21 days) has been shown to be inferior in metastatic disease [16] (although it was given in both arms).

5. Results from a comparison of doxorubicin followed by CMF to AC alone or CMF (Bonadonna regimen [6]) alone would be more applicable today.

Relevance

The sequential regimen used in this trial has widely influenced the adjuvant chemotherapy practise in Europe. Several cycles of anthracyclines are generally followed by several cycles of CMF in patients for whom anthracyclines are warranted, although a total of 12 cycles is not universally given. A recent trial (see related reference (2)) has suggested superiority of standard chemotherapy (AC or AC/paclitaxel) given every two weeks rather than every three weeks [17], again supporting the Gompertzian growth theory, and leading to a shift at least in the United States, to this dose dense approach.

Paper 5

Two months of doxorubicin–cyclophosphamide with and without interval reinduction therapy compared with 6 months of cyclophosphamide, methotrexate, and fluorouracil in positive-node breast cancer patients with tamoxifen-nonresponsive tumors: Results from the National Surgical Adjuvant Breast and Bowel Project B-15

Authors

Fisher B, Brown AM, Dimitrov NV, *et al.*

Reference

Journal of Clinical Oncology 1990; **8**:1483–1496

Summary

This large randomized trial compared disease-free survival (DFS) and overall survival (OS) in tamoxifen non-responsive node-positive breast cancer patients randomized to AC × 4 (60 mg/m^2 and 600 mg/m^2 d1 q21d), CMF × 6 (C 100 mg/m^2 p.o. d1–14, M 40 mg/m^2 d1,8 i.v., F 600 mg/m^2 d1,8 i.v. q28d), or AC × 4 followed by a 6-month break and then CMF × 3 (C 750 mg/m^2 i.v. d1, M 40 mg/m^2 d1,8 i.v., F 600 mg/m^2 d1,8 i.v. q28d). Patients were stratified for the number of positive nodes, level of progesterone receptor (PgR) positivity, and type of surgery. At 26 months median follow-up, 2194 eligible patients were analysed: DFS (AC 62%, CMF 63%, AC/CMF 68% $p = 0.5$), distant-DFS, and OS (AC 90.6%, CMF 90%, AC/CMF 90% $p = 0.8$) were similar for all three groups. AC was tolerated better in that it was of shorter overall duration and had less hematologic toxicity, nausea, diarrhea, weight gain, and hemorrhagic cystitis; however, this group experienced more alopecia and vomiting. In the two AC groups, dose reductions were not allowed: delays were instituted if the white blood cell (WBC) or platelet counts were too low to deliver the next cycle at the scheduled time. In the CMF-only arm, after a delay to allow hematologic recovery, subsequent doses were reduced to 75% if the WBC was between 2500 and 3500 or platelets were 75,000–100,000; 100% were given if WBC was ≥ 3500 and platelets were ≥ 100,000. The median delivered doses of C, M, and F were slightly lower in this group compared with A and C in the first 2 groups: 30–35% of patients in the CMF group did not receive at least 80% of drugs at the planned dose intensity, compared with only 11–15% in the two AC groups (for A and C).

Key message

Four cycles of AC provides equivalent DFS as 6 cycles of conventional CMF. The reintroduction of CMF several months after AC does not improve the outcome observed with AC alone. AC appears to require less treatment delay due to myelosuppression.

Why it's important

This trial provided justification for the use of AC $\times$ 4 or conventional CMF $\times$ 6 as equivalent adjuvant CT regimens in node-positive breast cancer. As a result, the majority of North American oncology centers adopted these as interchangeable regimens, selecting one or the other depending on individual preference and circumstance. A more recent trial [17] and the Oxford overview [5] have suggested that anthracycline-based regimens may provide additional benefit over CMF, particularly in node-positive disease, and the current trend is to favour anthracycline-based CT in this scenario. However AC $\times$ 4 and CMF $\times$ 6 are still frequently accepted as equivalent options in node-negative breast cancer. In North America, the result of this trial also largely led to the abandonment of the combination of several cycles of CMF following anthracycline-based CT.

Strengths

1. This was a large trial with uniform entry criteria, short accrual period, and few ineligible patients.

2. A power calculation was provided (10% DFS and 7% OS differences at 3 years).

Weaknesses

1. Dose reduction for hematologic toxicity was only instituted for the CMF arm, which undoubtedly accounts for the lower delivered dose intensity in this arm compared with the AC and AC/CMF arms.

2. Follow-up is too short to comment on survival differences for the three arms.

3. The potential importance of anthracycline cumulative dose was not investigated: although AC $\times$ 4 may be equivalent to CMF $\times$ 6, recent studies suggest that anthracycline regimens are superior to CMF [4]. Thus AC $\times$ 4 may not be as effective as longer courses with a higher total dose of anthracycline.

Relevance

This trial led to the acceptance in North America (predominantly) of AC (60/600 mg/m^2 i.v. d1 q21d $\times$ 4) as a standard adjuvant regimen. It is widely used today for both node-positive and negative breast cancer. Subsequent trials in high-risk disease have examined the value of increasing the total dose and/or the dose density (reducing the interval between cycles) of doxorubicin [18] or cyclophosphamide [19,20], although thus far neither strategy has proved to offer an advantage over conventional doses. The addition of taxanes to anthracycline-based adjuvant CT is an exciting current avenue of investigation. It is being addressed by several large co-operative trials, and early results of at least one offer some promise of superior DFS and OS with paclitaxel [18].

Paper 6

Randomized trial of intensive cyclophosphamide, epirubicin, and fluorouracil chemotherapy compared with cyclophosphamide, methotrexate, and fluorouracil in premenopausal women with node-positive breast cancer

Authors

Levine MN, Bramwell VH, Pritchard KI, *et al.* for the National Cancer Institute of Canada Clinical Trials Group

Reference

Journal of Clinical Oncology 1998; **16**:2651–2658

Summary

This adjuvant randomized trial demonstrated significantly better relapse-free survival (RFS: 63% vs. 53%, $p = 0.009$) and OS (77% vs. 70%, $p = 0.03$) for an anthracycline-containing regimen (CEF: cyclophosphamide, epirubicin, and 5-FU) over Bonadonna-CMF [5] in premenopausal breast cancer patients with involved axillary nodes. Patients had either lumpectomy with radiation (RT) or mastectomy, and were then randomized to 6 cycles of CMF or CEF. Study endpoints were RFS, OS, quality of life (QOL), and toxicity. Stratification was according to type of surgery (as above), estrogen receptor and progesterone receptor status, and number of involved nodes (1–3, 4–10, >10). The advantage of CEF was observed despite significantly greater toxicity (including 5 cases of acute myeloid leukemia, 4 of which were fatal) and lower delivered dose intensity (77% for CEF, 88% for CMF, $p = 0.0001$). Women with >3 positive nodes had more benefit from CEF (hazard ratio for RFS 1.41, 95% confidence interval [CI] 1.02–1.95; OS 82% CEF vs. 78% CMF) than women with 1–3 positive nodes (hazard ratio 1.26, 95% CI 0.91–1.74; OS 70% CEF vs. 58% CMF). QOL was lower with CEF; however, by 6 months after completion of CT, there was no difference in QOL scores for the two treatment groups.

Related reference   **(1)**   Carpenter JT, Velez-Garcia E, Aron BS, *et al.* Five-year results of a randomized comparison of cyclophosphamide, doxorubicin, and fluorouracil versus cyclophosphamide, methotrexate, and fluorouracil for node-positive breast cancer. *Proceedings of the American Society of Clinical Oncology* 1994; **13**:68a [abstr].

Key message

Anthracycline-based chemotherapy offers a RFS and OS advantage over CMF in node-positive operable breast cancer. However, given the increased toxicity and approximately 1.8% risk of secondary leukemia with CEF, the risk–benefit ratio is more balanced in the subgroup of women with >3 positive nodes, who have both a higher relapse risk and more significant benefit from CEF.

Why it's important

At the time that this trial was designed, substantial controversy existed over whether anthracycline-based adjuvant CT is superior to non-anthracycline-based CT. This study supports the selected use of anthracycline regimes like CEF in high-risk (node-positive) disease, where the clear benefit offsets the higher morbidity. Previous trials that failed to show a difference between CMF and anthracycline had lower anthracycline total dose and dose intensity [21–24], shorter follow-up [23], or gave anthracyclines only several months after the primary surgery and CMF [24]. The Oxford overview [5] found a small advantage with anthracyclines over CMF which was of borderline significance; however, this included node-negative patients, which may have diluted the advantage of anthracyclines in high-risk disease. Moreover, many of these trials had flawed designs. There is still controversy about whether node-negative breast cancer patients benefit substantially more from anthracycline-based CT, given a very small advantage demonstrated in one trial [12], and their low overall relapse risk. A recent trial has suggested that certain patient subsets, such as those whose tumors overexpress c-*erb*B-2, may have particular benefit from anthracycline-containing regimens [25].

Strengths

1. The distribution of baseline prognostic characteristics was similar in both groups.
2. The statistical hypothesis, sample size, and number of events needed (power calculation) were well defined.
3. QOL assessments were included prospectively.

Weakness

This trial was designed to compare dose-intense CEF to conventional dose CMF. However, only 77% of intended doses of cyclophosphamide, epirubicin, and 5-FU could be delivered due to hematologic toxicity, making it a difficult regimen to recommend for routine use in women with less than high relapse risk.

Relevance

This trial demonstrates the small but nevertheless real survival advantage of anthracycline-based adjuvant CT over CMF in high-risk (node-positive) breast cancer, which was also suggested by the Oxford overview [4]. As a result of this key trial, epirubicin became registered in the United States for adjuvant node-positive breast cancer therapy. Inclusion of this data, and other recent similar comparisons, in the 2000 Oxford overview will provide a greater patient number, perhaps eliminating any remaining doubt about this question. In multiple node-positive disease, the majority of clinicians favor anthracycline-based regimens in the absence of contraindications to anthracyclines.

Paper 7

Polychemotherapy for early breast cancer: An overview of the randomized trials

Authors

Early Breast Cancer Trialists' Collaborative Group

Reference

Lancet 1998; **352**:930–942

Summary

This is a comprehensive summary of randomized adjuvant poly-CT trials (about 30 000 women, 69 trials) of prolonged vs. no CT, anthracycline-containing regimens vs. CMF, and short vs. longer CT. Absolute improvements in 10-year overall survival for women <50 were 11% and 7% for node-positive and negative disease (baseline risk, no CT 42% and 71%), respectively, and 3% and 2%, respectively for women >50 (baseline risk 46% and 71%). No difference in overall survival was observed for >6 vs. ≤6 months of CT. Anthracycline-containing CT was associated with an 11% greater relative reduction in death over CMF; however, results from some recent large comparative trials were not available. CT-associated toxicity was not addressed, except all-cause mortality, which was similar in the CT-treated and untreated groups.

Related reference **(1)** Early Breast Cancer Trialists' Collaborative Group. Systemic treatment of early breast cancer by hormonal, cytotoxic, or immune therapy. *Lancet* 1992; **339**:1–15.

Key message

Three to six months of adjuvant CT using CMF or anthracycline-containing regimens significantly reduces relapse and death in node-negative and node-positive breast cancer. Given the smaller absolute benefit in older women (2–3%) compared with younger women (7–11%), a decision to offer CT should always take potential side-effects into consideration.

Why it's important

Following this publication, which updates data from 1992 [4], there can be no lingering doubt that adjuvant CT improves overall survival. This is of particular importance in node-negative breast cancer, where a controversy existed about the absolute benefit of CT given low recurrence risk and potential treatment-related morbidity. There are several subgroups for which the magnitude of the benefit of CT remains speculative, such as node-negative disease with good prognostic features, and elderly women with estrogen receptor-positive tumors.

Strength

The group has expressed commitment to regular periodic re-analysis of these and more recently published trials so that updated information will be made available and currently unresolved questions may become clearer.

Weakness

Because the trials are heterogeneous, limited subset analyses can be performed. Thus it is difficult to ascertain the magnitude of benefit of CT in all patient subgroups, and the incremental benefit of CT over tamoxifen in subgroups such as low risk postmenopausal women with estrogen receptor-positive tumors, for whom tamoxifen is clearly indicated.

Relevance

Together with the St Gallen consensus guidelines for risk stratification and adjuvant treatment [11], the results summarized in this paper can be used to guide the decision to offer a patient with early breast cancer adjuvant systemic therapy.

Paper 8

Meeting highlights: International Consensus Panel on the treatment of primary breast cancer

Authors

Goldhirsch A, Glick JH, Gelber RD, Senn HJ

Reference

Journal of the National Cancer Institute 1998; **90**:1601–1608

Summary

This document provides guidelines for adjuvant systemic therapy according to risk stratification, based on well studied evidence about prognostic factors and the benefits of available systemic adjuvant therapies, and compiled by a panel of 40 breast cancer experts. Adjuvant systemic therapy is not recommended for women with less than 10% recurrence risk over 10 years. For all others, risk is divided into node-negative low-, intermediate-, and high-risk disease, and node-positive disease. Degree of risk in node-negative breast cancer takes into consideration tumor size, histologic and nuclear grade, hormone receptor status, tumor invasion of lymphatic and vascular spaces, and patient age (Table 14.1). Treatment recommendations for each of these categories is given for pre-menopausal, postmenopausal, and elderly women separately, and takes into consideration the level and amount of evidence existing about various systemic modalities, and when possible, patient preference (Table 14.2). The consensus highlights that although the Oxford overview concluded that ovarian ablation improves overall survival compared to control in young women [26], recommendation for the routine use of this modality must await mature results of comparative trials to adjuvant CT [27–29]. Five years of adjuvant tamoxifen is recommended for all women with hormone receptor-positive breast cancer with the exception of low-risk node-negative breast cancer according to patient preference; more than 5 years remains investigational. Neoadjuvant CT and endocrine therapy are acknowledged to enhance breast conserving surgery but do not alter survival compared with adjuvant delivery of these modalities. Anthracycline-based therapy is considered slightly superior to, but slightly more toxic than CMF CT. Anthracycline–tamoxifen but not CMF–tamoxifen combinations are concluded to provide superior survival over single modality. New issues since the previous St Gallen consensus [30,31] include the emerging availability of genetic testing of women at risk of hereditary breast cancer, of chemopreventive agents for high-risk and postmenopausal women, of sentinel-node biopsy, of neoadjuvant CT and endocrine therapy, of improved local control with radiation after mastectomy in women with high local recurrence risk, and preliminary results of comparisons of CT to CT plus ovarian ablation in pre-menopausal women. The optimal treatment for the increasing incidence of ductal carcinoma *in situ*, the need for full axillary dissection in cases with microscopic invasion of the sentinel node, the role of biologic therapies, of chemoprevention and the need for predictive markers of response, such as hormone receptor status and c-*erb*B-2 overexpression, are highlighted as areas of ongoing investigation.

Related reference   **(1)**   The steering committee on Clinical Practice Guidelines for the care and treatment of breast cancer. Adjuvant systemic therapy for women with node-positive and node-negative breast cancer. *Canadian Medical Association Journal* 1998; **158**(Suppl 3):S43–51, S52–64.

Key message

By summarizing the wealth of available level I–II evidence, it is possible to provide general adjuvant treatment recommendations for premenopausal, postmenopausal, and elderly women with breast cancer according to the degree of recurrence risk.

Table 14.1 Risk categories for patients with node-negative breast cancer

Factors*	Minimal/low risk (has all listed factors)	Intermediate risk (risk classified between the other two categories)	High risk (has at least one listed factor)
Tumor size†	≤1 cm	>1–2 cm	>2 cm
Estrogen receptor (ER) and/or progesterone receptor (PgR) status‡	Positive	Positive	Negative
Grade§	Grade 1 (uncertain relevance for tumors ≤1 cm)	Grade 1–2	Grade 2–3
Age, y‖	≥35		<35

  * Some panel members also recognize lymphatic and/or vascular invasion as an important feature that indicates an increased risk.

  † It was generally agreed by the panel members that pathologic tumor size (i.e., size of the invasive component) was the most important prognostic factor for defining the additional risk or relapse.

  ‡ ER status and PgR status are important biologic characteristics that identify responsiveness to endocrine therapies.

  § Histologic and/or nuclear grade.

  ‖ Patients who develop breast cancer at a young age are considered to be at high risk of relapse, although an exact age threshold for this increased risk has not been defined.

Why it's important

This document and others like it [32,33] enable clinicians to develop a consistent and evidence-based approach to the adjuvant treatment of breast cancer. Given the volume and variable strength of evidence available for various treatments and risk factors, summary guidelines assist clinicians to make evidence-based recommendations to their patients, and outline areas that are still investigational and/or controversial.

Strength

This represents consensus by some of the leading experts in the field who are familiar and up-to-date with the evidence and areas where evidence is lacking.

Weaknesses

1. Guidelines are descriptive, based on summary of the literature, and not statistically based. Although they are widely used, summary guidelines convened by experts are considered level IV evidence, even when based on level I primary sources. [34].

2. When all evidence on a particular topic points to a similar conclusion, guidelines can make confident statements. When divergent results exist, the guideline statement is subject to the bias of the expert panel.

Table 14.2 Adjuvant treatment for patients with node-negative (A) and node-positive (B) breast cancer*

A. Node negative			
Patient group	**Minimal/low risk**	**Intermediate risk**	**High risk**
Premenopausal, ER- or PgR-positive	**None or tamoxifen**	**Tamoxifen ± chemotherapy†** Ovarian ablation‡ GnRH analogue‡	**Chemotherapy + tamoxifen†** Ovarian ablation‡ GnRH analogue‡
Premenopausal, ER- and PgR-negative	Not applicable	Not applicable	**Chemotherapy§**
Postmenopausal, ER- or PgR-positive	**None or tamoxifen**	**Tamoxifen ± chemotherapy†**	**Tamoxifen + chemotherapy†**
Postmenopausal, ER- and PgR-negative	Not applicable	Not applicable	**Chemotherapy§**
Elderly	**None or tamoxifen**	**Tamoxifen ± chemotherapy**	**Tamoxifen** If no ER and PgR expression: **chemotherapy**

B. Node positive	
Patient group	**Treatments**
Premenopausal, ER- or PgR-positive	**Chemotherapy + tamoxifen** **Ovarian ablation** (or GnRH analogue) ± tamoxifen‡ Chemotherapy ± ovarian ablation or (GnRH analogue) ± tamoxifen‡
Premenopausal, ER- and PgR-negative	**Chemotherapy§**
Postmenopausal, ER- or PgR-positive	**Tamoxifen + chemotherapy†**
Postmenopausal ER- and PgR-negative	**Chemotherapy§**
Elderly	**Tamoxifen** If no ER and PgR expression: **chemotherapy**

* ER = estrogen receptor: PgR = progesterone receptor: GnRH = gonadotropin-releasing hormone. Bold entries are treatments accepted for routine use or baseline in clinical trials.

† The addition of chemotherapy is considered an acceptable option based on evidence from clinical trials. Considerations about a low relative risk of relapse, age, toxic effects, socioeconomic implications, and information on patient's preference might justify the use of **tamoxifen alone**.

‡ Indicates treatments still being tested in randomized clinical trials.

§ The addition of tamoxifen following chemotherapy might be considered for patients whose tumors are classified as ER- and PgR-negative but which exhibit minimal/trace levels of either ER or PgR.

Relevance

Guidelines such as these are widely used by clinicians to guide their treatment recommendations. They enable the clinician to remain relatively up-to-date in the area of breast cancer therapy without having to read every randomized trial published in the field. However, it must be recognized that these guidelines are only published periodically and can become outdated fairly rapidly when new evidence emerges.

Paper 9

Dose and dose intensity of adjuvant chemotherapy for stage II, node-positive breast carcinoma

Authors

Wood WC, Budman DR, Korzun AH, *et al.*

Reference

New England Journal of Medicine 1994; **330**:1253–1259

Summary

By comparing three schedules of CAF (cyclophosphamide, doxorubicin, and 5-FU), this was the first study to prospectively demonstrate a threshold dose intensity of adjuvant CT for breast cancer below which disease-free and overall survival were compromised. The 3 arms were: (1) 4 × C 600 d1, A 60 d1, F 600 d1,8 q28d; (2) 6 × C 400 d1, A 40 d1, F 400 d1,8 q28d; (3) 4 × C 300 d1, A 30 d1, F 300 d1,8 q28d (doses given in mg/m^2). Ninety-five percent of the patients received at least 90% of their assigned doses; 22 patients received no treatment and were not included in the analysis (together with 21 patients with inadequate follow-up data). Both disease-free and overall survival were significantly poorer in group 3 (low dose intensity and low total dose arm) compared with groups 1 and 2; the differences between groups 1 and 2 were not significant. Benefits favoring the intermediate- and high-dose arms were seen in all subgroups (number of nodes, menopausal status, estrogen receptor status, T^m size, type of surgery). Toxicity was manageable and directly correlated with dose intensity. The disease-free and overall survival differences have been maintained through 9 years of follow-up [35], and the doses given in group 3 are now considered inadequate.

Related references **(1)** Bonadonna G, Valagussa P. Dose–response effect of adjuvant chemotherapy in breast cancer. *New England Journal of Medicine* 1981; **304**:10–15.

(2) Bonneterre J, Roche H, Bremond A, *et al.* Results of a randomized trial of adjuvant chemotherapy with FEC 50 vs. FEC 100 in high risk node-positive breast cancer Patients. *Proceedings of the American Society of Clinical Oncology* 1998; **17**:124a [abstr].

(3) Carmo-Pereira J, Costa FO, Henriques E, *et al.* A comparison of two doses of adriamycin in primary chemotherapy of disseminated breast carcinoma. *British Journal of Cancer* 1987; **56**:471–473.

Key message

There is a significant relationship between chemotherapy dose intensity, cumulative dose, and survival in early breast cancer. Regimens given at suboptimal doses negatively impact on breast cancer survival.

Why it's important

This was the first study to prospectively confirm the retrospective observation of a dose–response relationship [36] and a threshold effect of CT in early breast cancer. It settled the controversy of the lower limit of the risk–benefit ratio, resulting in a shift in attitude and practise, with attempts made to deliver the maximal intended doses possible.

Strengths

1. This was a prospective design with large patient cohort.
2. There was stratification for factors that could have skewed the results: menopausal status, number of positive nodes, estrogen receptor status.
3. Complementary primary therapy (mastectomy or lumpectomy plus radiotherapy, both with axillary node dissection) is still the standard of care today. Adjuvant tamoxifen for estrogen receptor-positive disease was added in all groups when its benefit became apparent.

Weakness

The article does not give the proportion of patients in each arm that received tamoxifen, a factor which may have influenced outcome if there was an imbalance between the arms.

Relevance

This study provided conclusive evidence that inadequate dose intensity and total dose of adjuvant chemotherapy compromised survival, and this was subsequently confirmed by several other trials [37,38]. The development of supportive care measures have largely focused on enabling delivery of adequate dose intensity chemotherapy by alleviating some of the associated toxicities (e.g. anti-emetics, oral analgesics, and hematopoietic growth factors). Additionally, the observed dose–response relationship provided the foundation for a generation of trials of higher-than-conventional dose intensities, aimed at exploring the other side of the dose–response curve.

Paper 10

Improved outcomes from adding sequential Paclitaxel but not from escalating Doxorubicin dose in an adjuvant chemotherapy regimen for patients with node-positive primary breast cancer

Authors

Henderson IC, Berry DA, Demetri GD, *et al.*

Reference

Journal of Clinical Oncology 2003; **21**:976–978

Summary

This large adjuvant trial in node-positive breast cancer explored two questions: first, whether increasing the dose intensity and total dose of anthracyclines in classic AC (doxorubicin and cyclophosphamide) CT improved DFS and OS; and second, whether these outcomes were improved by the addition of 4 cycles of paclitaxel (T) following 4 cycles of AC. Patients were randomized to three different doses of doxorubicin, 60, 75, or 90 mg/m^2, in combination with cyclophosphamide 600 mg/m^2, followed by either 4 cycles of paclitaxel 175 mg/m^2 or no further CT. At the interim analysis, with 18 months median follow-up, significantly superior DFS and OS was observed for the patients randomized to receive paclitaxel. DFS was 86% and 90% ($p = 0.008$) in the AC and AC + T arms, respectively, while OS was 95% and 97% ($p = 0.04$), respectively. In contrast, increasing the dose intensity and cumulative dose of anthracyclines had not, during that follow-up period, improved the DFS or OS. The prolongation of CT with paclitaxel had some associated side-effects; however, these were modest in incidence and severity.

Related references

(1) Bonadonna G, Valagussa P. Dose–response effect of adjuvant chemotherapy in breast cancer. *New England Journal of Medicine* 1981; **304**:10–15.

(2) Nabholtz JM, Pienkowski T, Mackey J, *et al.* Phase III trial comparing TAC (docetaxel, doxorubicin, cyclophosphamide) with FAC (5-fluorouracil, doxorubicin, cyclophosphamide) in the adjuvant treatment of node positive breast cancer (BC) patient: interim analysis of the BCIRB 001 study. *Proceedings of the American Society of Clinical Oncology* 2001: **36a**: abstract 141.

Key message

The risk of relapse and death from node-positive breast cancer and survival can be improved beyond the benefits observed with anthracycline-based CT by the addition of several cycles of a taxane. Escalation of anthracyclines beyond the conventional dose range does not appear to impact on DFS or OS, at least not early on in follow-up.

Why it's important

Having demonstrated significant activity in metastatic breast cancer [39–41], even after resistance to anthracycline [42], taxanes hold new promise of improving outcome in the adjuvant setting. Although they have relatively good tolerability, and no long-term sequelae, several septic deaths occurred in the paclitaxel arm, suggesting that it must be used cautiously in the adjuvant setting [43]. The taxanes is the first group of new drugs, that has resulted in improved DFS and OS in early breast cancer since the introduction of CMF and anthracyclines over 15 years ago. At least one other trial, the combination of taxotere with AC (TAC) has demonstrated superiority over FAC confirming the promising role of taxanes in the adjuvant management of breast cancer [44]. Other similar trials are ongoing, and it is hoped that they will confirm these findings. Long-term follow-up is necessary to determine whether OS is maintained and whether any long term sequelae can be anticipated..

This study also confirms the findings of several other trials [18,37,38,45,46] that increasing the dose intensity of anthracyclines beyond the conventional range does not appear to improve OS. New evidence, however, suggests that dose intensity may be of some advantage in certain sub-groups, such as in women with c-*erb*-B2-positive tumors [25].

Strengths

1. This is a large randomized trial with an elegant design that allows two questions to be answered simultaneously: the value of dose-intense anthracycline, and of adding a taxane.
2. The design incorporates the two most active drug classes in breast cancer.

Weaknesses

1. Confirmatory trials are needed along with longer term follow up to determine whether the survival advantage is robust and maintained.
2. A significant confounding factor is the longer duration of therapy in patients randomized to paclitaxel. This, rather than the unique activity of a taxane, may account for a large part of the superior outcome observed for this group.
3. Subset analysis suggested that the benefit of prolonged therapy may be confined to estrogen receptor-negative tumors, an important observation that requires prospective confirmation.

Relevance

Currently the adjuvant use of taxanes is considered experimental; however, numerous adjuvant node-positive trials are incorporating taxanes. These should provide level I evidence as to their potential advantage in just a few years. If their efficacy and toxicity results are similar, improved survival in early breast cancer will be confirmed, and future adjuvant CT regimens will routinely include taxanes for high-risk disease. The next challenges will be whether taxanes should be given to lower risk patients, and how to treat metastatic breast cancer patients who received the two most active drugs in the adjuvant setting.

Paper 11

High-dose chemotherapy and autologous bone marrow support as consolidation after standard-dose adjuvant therapy for high-risk primary breast cancer

Authors

Peters WP, Ross M, Vredenburgh J, *et al.*

Reference

Journal of Clinical Oncology 1993; **11**:1132–1143

Summary

In this large single-arm phase II study of high-risk breast cancer ($\geq$ 10 nodes positive), 85 patients were treated with standard-dose CAF for 3 cycles, followed by bone marrow harvest (with or without peripheral blood stem cell collection), a fourth CAF, and finally with high-dose chemotherapy (cyclophosphamide, cisplatin, and carmustine) and autologous bone marrow support (ABMS). All estrogen receptor-positive patients received tamoxifen, and locoregional radiotherapy was added to all patients after 3 locoregional recurrences were observed. The DFS and OS rates after 2.5 years median follow-up were considered substantially superior when compared to a historical population of high-risk breast cancer patients with similar characteristics ($\geq$ 10 nodes positive, $\leq$ 56 years old) who were treated with standard-dose CMF or CAF in clinical trials. A very thorough description of treatment-related toxicity made it clear that both morbidity (especially infectious and pulmonary) and mortality were high with this high-dose regimen. Post-transplant QOL assessment suggested no long-term sequelae from the treatment.

Related references (1) Peters W, Rosner G, Vredenburgh J, *et al.* A prospective, randomized comparison of two doses of combination alkylating agents (AA) as consolidation after CAF in high-risk primary breast cancer involving ten or more axillary lymph nodes (LN): preliminary results of CALGB 9082/SWOG 9114/NCIC MA-13. *Proceedings of the American Society of Clinical Oncology* 1999; **18**:1a [abstr].

(2) The Scandinavian Breast Cancer Study Group 9401. Results from a randomized adjuvant breast cancer study with high dose chemotherapy with CTC_b supported by autologous bone marrow stem cells versus dose escalated and tailored FEC therapy. *Proceedings of the American Society of Clinical Oncology* 1999; **18**:2a [abstr].

(3) Hortobagyi GN, Buzdar AU, Theriault RL, *et al.* Randomized trial of high-dose chemotherapy and blood cell autografts for high-risk primary breast carcinoma. *Journal of the National Cancer Institute* 2000; **92**:225–233.

Key message

High-dose chemotherapy at myeloablative doses followed by Autologous bone marrow stem cell support (ABMS), may increase disease-free survival among women with extreme-risk primary breast cancer compared with that which is observed after conventional-dose CT; however, there is increased treatment-related morbidity and mortality with this strategy.

Why it's important

This was the first published trial among a proliferation of single arm and randomized trials of high dose CT with AMBS in adjuvant high-risk breast cancer. This and like trials also fueled the drive among individual patients, particularly in North America, to demand and receive high-dose chemotherapy outside the controlled setting of a trial.

Strengths

1. This was a large phase II with relatively short accrual period of 4 years.
2. The induction regimen was standard for all patients, and included anthracyclines, which are considered the most active drugs in early breast cancer management.

Weaknesses

1. Some of the historical controls received CMF while others received anthracycline-based regimens, making this an inhomogeneous comparison population.
2. Exclusion of metastatic disease prior to entry into the trial included bone marrow biopsies, which were not required in the trials from which the control population is derived, thus some control patients may have had occult metastases which would have worsened their baseline prognosis.
3. There is no description of the statistical design used to select the patient number, and no description of how many historical controls were selected for each high-dose patient or whether the baseline characteristics of the two groups (beyond selecting women with >10 nodes positive and younger than 56) were in fact similar.
4. There was no baseline QOL data obtained to enable a true comparison of QOL before and after high-dose therapy.

Relevance

High-dose CT became a major research thrust for both adjuvant and metastatic disease from the late 1980s to the present day. Unfortunately, preliminary results from large RCTs [47–54] have failed to support the promising results observed with this large phase II trial, and investigators are now divided into two camps: those who believe that high-dose CT does not improve overall survival, and those who believe that alternative strategies, such as tandem transplants and up-front high-dose CT without standard dose induction, may be more effective and deserve exploration. Current trials exploring these strategies and many now include taxanes in the induction and/or control arms. Overall, however, there is a dying enthusiasm for this strategy of therapy in the breast cancer oncology community.

Paper 12

'Classical' CMF versus a 3-weekly intravenous CMF schedule in postmenopausal patients with advanced breast cancer. An EORTC Breast Cancer Co-operative Group Phase III Trial (10808)

Authors

Englesman E, Klijn JCM, Rubens RD, *et al.*

Reference

European Journal of Cancer 1991; **27**:966–970

Summary

This trial was designed following observations that many patients had difficulty tolerating and complying with 2 weeks of oral cyclophosphamide in the classic Bonadonna CMF regimen [6] which had become a standard schedule in both the advanced and adjuvant settings. Given that this schedule was selected more or less arbitrarily, this trial investigated whether an i.v. schedule, with all 3 drugs given day 1 (C 600 mg/m^2, M 40 mg/m^2, and F 600 mg/m^2) and recycled every 3 weeks, would be better tolerated and equally efficacious. Both regimens were given as first-line CT until progressive disease (PD) or excessive toxicity. The design called for 137 eligible patients per arm (274 total) in order to demonstrate a 15% difference in response. Although 332 patients were randomized, only 233 patients were evaluable for response (78 were ineligible and further 21 not evaluable). Nevertheless, the response was significantly lower in the 3-week than in the classical regimen, 29% and 48%, respectively, $p = 0.003$ (20.2% vs. 33.5% by intention to treat). Although duration of response in responding patients was similar, time to progression (TTP) ($p < 0.001$) and OS (17 vs. 12 months, $p = 0.02$) were longer in the classic CMF group. Hematologic toxicity necessitating dose reductions was higher in the classic group; however, only 11% and 8.5% of the patients in the classic and 3-week regimens, respectively, received less than 80% of the intended doses. Dose intensity of all 3 drugs was also higher in the classic regimen (C 2800 mg/m^2 vs. 1800 mg/m^2; M 160 mg/m^2 vs. 120 mg/m^2; F 2400 mg/m^2 vs. 1800 mg/m^2, after 2 CMF-classic and 3 CMF-3-weekly cycles, respectively), which is offered as the reason for the superior outcome in the former schedule.

Related references (1)	Tannock IF, Boyd NF, DeBoer G, *et al.* A randomized trial of two dose levels of cyclophosphamide, methotrexate, and fluorouracil chemotherapy for patients with metastatic breast cancer. *Journal of Clinical Oncology* 1988; **6**:1377–1387.
(2)	Goldhirsch A, Gelber RD. Understanding chemotherapy for breast cancer. *New England Journal of Medicine* 1994; **330**:1308–1309.

Key message

CMF given on day 1 every 3 weeks is inferior to the classic Bonadonna CMF schedule because both total dose and dose density are compromised.

Why it's important

The q3wk i.v. CMF regimen had been gaining a role as an acceptable alternative to Bonadonna CMF, in order to enhance patient compliance and minimize side-effects, particularly nausea attributed to prolonged oral C. This and a similar trial [55] provided the evidence that it was in fact inferior. These results also reinforced the need to give adequate dose intensity, despite slightly higher toxicity. Despite its importance, this evidence has been largely overlooked, and the q3wk regimen is still used both in clinical practice and as a standard arm in some randomized trials. Another popular regimen for patients who do not tolerate the classic CMF regimen is a modified regimen where $600\,mg/m^2$ of cyclophosphamide is given i.v. days 1 and 8, and the rest of the schedule is unaltered. Although this is widely assumed to be equivalent, since similar dose intensity is achieved, it has never been prospectively compared to the Bonadonna regimen.

The 3-week regimen has been used in several randomized comparisons to anthracycline-containing combinations and novel cytotoxic drugs in both the adjuvant and advanced settings, calling into question whether differences in efficacy observed are due to superiority of the comparison arms over CMF, or the use of sub-standard CMF regimen.

Strengths

1. The arms were well balanced for known prognostic factors and the eligibility criteria were fairly comprehensive.
2. Dose reductions due to toxicity were uniform for both treatment groups.
3. The statistical design of the study is laid out *a priori*, although a power calculation is missing.

Weaknesses

1. There was a high rate of ineligible patients (78 of 332, 23%) and an additional 21 patients not evaluable for response, thus 30% of all enrolled patients were not evaluated for the primary endpoint.
2. QOL and compliance assessments should have been a component of the trial design, considering that the two regimens might have proven to be equivalent in terms of response, and the goal was to establish whether a less toxic, equally effective regimen existed.

Relevance

This trial adds to the literature that supports a minimum total dose and dose intensity of CT below which survival in breast cancer is compromised [35,36]. It reinforces the need to provide supportive care for the associated side-effects of treatment rather than lowering the dose or altering the chemotherapy schedule wherever possible. Particularly in metastatic disease, when the goal of therapy is palliation, dose reductions are often made to maximize QOL and minimize side-effects. This study demontrates the need to balance these, given that even in the metastatic setting, overall survival can be compromised when substandard or inferior regimens are used.

Paper 13

Phase III trial of doxorubicin, paclitaxel and the combination of doxorubicin and paclitaxel as front-line chemotherapy for metastatic breast cancer: an intergroup trial (E1193)

Authors

Sledge Jr GW, Neuberg D, Bernardo P, *et al.*

Reference

Journal of Clinical Oncology, 2003; **21**:588–592

Summary

This randomized trial compared response and survival in metastatic breast cancer patients treated with either single-agent doxorubicin, paclitaxel, or the two combined at slightly lower doses, given as first-line CT. The response rate and time to treatment failure were identical in the doxorubicin- and paclitaxel-treated patients. Although the response rate and time to treatment failure were superior in the combination arm, survival was similar in all three arms. Twenty percent and 14% of the patients who were crossed over to paclitaxel and doxorubicin, respectively, responded after having progressed with the first drug assigned. QOL appeared to be similar in all three arms, but hematologic toxicity and injections were higher in the combination arm.

Related reference (1)   Paridaens R, Biganzoli L, Bruning P, *et al.* Paclitaxel versus doxorubicin as first-line single-agent chemotherapy for metastatic breast cancer: a European Organization for Research and Treatment of Cancer randomized study with cross-over. *Journal of Clinical Oncology* 2000; **18**:724–733.

Key message

In metastatic breast cancer, first-line paclitaxel is as effective as anthracyclines, which have historically been the most active drug class in this disease. Combination chemotherapy may have an advantage in terms of earlier and better symptom control in patients with bulky symptomatic disease based on the better response rate observed, however most combinations do not enhance overall survival over single-agent CT given at adequate doses. Efficacy is still observed when a taxane is given after anthracycline failure, and vice versa (20%, 14% response, respectively), confirming that these drugs are non-cross-resistant.

Why it's important

Cardiotoxicity limits the cumulative anthracycline dose that can be given, even in responding patients. Prior to the advent of taxanes, alternative therapies were less effective. This and similar studies [40,56,57] provide evidence that taxanes offer substantial non-cross-resistant activity in metastatic breast cancer, widening the treatment options available for this stage of disease and offering the potential to prolong survival.

There has been a long-standing debate as to whether combination CT is superior to single-agent CT in the metastatic setting. Combinations are routinely used in the adjuvant setting, but thus far, most trials have failed to demonstrate a superiority for combinations in metastatic breast cancer, particularly in comparison to single-agent taxanes [39,56,58].

Strength

At the time of publication, over 80% of the enrolled patients had died, making the date mature.

Weakness

The maximum number of doxorubicin cycles allowed was eight, while paclitaxel could be continued until progression. Tthe median number of cycles actually given is not stated; if significantly different, this could impact on the results.

Relevance

Taxanes are now accepted together with anthracyclines as the most effective cytotoxic drugs in metastatic breast cancer. A recent trial has demonstrated a survival advantage to taxotere plus capecitabine over taxotere alone [59], which is promising, and re-opens the question of combination versus single sequential CT. Metastatic trials comparing the combination of doxorubicin plus T (T being either paclitaxel or docetaxel) to standard AC or AC-like combinations are reaching completion [60–62] and mature results are eagerly awaited. Based on their success in the metastatic setting, taxanes are being examined in adjuvant therapy trials to determine whether combining them with anthracyclines provides superior results compared with classic adjuvant regimens like AC and CMF [63]. Their results are eagerly anticipated.

Paper 14*

Improving the quality of life during chemotherapy for advanced breast cancer. A comparison of intermittent and continuous treatment strategies

Authors

Coates A, Gebski V, Stat M, *et al.* for the Australian–New Zealand Breast Cancer Trials Group, Clinical Oncological Society of Australia

Reference

New England Journal of Medicine 1987; **317**:1490–1495

Summary

Three hundred and eight patients with metastatic breast cancer and no previous CT for metastatic disease were randomized to either AC (50/75 mg/m^2 every 21 days) or CMF–prednisone (Bonadonna regimen [6]) for either 3 cycles or until disease progression up to 18 months. Response, OS, and QOL were compared in the 4 arms, and in the grouped intermittent vs. continuous arms. There was no significant difference in response rate (RR) between AC- and CMF-treated patients. The combined RR in the intermittent and continuous groups were 32% and 49%, respectively (*p* = 0.02). There was a non-significant trend to superior survival in the continuous group (relative risk 1.3, 95% confidence intervals 0.99–1.6). QOL was better in the continuous group of terms of physical well-being, mood, appetite, and overall as judged by both the patient and physician, and better in the intermittent group for nausea and vomiting after the first 3 months (that is, once off CT).

Related reference   **(1)**   Muss HB, Case LD, Richards F, *et al.* Interrupted versus continuous chemotherapy in patients with metastatic breast cancer. *New England Journal of Medicine* 1991; **325**:1342–1348.

Key message

Three cycles of first-line CT produce worse RR, shorter time to progression (TTP), and a trend to lower OS as compared to the same regimen given until disease progression, or for a maximum of 18 months. Symptoms consistent with anxiety and depression (in the physical well-being, mood, and appetite domains) are less prominent in the patients who receive continuous CT.

---

* See also Paper 4 in Chapter 16.

Why it's important

There are no guidelines that address how long CT for metastatic breast cancer should be given; thus various strategies are practised among clinicians: continuously until progression; for a pre-defined number of cycles, or for several cycles after best response. The suggestion made by this trial is that CT given continuously may enhance survival duration compared with CT given intermittently. However, the choice of only 3 cycles in the intermittent arm raises the possibility that this does not reflect an adequate amount of 'intermittent' therapy, given that patients who had partial responses or stable disease might have continued to respond with slightly longer therapy, and given that few clinicians would give less than 4–6 cycles of intermittent therapy in routine practise. Muss *et al.* [64] compared first-line FAC for 6 cycles to CMF-prednisone, given until progression or a maximum of 12 months, and demonstrated equivalent survival among 250 patients (19.6 and 21.1 months, respectively $p = 0.68$), despite shorter TTP in the CAF arm. The study by Ejlertsen *et al.* [65], reported longer OS for 18 vs. 6 months of CEF; however, the results are confounded because all women received continuous tamoxifen (and ovarian ablation in premenopausal women). The remaining two randomized comparisons of intermittent and continuous CT [66,67] allowed previous CT for metastatic disease, were smaller, and were negative for OS differences. A meta-analysis [68] of four of these trials reported an OS advantage for more prolonged CT ($p = 0.01$); however, given that a large negative trial was not included [64], it is difficult to be confident about this conclusion. Thus it would seem from the available evidence that the advantage of continuous over intermittent first-line CT in metastatic breast cancer would be to enhance mood, appetite, and well-being at the expense of increased nausea.

Strength

There were well-balanced patient groups, only 2 ineligible and 1 lost patient, and survival was reported when the majority of deaths (90%) had occurred such that results are unlikely to change with further follow-up.

Weaknesses

1. Only 3 CMF or AC cycles were given in the intermittent arm, which may have been an insufficient total dose of 'intermittent' therapy.
2. Fatigue, which is a common complaint among patients receiving CT, was not measured in the QOL assessments. It is not clear that the QOL instruments used had been previously validated.

Relevance

The available evidence would suggest that survival is similar when first-line CT is given intermittently or continuously for metastatic breast cancer. Thus treatment duration can be individualized according to a patient's preference and tolerance.

Paper 15*

Conventional-dose chemotherapy compared with high-dose chemotherapy plus autologous hematopoietic stem-cell transplantation for metastatic breast cancer

Authors

Stadtmauer EA, O'Neill A, Goldstein LJ, *et al.* for the Philadelphia Bone Marrow Transplantation Group

Reference

New England Journal of Medicine 2001; **342**: 1069–1076

Summary

Five hundred and fifty-three metastatic breast cancer patients with no previous CT for metastatic disease were treated with 4–6 cycles of CAF. Responders (complete [CR] or partial [PR] response) were eligible for randomization to high-dose CT (HDCT) with stem cell transplant/support (SCT) or maintenance CMF. Of 310 responders, 199 were eligible and consented to randomization. Of these, 15 were found to be ineligible; 9 others with minor protocol violations were included in the analysis (total 184:101 HDCT, 83 CMF). The design allowed detection of a doubling in median OS using HDCT, with 85% power and an α error of 0.05. Stratification was for CR vs. PR, age, visceral disease, and estrogen receptor status. Final analysis, after 114 deaths and a median of 3 years follow-up, demonstrated no differences in median overall survival (24 m, 26 m, $p = 0.14$), TTP (9.6 m, 9.0 m, $p = 0.3$), 3-year progression-free survival (PFS) (6%, 12%, $p = 0.3$) or 3-year OS (32%, 38%,) for the HDCT and CMF arms, respectively. The proportion of PRs that converted to CRs with subsequent treatment was the same in both arms. Toxicity was higher with HDCT, although this was generally short-lived; there was one toxic death.

Related references   **(1)**   Lotz JP, Curé H, Janvier M, *et al.* High-dose chemotherapy (HD-CT) with hematopoietic stem cells transplantation (HSCT) for metastatic breast cancer (MBC): results of the French protocol PEGASE 04. *Proceedings of the American Society of Clinical Oncology* 1999; **18**:43a [abstr].

          (2)   Peters WP, Jones RB, Vredenburgh J, *et al.* A large prospective, randomized trial of high-dose combination alkylating agents (CPB) with autologous cellular support (ABMS) as consolidation for patients with metastatic breast cancer achieving complete remission after intensive doxorubicin-based induction therapy (AFM). *Proceedings of the American Society of Clinical Oncology* 1996; **15**:121 [abstr].

---

*See also Paper 12 in Chapter 16.

Key message

First-line HDCT with SCT following a response to induction anthracycline-based CT does not improve TTP or OS in metastatic breast cancer.

Why it's important

Based on promising non-randomized trials, HDCT with SCT gained widespread use within and outside (particularly in North America) the clinical trial over the last 15 years. Results of randomized trials are now conclusively demonstrating minimal additional benefit of high-dose over conventional CT in patients who respond to induction CT [52–54]. In this trial, only 7% of PRs converted to CRs with further therapy (similar percentage in each arm), and the TTP was within the range seen after 4–6 cycles of first line CT for MBC, suggesting that there may be little advantage of *any* CT (conventional or HDCT) after a response has been achieved with an adequate duration of an anthracycline-based regimen. This is supported by randomized trials, which as a whole have failed to show superiority of continuous over adequate intermittent therapy [64–69].

Strengths

1. The induction regimen was anthracycline-based, which, together with more recently available taxanes, is considered the most active regimen in metastatic breast cancer.
2. The 3-year PFS of 6% and 12% means that results are mature and unlikely to change significantly with further follow-up.

Weaknesses

1. Long (7 year) enrolment period with high attrition rate from enrolment to randomization, even among responding patients.
2. There was no QOL assessment in this study.
3. The statistical design was based on a doubling of median survival, which is rather optimistic for any new therapy in the metastatic setting.

Relevance

Several trials (Belgian, Anglo-Celtic [EBDIS], NCIC [MA-16], and French [PEGASE 03]) are still open; they all give induction CT prior to HDCT. In three, only responders are randomized, while in EBDIS, all eligible patients not progressing during induction are randomized. Increasingly, the strategy of induction CT is being questioned as ineffective. Whether the enthusiasm for HDCT will collapse, or whether different strategies will be explored, including upfront HDCT without induction (a strategy designed to reduce the emergence of multi-drug resistance) and multiple cycles of HDCT (to enhance total cell kill), remains to be seen.

Paper 16

ErbB-2, p53, and efficacy of adjuvant therapy in lymph node-positive breast cancer

Authors

Thor AD, Berry DA, Budman DR, *et al.*

Reference

Journal of the National Cancer Institute 1998; **90**:1346–1360

Summary

Tumor blocks for 992 (64%) node-positive breast cancer patients enrolled in an adjuvant CALGB trial of 3 different CAF doses (CALGB 8541) were assessed for c-*erb*B-2 (HER2/*neu*) with a monoclonal antibody (CB-11; positive test ≥50% membrane staining) and a test of gene amplification. *p53* status (positive test ≥1% staining) was also assessed by immunohistochemistry (IHC). In the parent trial, OS was lower for patients in the low-dose arm. This study sought to validate the previously generated hypothesis among 397 patients [70], that for c-*erb*B-2-positive tumors, OS is improved with high-dose CAF, and thus these tumors may be uniquely sensitive to anthracycline dose intensity. An independent correlation between c-*erb*B-2 status, *p53* status, and outcome (DFS and OS) was evident when known prognostic factors were included in multivariate analysis. For all patients (sets A [hypothesis set] + B [validation set]), IHC and gene amplification for c-*erb*B-2 were well correlated. Both were independently associated with poorer DFS ($p = 0.004$) and OS ($p < 0.001$), as were the number of positive nodes, no tamoxifen use, T^m size, and *p53*-positivity ($p < 0.04$ for DFS, $p = 0.02$ for OS). Median follow-up for set A+B was 9.3 years. A test of interaction between CAF dose and c-*erb*B-2 status demonstrated significantly better DFS and OS for women with c-*erb*B-2-positive tumors treated with high- and moderate-dose CAF, while for patients with c-*erb*B-2-negative tumors, outcome was similar regardless of CAF dose (set A+B). This interaction was not significant for set B alone; however, patients with c-*erb*B-2-positive tumors and low-dose CAF in this set had significantly worse baseline prognostic factors than their counterparts in set A; when these were adjusted for, the interaction between CAF dose and c-*erb*B-2 positivity emerged. The opposite interaction was observed between *p53* status and CAF dose: patients with *p53*-negative tumors had a superior OS with high-dose CAF than those with *p53*-positive tumors. Ten-year OS for *p53*-negative, c-*erb*B-2-positive patients was 90% with high-dose and 39% with low-dose CAF ($n = 34, 33$, respectively).

Related reference **(1)** Paik S, Bryant J, Park C, *et al.* ErbB-2 and response to doxorubicin in patients with axillary lymph node-positive, hormone receptor-negative breast cancer. *Journal of the National Cancer Institute* 1998; **90**:1361–1370.

Key message

Overexpression of c-*erb*B-2, a transmembrane tyrosine kinase receptor with growth stimulatory properties, may be a marker of unique sensitivity to anthracycline dose intensity.

Why it's important

The CALGB 8541 study demonstrated that doses below what are now considered conventional are associated with inferior outcome in early breast cancer [35], while other studies have failed to show an advantage for higher-than-conventional doses [18–20]. This study, however, suggests that there may be a narrow population for which dose intensity offers a therapeutic advantage. Correlation of outcome by both c-*erb*B-2 status and dose intensity in already completed randomized trials of anthracycline and cyclophosphamide dose intensification may help to confirm this observation; prospective trials are also warranted.

Strength

Patient and disease characteristics were similar in the 3 CAF groups of this series and the parent 8541 study. Thus although only 64% of the tumor blocks were collected, the proportion and distribution of known prognostic factors were representative of the parent study.

Weakness

The distribution of some patient and tumor characteristics in set A was different than in set B, thus using B as a validation set poses some problems; tamoxifen allocation in the latter part of the trial contributed to this discrepancy.

Relevance

This and like studies mark a shift in the approach to adjuvant CT. Like the role of estrogen receptor in selecting candidates for hormone therapy, mounting evidence suggests that c-*erb*B-2, and possibly *p53*, may enable tailoring of a CT regimen to the individual tumor. Both are being investigated prospectively to confirm their predictive value. Refinement of systemic CT, not only by prognostic profile, but also by understanding a tumor's unique sensitivity to cytotoxic drugs, is being increasingly recogized as an important adjunct to improving the current cure rate of early breast cancer.

Paper 17

Final results of a randomized phase III trial comparing cyclophosphamide, epirubicin, and fluorouracil with a dose-intensified epirubicin and cyclophosphamide + filgrastim as neoadjuvant treatment in locally advanced breast cancer: an EORTC-NCIC-SAKK multicenter study

Authors

Therasse P, Mauriac L, Welnicka-Jaskiewicz M, *et al.*

Reference

Journal of Clinical Oncology 2003; **21**:843–850

Summary

This multicenter, multigroup phase III clinical trial compared PFS and OS in locally advanced (LABC) and inflammatory (IBC) breast cancer patients randomized to two epirubicin-containing regimens, one at a conventional dose (arm A, epirubicin $60\,mg/m^2$ d1,8 q28d $\times$ 6), the other at a dose that was dense and intense (arm B, epirubicin $120\,mg/m^2$ q14d $\times$ 6). After 5.5 years median follow up, there have been 277 events among 448 randomized patients. No difference in PFS was apparent. No survival advantage was seen for CEF (34 months) or EC (33.7 months), p = 0.68. Toxicity in arm B was manageable in an outpatient setting. QOL, which was reported separately [71], was inferior for arm B during the first 3 months, but by one year there were no differences.

Related reference (1)

O'Reilly SE, Gelmon KA, Tolcher AW, *et al.* Comparison of outcomes in high risk, locally advanced and inflammatory breast cancer treated with investigational high dose chemotherapy (Quartet) versus recipients of standard doxorubicin-based regimens. *Proceedings of the American Society of Clinical Oncology* 1999; **18**:85a [abstr].

Key message

Dose-intense anthracycline-based CT is well tolerated but not superior to conventional CT in locally advanced and inflammatory disease (in terms of PFS).

Why it's important

Five-year OS in LABC and IBC is 25–30% despite multimodal adjuvant therapy. Many strategies have been examined in attempt to improve these OS and PFS figures. Other trials examining dose-intense regimens have also failed to show an advantage for dose-intense CT [72]. Compared with adjuvant CT, neoadjuvant CT can enhance breast conserving surgery, but does not enhance OS [73,74]. Another randomized trial compared four strategies: locoregional radiotherapy (RT) alone, RT + hormone therapy, RT + CT, and RT with hormone and CT [75]. Similar PFS was reported in the arms that received either CT or hormone therapy, underscoring the important contribution of endocrine therapy. No arm demonstrated a clear OS advantage; however, the sample size is relatively small (363) for 4-arm comparison. Thus, improvements in OS over that achieved with conventional multimodal therapy in LABC and IBC remain elusive.

Strengths

1. This was an efficient intergroup collaboration with short accrual period and large trial size.
2. There was similar endocrine therapy (tamoxifen) in both arms.

Weaknesses

Locoregional therapy was flexible and it is not clearly stated what components were mandatory and whether the distribution of different locoregional therapies was similar in the two arms. Locoregional therapy is known to enhance outcome [76, 77] and so this may be important.

Relevance

Although this trial failed to show a benefit of dose-intense CT in LABC and IBC, it did effectively tackle a particular problem of trials which target small patient populations. In this setting, clinical trials of a size sufficient to effectively test a treatment strategy are often difficult to perform. Long accrual periods mean that modalities tested are often outdated by the time results are disseminated; smaller trials leave uncertainty about whether novel approaches are no better or just appear so due to lack of study power. Some studies have grouped locally advanced and metastatic patients together, which is an unsatisfactory solution [78]. Although meta-analyses were designed to overcome this problem, they group data from trials with different treatments and designs which weakens their conclusions, and they lend themselves to limited subset analyses. This trial was unique because participation from several different multinational cooperative groups enabled the accrual of a large number of patients with an uncommon condition in a relatively short period (448 patients, 3 years). This spirit of cooperation was embraced by the Breast International Group (BIG), created specifically to enable cooperative groups which already exist (such as in the US, Canada, Australia and New Zealand, and Europe) to join together in the execution of large clinical trials in relatively short time periods, which is critical to demonstrate small but nevertheless important improvements over current adjuvant and metastatic therapies. Multinational and multi-cooperative group collaboration represents the quickest and most efficient mechanism to propel the science forward.

References

[1] Nissen-Meyer R, Kjellgren K, Mansson B. Preliminary report from the Scandinavian Adjuvant chemotherapy Study Group. *Cancer Chemotherapy Report* 1971; **55**:561–566.

[2] Fisher B, Carbone P, Economou SG, *et al.* L-Phenylalanine mustard (L-PAM) in the management of primary breast cancer: a report of early findings. *New England Journal of Medicine* 1975; **292**:117–122.

[3] Bonadonna G, Valagussa P, Moliterni A, *et al.* Adjuvant cyclophosphamide, methotrexate, and fluorouracil in node-positive breast cancer. The results of 20 years of follow-up. *New England Journal of Medicine* 1995; **332**:901–926.

[4] Early Breast Cancer Trialists' Collaborative Group. Systemic treatment of early breast cancer by hormonal, cytotoxic, or immune therapy. *Lancet* 1992; **339**:1–15.

[5] Early Breast Cancer Trialists' Collaborative Group. Polychemotherapy for early breast cancer: an overview of the randomised trials. *Lancet* 1998; **352**:930–942.

[6] Bonadonna G, Brusamolino E, Valagussa P, *et al.* Combination chemotherapy as an adjuvant treatment in operable breast cancer. *New England Journal of Medicine* 1976; **294**:405–410.

[7] Bonadonna G, Rossi A, Valagussa P, *et al.* The CMF program for operable breast cancer with positive axillary nodes. Updated analysis on the disease-free interval, site of relapse and drug tolerance. *Cancer* 1977; **39**:2904–2915.

[8] Fisher B, Bauer M, Margolese R, *et al.* Five-year results of a randomized clinical trial comparing total mastectomy and segmental mastectomy with or without radiation in the treatment of breast cancer. *New England Journal of Medicine* 1985; **312**:665–673.

[9] Fisher B, Dignam J, Mamounas EP, *et al.* Sequential methotrexate and fluorouracil for the treatment of node-negative breast cancer patients with estrogen receptor-negative tumors: eight-year results form National Surgical Adjuvant Breast and Bowel Project (NSABP) B-13 and first report of findings from NSABP B-19 comparing methotrexate and fluorouracil with conventional cyclophosphamide, methotrexate, and fluorouracil. *Journal of Clinical Oncology* 1996; **14**:1982–1992.

[10] Fisher B, Dignam J, DeCillis DL, *et al.* The worth of chemotherapy and tamoxifen (TAM) over TAM alone in node-negative patients with estrogen-receptor (ER) positive invasive breast cancer (BC): first results from NSABP B-20. *Proceedings of the American Society of Clinical Oncology* 1997; **16**: 1a [abstr].

[11] Goldhirsch A, Glick JH, Gelber RD, Senn HJ. Highlights: international consensus panel on treatment of primary breast cancer. *Journal of the National Cancer Institute* 1998; **90**:1601–1608.

[12] Hutchins L, Green S, Ravdin P, *et al.* CMF versus CAF with and without tamoxifen in high-risk node-negative breast cancer patients and a natural history follow-up study in low-risk node-negative patients: first results of Intergroup trial INT 0102. *Proceedings of the American Society of Clinical Oncology* 1998; **17**:1a [abstr].

[13] Thomssen C, Prechtl A, Polcher M, *et al.* Interim-analysis of a randomized trial on risk-adapted adjuvant chemotherapy in node-negative breast cancer patients guided by the prognostic factors uPA and PAI-1. *Breast Cancer Research and Treatment* 1999; **57**:25 [abstr].

[14] Bonadonna G, Zambetti M, Valagussa P. Sequential or alternating doxorubicin and CMF regimens in breast cancer with more than three positive nodes. Ten-year results. *Journal of the American Medical Association* 1995; **273**:542–547.

[15] Norton L. Evolving concepts in the systemic drug therapy of breast cancer. *Seminars in Oncology* 1997; **24**(Suppl 10):3–10.

[16] Englesman E, Klijn JCM, Rubens RD, *et al.* 'Classical' CMF versus a 3-weekly intravenous CMF schedule in postmenopausal patients with advanced breast cancer. An EORT Breast Cancer Co-operative Group Phase III Trial (10808). *European Journal of Cancer* 1991; **27**:966–970.

[17] Citron M, Berry D, Cirrincione C, *et al.* Superiority of dose-dense (DD) over conventional scheduling (CS) and equivalence of sequential (SC) vs. combination adjuvant chemotherapy (CC) for node-positive breast cancer (CLAGB 9741, INT C9741). *Breast Cancer Research and Treatment* 2002; **76** (Supp 1): S32, abstract 15.

[18] Henderson IC, Berry D, Demetri G, *et al.* Improved disease-free (DFS) and overall survival (OS) from the addition of sequential paclitaxel (T) but not from the escalation of doxoru-

bicin (A) dose level in the adjuvant chemotherapy of patients (pts) with node-positive primary breast cancer (BC). *Proceedings of the American Society of Clinical Oncology* 1998; **17**:101a [abstr 390A].

[19] Fisher B, Anderson S, Wickerham DL, *et al.* Increased intensification and total dose of cyclophosphamide in a doxorubicin-cyclophosphamide regimen for the treatment of primary breast cancer: findings from National Surgical Adjuvant Breast and Bowel Project B-22. *Journal of Clinical Oncology* 1997; **15**:1858–1869.

[20] Fisher B, Anderson S, DeCillis A, *et al.* Further evaluation of intensified and increased total dose of cyclophosphamide for the treatment of primary breast cancer: findings from National Surgical Adjuvant Breast and Bowel Project B-25. *Journal of Clinical Oncology* 1999; **17**:3374–3388.

[21] Carpenter JT, Velez-Garcia E, Aron BS, *et al.* Five-year results of a randomized comparison of cyclophosphamide, doxorubicin, and fluorouracil versus cyclophosphamide, methotrexate, and fluorouracil for node-positive breast cancer. *Proceedings of the American Society of Clinical Oncology* 1994; **13**:68 [abstr].

[22] Coombes RC, Bliss JM, Wils J, *et al.* Adjuvant cyclophosphamide, methotrexate, and fluorouracil versus fluorouracil, epirubicin, and cyclophosphamide chemotherapy in premenopausal women with axillary node-positive operable breast cancer. *Journal of Clinical Oncology* 1996; **14**:35–45.

[23] Fisher B, Brown AM, Dimitrov NV, *et al.* Two months of doxorubicin-cyclophosphamide with and without interval reinduction therapy compared with six months of cyclophosphamide, methotrexate, and fluorouracil in positive-node breast cancer patients with tamoxifen-nonresponsive tumors: Results from the National Surgical Adjuvant Breast and Bowel Project B-15. *Journal of Clinical Oncology* 1990; **8**:1483–1496.

[24] Moliterni A, Bonadonna G, Valagussa P, *et al.* Cyclophosphamide, methotrexate, and fluorouracil with and without doxorubicin in the adjuvant treatment of resectable breast cancer with one to three positive axillary nodes. *Journal of Clinical Oncology* 1991; **9**:1124–1130.

[25] Thor AD, Berry DA, Budman DR, *et al.* ErbB-2, p53, and efficacy of adjuvant therapy in lymph node-positive breast cancer. *Journal of the National Cancer Institute* 1998; **90**:1346–1360.

[26] Early Breast Cancer Trialists' Collaborative Group. Ovarian Ablation in early breast cancer: overview of the randomised trials. *Lancet* 1996; **348**:1189–1196.

[27] Ejlertsen B, Dombernowsky P, Mouridsen HT, *et al.* Comparable effect of ovarian ablation and CMF chemotherapy in premenopausal hormone receptor positive breast cancer patients. *Proceedings of the American Society of Clinical Oncology* 1999; **18**:66a [abstr 248].

[28] Jakesz R, Hausmaninger H, Samonigg H, *et al.* Comparison of adjuvant therapy with tamoxifen and goserelin versus CMF in premenopausal stage I and II hormone-responsive breast cancer patients: four-year results of Austrian Breast Cancer Study Group (ABCSG). *Proceedings of the American Society of Clinical Oncology* 1999; **18**:67a [abstr 250].

[29] Davidson N, O'Neill A, Vukov A, *et al.* Effect of chemohormonal therapy in premenopausal, node positive, receptor positive breast cancer: An Eastern Cooperative Oncology Group phase III Intergroup trial. *Proceedings of the American Society of Clinical Oncology* 1999; **18**:67a [abstr 249].

[30] Goldhirsch A, Wood WC, Senn H-J, Gelber RD. International consensus panel on the treatment of primary breast cancer. *European Journal of Cancer* 1995; **31A**:1754–1759.

[31] Glick JH, Gelber RD, Goldhirsch A, Senn HJ. Adjuvant therapy of primary breast cancer. *Annals of Oncology* 1992; **3**:801–807.

[32] Adjuvant systemic therapy for women with node-positive breast cancer. The steering committee on Clinical Practice Guidelines for the care and treatment of breast cancer. *Canadian Medical Association Journal* 1998; **158**(Suppl 3):S52–64.

[33] Adjuvant systemic therapy for women with node-negative breast cancer. The steering committee on Clincal Practice Guidelines for the care and treatment of breast cancer. *Canadian Medical Association Journal* 1998; **158**(Suppl 3): S43–51.

[34] Sackett DL, Haynes RB, Guyatt GH, Tugwell P. *Clinical Epidemiology: a Basic Science for Clinical Medicine.* 2nd edn. Boston: Little, Brown, 1991.

[35] Budman DR, Berry DA, Cirrincione CT, *et al.* Dose and dose intensity as determinants of outcome in the adjuvant treatment of breast cancer. *Journal of the National Cancer Institute* 1998; **90**:1205–1211.

[36] Bonadonna G, Valagussa P. Dose–response effect of adjuvant chemotherapy in breast cancer. *New England Journal of Medicine* 1981; **304**:10–15.

[37] Fumoleau P, Kerbrat P, Romestaing P, *et al.* Randomized trial comparing six versus three cycles of epirubicin-based adjuvant chemotherapy in premenopausal, node-positive breast cancer patients; 10-year follow-up results of the French Adjuvant Study Group 01 trial. *Journal of Clinical Oncology* 2003, **21**:298–305.

[38] Bonneterre J, Roche H, Bremond A, *et al.* Results of a randomized trial of adjuvant chemotherapy with FEC 50 vs. FEC 100 in high risk node-positive breast cancer patients. *Proceedings of the American Society of Clinical Oncology* 1998; **17**:124a [abstr].

[39] Bishop JF, Dewar J, Toner GC, *et al.* Initial Paclitaxel improves outcome compared with CMFP combination chemotherapy as front-line therapy in untreated metastatic breast cancer. *Journal of Clinical Oncology* 1999; **17**:2355–2364.

[40] Paridaens R, Biganzoli L, Bruning P, *et al.* Paclitaxel versus doxorubicin as first-line single-agent chemotherapy for metastatic breast cancer: a European Organization for Research and Treatment of Cancer randomized study with cross-over. *Journal of Clinical Oncology* 2000; **18**:724–733.

[41] Piccart MJ, DiLeo A. Future perspectives of docetaxel (Taxotere) in front-line therapy. *Seminars in Oncology* 1997; **4**(suppl 10):S10–33.

[42] O'Reilly SM, Moiseyenko V, Talbot DC, *et al.* A randomized phase II study of Xeloda™ (capecitabine) vs. paclitaxel in breast cancer patients failing previous anthracycline therapy. *Proceedings of the American Society of Clinical Oncology* 1998; **17**:163a [abstr 627].

[43] Oncology Drug Advisory Committee (ODAC), a branch of the US Food and Drug Administration (FDA). Data presented to ODAC meeting in 1999, and which is also summarized in the Bristol-Myers Squibb website for Taxol (http://www.taxol.com/txpi.html). This data has not been published elsewhere.

[44] Nabholtz JM, Pienkowski T, Mackey J, *et al.* Phase III trial comparing TAC (docetaxel, doxorubicin, cyclophosphamide) with FAC (5-fluorouracil, doxorubicin, cyclophosphamide) in the adjuvant treatment of node positive breast cancer (BC) patient: interim analysis of the BCIRB 001 study. *Proceedings of the American Society of Clinical Oncology* 2001: **36a**: abstract 141.

[45] Del Mastro L, Garrone O, Sertoli MR, *et al.* A pilot study of accelerated cyclophosphamide, epirubicin and 5-fluorouracil plus granulocyte colony stimulating factor as adjuvant therapy in early breast cancer. *European Journal of Cancer* 1994; **30A**:606–610.

[46] Di Leo A, Larsimont D, Beauduin A, *et al.* CMF or anthracycline-based chemotherapy for node-positive breast cancer patients: 4 year results of a Belgian randomised clinical trial with predictive markers analysis. *Proceedings of the American Society of Clinical Oncology* 1999; **18**:69a [abstr].

[47] Hortobagyi GN, Buzdar AU, Theriault RL, *et al.* Randomized trial of high-dose chemotherapy and blood cell autografts for high-risk primary breast carcinoma. *Journal of the National Cancer Institute* 2000; **92**: 225–233.

[48] Hortobagyi GN, Buzdar AU, Theriault RL, *et al.* Randomized trial of high-dose chemotherapy and blood cell autografts for high-risk primary breast carcinoma. *Journal of the National Cancer Institute* 2000; **92**:225–233.

[49] Peters W, Rosner G, Vredenburgh J, *et al.* A prospective, randomized comparison of two doses of combination alkylating agents as cosolidation after AC in high-risk primary breast cancer involving ten or more axillary lymph nodes: Preliminary Results of CALGB 9082/SWOG 9114/NCIC MA-13. *Proceedings of the American Society of Clinical Oncology* 1999; **18**:1a [abstr].

[50] The Scandinavian Breast Cancer Study Group 9401. Results from a randomized adjuvant breast cancer study with high dose chemotherapy with CTCb supported by autologous bone marrow stem cells versus dose escalated and tailored FEC therapy. *Proceedings of the American Society of Clinical Oncology* 1999; **18**:2a [abstr].

[51] Rodenhuis S, Richel DJ, van der Wall E, *et al.* Randomised trial of high-dose chemotherapy and haemopoietic progenitor-cell support in operable breast cancer with extensive axillary lymph-node involvement. *Lancet* 1998; **352**:515–521.

[52] Stadtmauer EA, O'Neill A, Goldstein LJ, *et al.* Conventional-dose chemotherapy compared with high-dose chemotherapy plus autologous hematopoietic stem-cell transplantation for metastatic breast cancer. Philadelphia Bone Marrow Transplant Group. *New England Journal of Medicine* 2000; **342**:1069–2076.

[53] Lotz JP, Curé H, Janvier M, *et al.* High-dose chemotherapy (HD-CT) with hematopoietic stem cells transplantation (HSCT) for metastatic breast cancer (MBC): results of the French protocol PEGASE 04. *Proceedings of the American Society of Clinical Oncology* 1999; **18**:43a [abstr].

[54] Peters WP, Jones RB, Vredenburgh J, *et al.* A large, prospective, randomized trial of high-dose combination alkylating agents (CPB) with autologous cellular support (ABMS) as consolidation for patients with metastatic breast cancer achieving complete remission after intensive doxorubicin-based induction therapy (AFM). *Proceedings of the American Society of Clinical Oncology* 1999; **15**:121 [abstr 149].

[55] Tannock IF, Boyd NF, DeBoer G, *et al.* A randomised trial of two dose levels of cyclophosphamide, methotrexate, and fluorouracil chemotherapy for patients with metastatic breast cancer. *Journal of Clinical Oncology* 1988; **6**:1377–1387.

[56] Nabholtz JM, Senn HJ, Bezwoda WR, *et al.* Prospective randomized trial of docetaxel versus mitomycin plus vinblastine in patients with metastatic breast cancer progressing despite anthracycline-containing chemotherapy. *Journal of Clinical Oncology* 1999; **17**:1413–1424.

[57] Chan S, Friedrichs K, Noël D, *et al.* Prospective randomized trial of docetaxel versus doxorubicin in patients with metastatic breast cancer. *Journal of Clinical Oncology* 1999; **17**:2341–2354.

[58] Joensuu H, Holli K, Heikkinen M, *et al.* Combination chemotherapy versus single-agent therapy as first- and second-line treatment in metastatic breast cancer: a prospective randomized trial. *Journal of Clinical Oncology* 1998; **16**: 3720–3730.

[59] O'Shaugnessy J, Miles D, Vukelja S, *et al.* Superior survival with capecitabine plus docetaxel combination therapy in anthracycline-pretreated patients with advanced breast cancer: phase III trial results. *Journal of Clinical Oncology*, 2002; **20**:2812–2823.

[60] Nabholtz JM, Falkson C, Campos D, *et al.* Docetaxel and doxorubicin compared with doxorubicin and cyclophosphamide as first-line chemotherapy for metastatic breast cancer: results of a randomized, multicenter, phase III trial. *Journal of Clinical Oncology* 2003, **21**:968–975.

[61] Muller V, Bauknecht T, du Bois A, *et al.* Results of a randomized multicenter phase III trial comparing epirubicin and paclitaxel with epirubicin and cyclophosphamide as first line chemotherapy in patients with metastatic breast cancer. *Breast Cancer Research and Treatment* 1999; **57**:84 [abstr 331].

[62] Biganzoli L, Cufer T, Bruning P, *et al.* Doxorubicin and paclitaxel versus doxorubicin and cyclophosphamide as first-line chemotherapy in metastatic breast cancer: The European Organization for Research and Treatment of Cancer 10961 Multicenter Phase III Trial. *Journal of Clinical Oncology* 2002; **20**:3114–3121.

[63] Sledge GW. Adjuvant chemotherapy: shifting rules, shifting roles. In: *American Society of Clinical Oncology Education Book*, 1999: 208–210.

[64] Muss HB, Case LD, Richards F, *et al.* Interrupted versus continuous chemotherapy in patients with metastatic breast cancer. *New England Journal of Medicine* 1991; **325**:1342–1348.

[65] Eljetsen B, Pfeiffer P, Pedersen D, *et al.* Decreased efficacy of cyclophosphamide, epirubicin, and 5 fluorouracil in metastatic breast cancer when reducing treatment duration from 18 to 6 months. *European Journal of Cancer* 1993; **29A**:527–531.

[66] Gregory RK, Powles TJ, Chang JC, *et al.* A randomised trial of six versus twelve courses of chemotherapy in metastatic carcinoma of the breast. *European Journal of Cancer* 1997; **33**:2194–2197.

[67] Harris AL, Cantwell BMJ, Carmichael J, *et al.* Comparison of short-term and continuous chemotherapy (mitozantrone) for advanced breast cancer. *The Lancet* 1990; **335**:186–190.

[68] Stockler M, Wilcken N, Coates A. Chemotherapy for metastatic breast cancer – When is enough enough? *European Journal of Cancer* 1997; **33**:2147–2148.

[69] Coates A, Gebski V, Stat M, *et al.* Improving the quality of life during chemotherapy for advanced breast cancer. A comparison of intermittent and continuous treatment strategies. *New England Journal of Medicine* 1987; **317**:1490–1495.

[70] Muss HB, Thor AD, Berry DA, *et al.* c-*erb*B-2 expression and response to adjuvant therapy in women with node-positive early breast cancer. *New England Journal of Medicine* 1994; **330**:1260–1266.

[71] Therasse P, Mauriac L, Welnicka M, *et al.* The added value of the combined evaluation of clinical efficacy, quality of life and cost-effectiveness in a randomized phase III study. Results of an EORTC–NCIC–SAKK neoadjuvant trial in patients with locally advanced breast cancer (LABC). Proceedings of The European Cancer Conference 1999. *European Journal of Cancer* 1999; **35**(suppl 4):S313 [abstr 1255].

[72] O'Reilly SE, Gelmon KA, Tolcher AW, *et al.* Comparison of outcomes in high risk, locally advanced and inflammatory breast cancer treated with investigational high dose chemotherapy (Quartet) versus recipients of standard doxorubicin-based regimens. *Proceedings of the American Society of Clinical Oncology* 1999; **18**:85a [abstr 323].

[73] Mauriac L, MacGrogan G, Avril A, *et al.* Neoadjuvant chemotherapy for operable breast carcinoma larger than 3 cm: a unicentre randomized trial with a 124-month median follow-up. *Annals of Oncology* 1999; **10**:47–52.

[74] Makris A, Powles TJ, Ashley SE, *et al.* A reduction in the requirements for mastectomy in a randomized trial of neoadjuvant chemoendocrine therapy in primary breast cancer. *Annals of Oncology* 1998; **9**:1179–1184.

[75] Bartlink H, Rubens RD, van der Schueren E, Sylvester R. Hormonal therapy prolongs survival in irradiated locally advanced breast cancer: a European Organization for Research and Treatment of Cancer Randomized Phase III Trial. *Journal of Clinical Oncology* 1997; **15**:207–215.

[76] Ragaz J, Jackson SM, Le N, *et al.* Adjuvant radiotherapy and chemotherapy in node-positive premenopausal women with breast cancer. *New England Journal of Medicine* 1997; **337**:956–962.

[77] Overgaard M, Hansen PS, Overgaard J, *et al.* Postoperative radiotherapy in high-risk premenopausal women with breast cancer who receive adjuvant chemotherapy. Danish Breast Cancer Cooperative Group 82b Trial. *New England Journal of Medicine* 1997; 337(14): 949–955.

[78] Smith RE, Brown AM, Mamounas EP, *et al.* Randomized trial of 3-hour versus 24-hour infusion of high-dose paclitaxel in patients with metastatic or locally advanced breast cancer: National Surgical Adjuvant Breast and Bowel Project Protocol B-26. *Journal of Clinical Oncology* 1999; **17**:3403–3411.

CHAPTER 15

Psychosocial aspects

LESLEY FALLOWFIELD

Introduction

Psychosocial oncology is a relatively new sub-specialty of cancer; therefore the number of truly seminal papers worthy of inclusion in this series of classic papers is small compared to those in other chapters in this book. Although there have been many accounts of the psychological dysfunction experienced by women following their diagnosis and treatment in the 20th century, many of these were either anecdotal, descriptive studies, or failed to use robust assessments and scientifically sound methodology. The earliest papers tended to focus on (i) how patients responded psychologically to the radical surgery being pursued to obtain cure, (ii) attempts to establish the types of premorbid personality patterns that either predisposed women to develop cancer or influenced survival, and (iii) efforts to provide supportive interventions. Consequently, I have chosen four seminal papers that examine these three areas in a more scientific fashion; they definitely did influence practice or thinking and led to an expansion of exciting and innovative research by investigators in both the physical and social sciences.

Paper I

Psychological response to breast cancer: Effect on outcome

Authors

Greer S, Morris T, Pettingale KW

Reference

Lancet 1979; **ii**:785–787

Summary

This influential paper was the first report from a prospective longitudinal study of an initial sample of 69 women with early-stage breast cancer, examining the relationship between psychological response to diagnosis and treatment and survival. Women were assessed at 3 and 12 months postoperatively, then annually for a further 4 years. Standardized psychological tests were used to determine depression (Hamilton Rating Scale), hostility (Caine & Foulds), personality (Eysenck Personality Inventory), intelligence (Mill Hill Vocabulary Scale). Women were also interviewed 3 months postoperatively and asked about their perceptions of the seriousness of their disease, attitudes to breast cancer and how their lives had been affected. The authors grouped the psychological responses to this into four mutually exclusive categories:

- **Denial**. Women appeared to reject that they had breast cancer, exemplified by responses such as '*it wasn't serious, they took off my breast as a precaution*'. They seemed reluctant to discuss the subject but were not overtly distressed.
- **Fighting spirit**. Women were highly optimistic about their outlook and had high information needs. They showed a determination to conquer the disease '*I can fight it and defeat it*' and also showed little overt signs of emotional distress.
- **Stoic acceptance**. Women just tried to get on with their lives as usual and made few requests for further information. They were initially distressed but their stoicism reduced this over 3 months. '*I know it's cancer, but I've just got to carry on as normal*'.
- **Helplessness/hopelessness**. Women in this category seemed totally overwhelmed by the fact that they had cancer. They had constant intrusive thoughts about dying and had given up hope that anything could be done. This reaction had been present since operation. '*There is nothing that they can do—I'm finished*'.

Attrition due to cancer and non-cancer-related deaths left 57 women available for assessment at 5 years. The authors found a statistically significant association between the initial psychological responses of women at 3 months and outcomes at 5 years. Recurrence-free survival was more apparent in women who had responded with denial or fighting spirit than in those who had been classified as exhibiting stoic acceptance or helplessness/hopelessness.

Related references (1) Pettingale KW, Morris T, Greer S, Haybittle J. Mental attitude to cancer: an additional prognostic factor. *Lancet* 1985; **i**:750.

(2) Greer S, Morris T, Pettingale KW, Haybittle J. Psychological response to breast cancer and 15 year outcome. *Lancet* 1990; **i**:49–50.

(3) Watson M, Haviland JS, Greer S, Davidson J, Bliss JM. Influence of psychological response on survival in breast cancer: a population based cohort study. *Lancet* 1999; **354**:1331–1336.

Key message

The coping strategies used by women with breast cancer may influence recurrence-free survival.

Why it's important

This paper provided some of the earliest empirical evidence that psychological factors are associated with outcome in breast cancer. The report together with the 10- and 15-year follow-up publications stimulated a renewed interest in psychoneuroimmunology among psychologists, clinicians and other scientists. Unfortunately, the results were also embraced enthusiastically by the lay press and alternative therapists who extrapolated far beyond the data presented and established psychological programmes with the aim of helping patients to cure their own cancer through adoption of a fighting spirit and other dietary nostrums. (The fact that denial had an equally favourable influence on outcome seemed conveniently ignored.) The authors repeatedly expressed caution about over-interpretation of their results, which required replication in bigger studies. They also called for further psychobiological research to identify biological mechanisms mediating the psychological factors influencing outcome in cancer.

Strength

This was the first prospective study of psychological response *vis-à-vis* outcome in women with early-stage disease with long-term follow-up.

Weaknesses

1. A small sample of patients was analysed, which, with attrition over time, reduced statistical power.
2. Information about nodal status was not collected routinely in the 1970s; therefore no adjustments are made for this important prognostic variable.
3. Assessment of psychological response was made via a brief open-ended question not a psychometrically validated questionnaire.

Relevance

A reductionist biomedical model of breast cancer does not satisfactorily explain the behaviour of the disease. This paper drew attention to the need to reconstruct biomedical theoretical frameworks to include states of mind. A biopsychosocial model is needed if we are to advance our understanding of breast cancer and its treatment to take account of the complex interactions that plausibly exist between mind and body.

Paper 2

Effect of psychosocial treatment on survival of patients with metastatic breast cancer

Authors

Speigel D, Bloom JR, Kraemer HC, Gottheil E

Reference

Lancet 1989; **ii**:888–891

Summary

In this important study, Spiegel and his colleagues reported 10-year follow-up data from a prospective randomized trial of group therapy in women with metastatic breast cancer. In a previous paper (related reference 1), Spiegel *et al.* had presented results showing that a supportive group intervention that included professionally led peer group support, emotional expression, relaxation therapy and autohypnosis produced psychological benefits. The treatment group ($N = 50$) had significantly lower scores on the Profile of Mood States (POMS), fewer maladaptive coping responses and were less phobic than the control group ($N = 36$), and had less pain.

The original study was designed to examine the effects of group support on psychological well-being but 10 years post-intervention, Spiegel *et al.* examined death records to investigate the impact on disease progression and mortality. At randomization, both groups appeared reasonably well matched in terms of age, amount of previous or subsequent surgery, radiotherapy, and cytotoxic and hormonal therapy. However, there was a modest, non-significant difference in initial staging of the disease before the development of metastasis, which slightly favoured the support group patients. At 10 years, 83 patients had died and 3, from the treatment arm, were still alive. There was a statistically significant difference in mean survival favouring the intervention group: 36.6 (SD 37.6) months versus 18.9 (SD 10.8) months for the control group. The time from first reported metastasis till death was also longer in the treatment group.

Related references **(1)** Speigel D, Bloom JR, Yalom I. Group support for patients with metastatic cancer. A randomized prospective outcome study. *Archives of General Psychiatry* 1981; **38**:527–533.

(2) Fox BH. A hypothesis about Spiegel *et al.*'s 1989 paper on psychosocial intervention and breast cancer survival. *Psycho-Oncology* 1998; **7**:361–370.

(3) Spiegel D, Kraemer HC, Bloom JR. A tale of two methods of randomisation versus matching trials in clinical research. *Psycho-Oncology* 1998; **7**:371–375.

(4) Fawzy FI, Fawzy NW, Hyun CS, *et al.* Malignant melanoma. Effects of an early structured psychiatric intervention, coping, and affective state on recurrence and survival 6 years later. *Archives of General Psychiatry* 1993; **50**:681–689.

(5) Kogon MM, Biswas A, Pearl D, Carlson RW, Spiegel D. Effects of medical and psychotherapeutic treatment on the survival of women with metastatic breast cancer. *Cancer* 1997; **80**:225–230.

Key message

This study provides objective evidence that psychological interventions influence psychological well-being and may influence disease progression and survival.

Why it's important

There have been many studies demonstrating that group therapy in patients with cancer produce psychological benefits, which include better adjustment, improved mood and less pain. Spiegel *et al.*'s was the first employing a randomized prospective design, demonstrating the effects on progression and mortality. The study has been subjected to considerable criticism (see related reference 2), mainly centred on methodological concerns, the study population sampled and subsequent analyses. Most of the criticisms have been countered well by Spiegel (see related reference 3). Furthermore, of the published randomized trials examining the effect of various types of psychotherapeutic intervention on survival in cancer (see e.g. related reference 4), the majority lend further support to Spiegel's findings. Like the research by Steven Greer and colleagues described in Paper 1, Spiegel's work has been over-extrapolated by others. However, close examination of his publications reveals that he himself has always taken a cautious view of the results and been an enthusiastic supporter of major replication trials not only by his own group but by others world-wide. He emphasized that the initial study had improvements in quality of life parameters as the primary outcome variable. The survival findings were an important observation worthy of report but these observations needed to be subjected to rigorous investigation in replication studies powered with survival as an *a priori* outcome measure. Such studies are currently being undertaken.

Strengths

1. This was the first randomized trial of professionally led psychotherapeutic support groups.
2. It was a clearly described intervention based on sound psychotherapeutic concepts which could be taught to others and tested.
3. It stimulated further work by the author and others in a quest for plausible psychoendocrine and psychoneuroimmunological explanations for improved survival following psychological intervention.
4. The supportive/expressive group therapy developed and utilized in this landmark study differed from other popular approaches, where patients were encouraged to fight their cancer, and therefore assume responsibility for poor outcomes. Spiegel's approach urged patients to face the fact of their cancer and to confront the reality of death. The focus was always on living better, not longer.

Weaknesses

1. The study was not originally designed to test the impact of intervention on survival.
2. Psychotherapy might have had a positive influence on medical outcomes such as survival due to improved compliance, better nutrition, physical activity, etc. This fact was acknowledged by the authors and subsequently examined (see related reference 5). The treatment effect was found to be independent of subsequent medical care.
3. The impact of the 'charisma' of the therapist is difficult to assess and might be hard to replicate; however, a variety of leaders conducted the groups in the original trial.

Relevance

This study stimulated considerable interest in the possibility of improving not only the quality but also the quantity of patients' lives through psychological approaches. Demands that psychosocial support be incorporated as an integral part of cancer care gained added impetus. Although some have queried the sample populations, methodology and data analysis used in this and subsequent studies, a good enough case has been made from available evidence that mind–body interactions do have some influence on cancer progression. However, none of this work is likely to gain the attention of most clinicians until the complex biological pathways mediating the effects have been established.

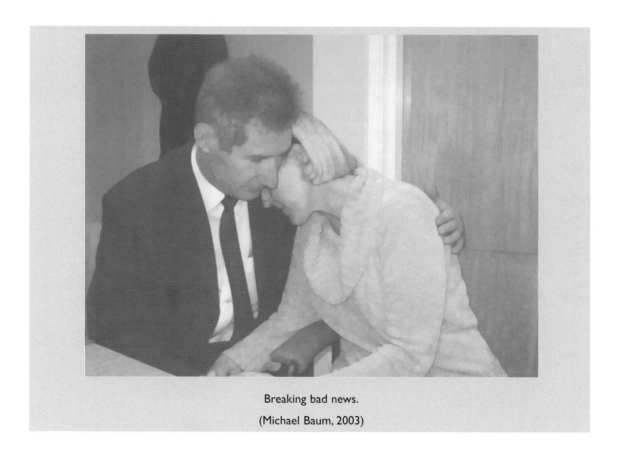

Breaking bad news.

(Michael Baum, 2003)

Paper 3

Effect of counselling on the psychiatric morbidity associated with mastectomy

Authors

Maguire P, Tait A, Brooke M, Thomas C, Sellwood R

Reference

British Medical Journal 1980; **281**:1454–1456

Summary

This seminal paper was the first properly controlled trial designed to determine the putative benefits of counselling, in particular the ability of a specialist nurse to prevent the psychiatric morbidity associated with mastectomy. Seventy-five women received counselling pre- and post-surgery and were visited by the specialist nurse at home and follow-up clinics to monitor their progress. A control group of 77 women received normal surgical unit care. Psychological morbidity was assessed by a trained interviewer using a standardized, semi-structured psychiatric interview, the Present State Examination (PSE), shortly after surgery and then at 3, 12 and 18 months later. Although the counselling failed to prevent psychiatric morbidity, regular monitoring by the nurse meant that problems were recognized and 76% of those needing psychiatric help were referred on. By contrast, only 15% of the control group who merited referral had their psychological diffculties recognized and as a result received help. At 12–18 months post-surgery, psychiatric morbidity was less in the counselled group (12%) than in the controls (39%), probably due to their referral on for appropriate help.

Related references **(1)** Watson M. *Breast Cancer in Cancer Patient Care: Psychosocial Treatment Methods*. Cambridge: Cambridge University Press, 1991: 220–237.

(2) Meyer TJ, Mark MM. Effects of psychosocial interventions with adult cancer patients; a meta analysis of randomised experiments. *Health Psychology* 1995; **14**:101–108.

(3) McArdle JM, George WD, McArdle CS, *et al.* Psychological support for patients undergoing breast cancer surgery: a randomised study. *British Medical Journal* 1996; **312**:813–816.

Key message

Women with breast cancer experience psychological dysfunction that is rarely recognized during routine clinics. The nature of this psychiatric morbidity is such that counselling alone may not be sufficient to prevent the problems, but regular monitoring by trained nurses means that patients who merit psychiatric intervention are referred on at an early stage.

Why it's important

This study reinforced findings from earlier reports that women diagnosed with breast cancer who undergo mastectomy needed specialist psychological support. It influenced calls for the appointment of specialist breast nurses and counsellors in the UK and many other countries. It also showed the importance of evaluating the efficacy of supportive interventions for women with breast cancer.

Strengths

1. This was a methodologically sound study of interventions to either prevent or ameliorate psychological problems experienced by women with breast cancer.
2. The study utilized a control group, randomization and standardized measures of social adjustment and psychiatric morbidity.

Weaknesses

1. Counselling did not prevent problems occurring, although subsequent reports and a meta-analysis have shown the efficacy of psychosocial and educational interventions, such as counselling.
2. The nature of the counselling and the level of expertise in counselling skills that specialist nurses had at this time were not fully described in the report, although it is clear that the nurses were given 3 months' training in psychological assessment and interviewing.

Relevance

Research such as this was responsible for the creation of specialist counselling posts in breast cancer units and stimulated considerable interest in the feasibility of offering different counselling interventions. Given the high prevalence of psychological and sexual dysfunction associated with breast cancer, clinicians and nurses should possess the assessment skills to recognize morbidity; if they lack expertise in treating such problems themselves then specialist referral services are needed. The primary author of the paper, Peter Maguire, pioneered the development of multidisciplinary training workshops in counselling skills. His training model has been copied and adapted by others throughout the world.

Paper 4

Effect of breast conservation on psychiatric morbidity associated with diagnosis and treatment of early breast cancer

Authors

Fallowfield LJ, Baum M, Maguire GP

Reference

British Medical Journal 1986; **293**:1331–1334

Summary

This important and controversial study was the first randomized trial designed to determine the psychological benefits of breast conserving surgery and radiotherapy compared with mastectomy. A total of 101 women with early (stage I or II) breast cancer who had expressed no strong preference for surgical treatment were randomized to either mastectomy or breast conservation. Psychiatric morbidity was assessed primarily via a standardized semi-structured interview (the Present State Examination). The mean time from operation to interview was 15.8 months (SD 7.25). According to DSM-III diagnostic criteria, 21% of the women with mastectomy had a depressive illness and 26% an anxiety state. Among the breast conservation group 27% had depression and 31% anxiety. Overall, an affective disorder of depression, anxiety or both was present in 33% of mastectomy patients and 38% of those treated with breast conserving techniques. Sexual dysfunction was also high, with 38% of previously sexually active women reporting a lack of sexual interest post-surgery.

Related references

(1) Fallowfield LJ, Hall A, Maguire GP, Baum M. Psychological outcomes of different policies in women with early breast cancer outside a clinical trial. *British Medical Journal* 1990; **301**:575–580.

(2) Fallowfield LJ, Hall A, Maguire GP, Baum M, A'Hern RP. A question of choice: results of a prospective 3-year follow-up study of women with breast cancer. *Breast* 1994; **3**:202–208.

(3) Maunsell E, Brisson J, Deschenes L. Psychological distress after initial treatment for breast cancer. *Cancer* 1992; **70**:120–125.

(4) Moyer A. Psychosocial outcomes of breast-conserving surgery versus mastectomy: a meta-analytic review. *Health Psychology* 1997; **16**:284–298.

Key message

Breast conserving surgery does not in itself protect women from psychological and sexual dysfunction. All women with breast cancer, irrespective of surgical treatment received, are at significant risk of psychiatric morbidity which is unremitting without treatment.

Why it's important

Prior to the publication of this study, there were numerous reports in both the lay and the medical press suggesting that the psychological trauma experienced by women with breast cancer was due to the mutilating effects of breast amputation and concomitant loss of body image, self-esteem and feelings of femininity. This study, with its counterintuitive results, highlighted the fact that whatever surgical treatment was offered, women still had to cope with the diagnosis of having a life-threatening disease. Following publication many other studies were conducted and most reported similar findings, that is, little evidence that breast conserving procedures conveyed any benefits in terms of protection from psychosexual dysfunction.

Strength

This was the first randomized evidence that mastectomy was not responsible for all the psychiatric morbidity seen in breast cancer.

Weaknesses

1. There were methodological problems of small sample size and retrospective design.
2. Women prepared to be randomized might not be typical of the general population of women with breast cancer.
3. If women are given choice of surgical options, the benefits of breast conservation might be more apparent. (This was explored in later studies by Fallowfield *et al.* (related references 1 and 2) and found not to be true.)
4. The study findings applied to the 1980s ,when many clinicians were less confident about the safety of breast conservation. Following results of randomized controlled trials throughout the world, women can now feel more confident that breast conservation does not compromise survival.

Relevance

This study showed how important it is to conduct scientific evaluation of seemingly intuitively reasonable assumptions about causal factors contributing to psychological distress. It showed that all women with breast cancer should have access to supportive interventions such as specialist nurse counsellors, not just those who have had a mastectomy. The research stimulated a plethora of further studies for at least 15 years examining the origins and maintaining factors for psychological morbidity following the diagnosis of breast cancer. Although effective breast conserving surgical techniques for early-stage disease were developed to improve breast cancer patients' quality of life, the overwhelming majority of studies continued to report that psychological morbidity was high: 25–30% depending on the assessments chosen. However, a more recent meta-analysis (related reference 4) which summarized the findings of 40 publications suggests that better techniques and improved specialist medical and nursing care for patients might be starting to demonstrate benefits. Mean weighted effect sizes were calculated for six psychosocial outcomes and revealed modest advantages for breast conserving surgery for psychological, marital–sexual and social adjustment, body/self-image, and cancer-related fears and concerns.

CHAPTER 16

Advanced disease and symptom control

KATHLEEN I PRITCHARD

Introduction

The request to select a small group of publications that represent classics in the area of advanced disease and symptom control of breast cancer has proved a fascinating and inspiring assignment. We are all excited by improvements in screening, diagnosis, and adjuvant therapy of breast cancer, but in day-to-day practice, we perhaps do not appreciate some of the encouraging changes that have also occurred in the management of metastatic disease.

While many other papers could have been included, I have selected publications that have changed our thinking about the management of metastatic disease and/or have provided practical advances resulting in improved tumour control, quality of life, and even survival in the metastatic setting. I was somewhat surprised to reflect on how much some of these advances have changed the day-to-day management of metastatic breast cancer, and, more importantly, the quality of life of the women who live with it.

It is also interesting to realize that, although appreciation of quality of life, better pain control, and better communication and attitudes towards patients in the 'palliative' situation have undoubtedly provided gains in the treatment of women with metastatic breast cancer, many of the most important and practical advances have been made by better approaches to tumour control.

I also chose to cite the 'ultimate classic' breast cancer publication, that of GT Beatson, not only because it opened the door to understanding the hormone-dependent biology of breast cancer but also because it led to the availability of a series of hormonal therapies that, together with the bisphosphonates, have I believe provided the greatest advances for women living with metastatic breast cancer today.

The opportunity to reflect and review the history of treatment in this area has made it both a pleasure and a challenge to write this chapter.

Paper 1*

On the treatment of inoperable cases of carcinoma of the mamma: Suggestions for a new method of treatment, with illustrative cases

Author

Beatson GT

Reference

Lancet 1896; **ii**:104–107

Summary

This delightful and pivotal paper was the first description of hormonal therapy for breast cancer. This report, which was actually presented by Beatson at the University of Edinburgh, summarizes the treatment of two women: one with locally advanced breast cancer operated on for cure following two pregnancies, who developed a local recurrence and in whom removal of the ovaries resulted in a nearly complete clinical response, and one with locally advanced breast cancer in whom oophorectomy resulted in a major partial response.

Related references

(1)   Schinzinger A. Ueber carcinoma mammae. *Verh Dtsch Ges Chir* 1889; **18**:28–29.

(2)   Huggins C, Bergenstahl DM. Inhibition of human mammary and prostatic cancer by adrenalectomy. *Cancer Research* 1952; **12**:134–141.

Key message

This was the first description of the concept of ovarian control over breast cancer based on clinical observations related to lactation made in sheep, cows and rabbits. The author then goes on to carry out experimental ovarian ablation in several patients, showing that this hormonal manoeuvre could result in major regression of disease in young premenopausal women.

---

* See also Paper 1 in Chapter 13.

Why it's important

In this fascinating if somewhat rambling report, Beatson described his construct of breast cancer. He speculated as to whether it is a disease of purely local origin or actually a blood disease with the breast tumour as the local manifestation of a blood affection. Beatson had spent time in the country caring for a man whose 'mind was affected', and while there had much leisure time. Observing lactation practices in sheep and cows in the area, he observed that secretion of milk was not affected by section of the sympathetic or of the spinal nerves, but learned that removal of the ovaries of a cow after calving would provide a continuous supply of milk. Although the concept of hormones was totally not understood at this time, Beatson reported great interest in 'one organ holding the control over the secretion of another and separate organ'. With this concept in mind, and with the permission of the patients and their husbands, he subsequently offered the experi mental treatment of ovarian removal to several women with locally recurrent and metastatic breast cancer, resulting in marked regression of the disease, which was otherwise considered incurable at that time.

What is most interesting about this paper is not only that Beatson described the concept of hormonal control of breast cancer from clinical observations in cows and sheep, but that he then carried out experimental oophorectomy, first in rabbits (for control of lactation only) and then (with informed consent) in women with otherwise incurable breast cancer.

Strength

This paper represents 'bedside to bench to bedside' research at its best. It is particularly remark-able at a time when the concept of hormones was not understood and breast cancer was considered either an infectious or a local disease.

Weakness

Beatson described only vaguely the denominator of patients from which these women were drawn. A colleague who has reviewed his original papers in the Edinburgh Library tells me that there were actually more patients who did not respond, and that overall response to ovarian ablation in this setting occurred in about one-third of the patients. Even more fascinating!

Relevance

At present, endocrine therapy for breast cancer remains the most effective and least toxic systemic treatment available for breast cancer. Beatson's paper was also key to the development of endocrine manipulations in prostate cancer, and has continued to influence the care of women with breast cancer to the present day.*

---

* See the discussion of Paper 1 in Chapter 13.

Paper 2

Evaluation of quality of life in patients receiving treatment for advanced breast cancer

Authors

Priestman TJ, Baum M

Reference

Lancet 1976; **i**:899–900

Summary

In this groundbreaking paper, Priestman and Baum introduced the use of the linear analogue self-assessment (LASA) tool to measure the subjective effects of treatment in women with advanced breast cancer. This paper introduced the concept that a simple technique could monitor the subjective benefit of treatment and compare in a readily comprehensible, convenient, and reliable way the subjective toxicities of different therapies. This paper was also one of the first to show that the subjective toxicity of cytotoxic chemotherapy (i) might not be related to patient age and (ii) actually diminished with successive courses of drugs.

Related reference   (1)

Gelber RD, Cole RF, Gelber S, Goldhirsch A. Comparing treatments using quality-adjusted survival: the Q-TwiST method. *American Statistician* 1995; **49**:161–169.

Key message

This paper was the first to show that a simple quality-of-life tool could provide reliable results that truly reflected important measures of patient well-being. It led to the introduction of routine quality-of-life measurements in many clinical trials.

Why it's important

The LASA tool and a variety of other techniques for measuring quality of life have been used since this time to compare both relatively similar (see Papers 4 and 6) and quite different (see Papers 5 and 12) types of therapeutic approaches. Furthermore, this paper helped to establish the concept that quality of life might be an even more reliable and more relevant endpoint than more 'traditional' endpoints such as response rate and duration. This has made us more aware, in the clinical setting, of the importance of balancing tumour shrinkage with patient quality of life.

Strength

This paper provided a description of a simple reliable tool for measurement of quality of life.

Weakness

It is felt by some that quality-of-life measures have not added a great deal to measurements of toxicity. Quality-of-life data are difficult to collect in trials for metastatic disease, and missing data create many problems in analysis.

Relevance

In spite of the above issues, measurement of quality of life has influenced both clinical trials research and patient care in major ways. Emphasis on the importance of quality of life has clearly produced positive results in both of these areas.

Paper 3

Anti-oestrogen therapy for breast cancer – A report on 300 patients treated with tamoxifen

Authors

Ward HWC, Arthur K, Banks AJ, *et al.*

Reference

Clinical Oncology 1978; **4**:11–17

Summary

In this often-cited paper, Ward and colleagues described tumour responses in up to 72% of cases (104 of 145), from the administration of 20 mg of tamoxifen twice daily, in women not previously treated with hormonal manipulation. Continued response of more than 2 years in 10% of cases (21of 203) was reported. Responses rates were described to be higher in women treated with 20 mg twice daily, up to 72% (104 of 145) versus 60% for 10 mg twice daily (22of 37).

Related references **(1)** Ward HWC. Anti-oestrogen therapy for breast cancer; a trial of tamoxifen at two dose levels. *British Medical Journal* 1973; **i**:3–4.

  (2) Cole MP, Jones CT, Todd IDH. A new anti-oestrogenic agent in late breast cancer. An early clinical appraisal of ICI 46,474. *British Medical Journal* 1971; **25**:270–275.

  (3) Cole MP, Jones CTA, Todd IDH. The treatment of advanced carcinoma of the breast with the anti-oestrogenic agent tamoxifen (ICI 46,474) – a series of 96 patients. *Advances in Antimicrobial and Antineoplastic Chemotherapy* 1972; **2**:529–531.

Key message

This report established substantial response rates to tamoxifen as endocrine therapy in post-menopausal women with metastatic breast cancer. It reported subset observations on dosage and on response in 2 of 6 premenopausal women.

Why it's important

This was the first major report of clinical response to tamoxifen. Expanding on an earlier report by Ward (related reference 1), it clearly established tamoxifen as a major non-toxic endocrine agent for the treatment of postmenopausal women with metastatic breast cancer and opened the door to the use of tamoxifen in premenopausal women.

Strength

This paper was a large (for its time) report of response to a single agent in metastatic breast cancer, and clearly described responses in a variety of subgroups. While not hypothesis-confirming, these subset observations were surprisingly accurate in terms of what is known today about response to tamoxifen.

Weakness

This paper mixed different response categories in a somewhat confusing fashion, although all of the data can be extracted as needed. It suggested that the dose of 40 mg daily is better than 20 mg, without any attention to whether this finding was statistically significant.

Relevance

This paper forms the basis for a huge number of trials in the metastatic and adjuvant treatment of breast cancer. Tamoxifen remains a mainstay in the treatment of women with breast cancer today, because of its efficacy and extremely low toxicity.

Paper 4*

Improving the quality of life during chemotherapy for advanced breast cancer. A comparison of intermittent and continuous treatment strategies

Authors

Coates A, Val Gebski MS, Bishop JF, *et al.* for the Australian–New Zealand Breast Cancer Trials Group, Clinical Oncological Society of Australia

Reference

New England Journal of Medicine 1987; **317**:1490–1495

Summary

This randomized trial compared continuous chemotherapy administered to the point of disease progression with intermittent therapy in which treatment was given for three cycles, stopped, and then repeated for three more cycles only when evidence of disease progression occurred. The chemotherapy in each treatment arm was doxorubicin combined with cyclophosphamide (AC) or cyclophosphamide combined with methotrexate, 5-fluourouracil, and prednisone (CMFP). Continuous therapy resulted in a significantly better response rate ($p = 0.02$), a significantly longer time to disease progression (relative risk 1.8, 95% confidence interval (CI) 1.4–2.4) and a trend toward longer survival (relative risk 1.3, 95% CI 0.99–1.6). Furthermore, quality of life, which improved significantly during the first three cycles in both treatment arms, was thereafter better with continuous therapy. Continuous therapy was associated with better scores for physical well-being, mood, and appetite, and for quality of life indices as indicated by the patient and the physician.

Related reference **(1)** Plotkin D, Waugh WJ. Hypothesis: discontinuous chemotherapy for advanced breast cancer. *American Journal of Clinical Oncology* 1983: **6**:375–379.

Key message

This study clearly showed that continuous chemotherapy, rather than treating briefly and waiting for progression before treating again, not only resulted in significantly better response and time to progression, but also improved quality of life in the metastatic setting.

Why it's important

Prior to this, it was often felt that, although chemotherapy might cause disease shrinkage or even contribute to slightly prolonged survival, it did not result in improved quality of life. This trial was therefore somewhat revolutionary in suggesting that continuing chemotherapy not only resulted in improvement of traditional endpoints, but also improved quality of life. It led to the recognition that tumour shrinkage, particularly in patients who were symptomatic from metastatic breast cancer, actually resulted in better quality of life.

---

* See also Paper 14 in Chapter 14.

Strength

This large randomized trial tested an important question and overturned previous dogma.

Weakness

The 'standard' arm in this study, namely three cycles of chemotherapy, was not really standard. A randomized trial comparing perhaps six cycles of therapy with continuous therapy might have provided a more standard control and therefore tested a more practical question. Another useful design could have been to treat to maximum tumour shrinkage and then stop, versus continuing therapy.

Relevance

Dosage of chemotherapy for metastatic disease varies in different parts of the world, even today. Because of trials such as this, however, clinicians are aware that causing tumour shrinkage in women with symptomatic metastatic disease will also clearly improve quality of life and that stopping therapy and letting the disease once again progress may not be the optimal approach.

Paper 5

A randomized trial of two dose levels of cyclophosphamide, methotrexate, and fluorouracil chemotherapy for patients with metastatic breast cancer

Authors

Tannock IF, Boyd NF, DeBoer G, *et al.*

Reference

Journal of Clinical Oncology 1988; **6**:1377–1387

Summary

In this trial, 133 women without prior chemotherapy for metastatic disease were randomly assigned to receive one of two different dose levels of CMF (cyclophosphamide, methotrexate, and 5-fluorouracil (5-FU)) administered intravenously every 3 weeks. On the high-dose arm, the prescribed doses were $600 \, mg/m^2$ of cyclophosphamide and 5-FU and $40 \, mg/m^2$ of methotrexate, with escalation if possible. Doses on the lower-dose arm were $300 \, mg/m^2$ of cyclophosphamide and 5-FU, respectively, and $20 \, mg/m^2$ of methotrexate without escalation. Patients who failed to respond to lower-dose CMF were crossed over to the higher-dose arm. Patients randomized to the higher-dose arm had longer survival (median survival 15.6 months versus 12.8 months) from initiation of chemotherapy ($p = 0.026$ by log-rank test), but the effect of dose was of borderline significance ($p \approx 0.12$) when adjusted using the Cox proportional hazard model for chance imbalance between the two arms in the time from first relapse to randomization. Response rates for patients with measurable disease were 30% (16 of 53) in the higher-dose arm and 11% (6 of 53) in the lower-dose arm. Only 1 of 37 patients responded on crossover from the lower- to the higher-dose arm. Patients experienced more vomiting, myelosuppression, conjunctivitis, and alopecia when receiving higher doses of chemotherapy. Linear analogue self-assessment scales confirmed greater toxicity in the immediate post-treatment period, but also a trend to improvement in general health and in some disease-related indices in patients receiving higher-dose chemotherapy.

Related reference   (1)   Hortobagyi GN, Bodey GP, Buzdar AU, *et al.* Evaluation of high-dose versus standard FAC chemotherapy for advanced breast cancer in protected environment units: a prospective randomized study. *Journal of Clinical Oncology* 1987; **5**:354–364.

Key message

This clinical trial demonstrated that patients randomized to higher-dose CMF chemotherapy had somewhat longer survival than those randomized to lower-dose CMF, and that tumour response and time to progression were significantly better for the higher-dose therapy. Although greater toxicity was seen in the higher-dose arm, results from at least a subset of patients suggested that more global health status measures were not adversely affected by this greater toxicity. Thus, this trial suggested greater palliation (longer survival without adverse effect on quality of life) from the use of the higher dose of chemotherapy.

Why it's important

This trial was one of the first demonstrations that higher-dose therapy was actually superior in terms of survival to lower-dose therapy, without any trade-off of lower quality of life. This paper also demonstrated overall failure (only 1 in 37) of response from crossover to higher-dose therapy after the use of lower-dose therapy.

Strength

This was a simple and original test of the role of higher- versus lower-dose standard chemotherapy in the treatment of metastatic breast cancer.

Weakness

Even the higher-dose therapy in this trial may be at the lower range of chemotherapy doses delivered in some other trials (see related reference 1). Quality-of-life data were only collected in a small subset of patients.

Relevance

This trial showed that reasonable doses of chemotherapy must be delivered to obtain optimal results – even in metastatic disease, where palliation is paramount. This hypothesis was quite controversial at the time at which this study was undertaken and published. Thus, this outcome was worthwhile and has been adopted in clinical practice.

Paper 6

Interrupted versus continuous chemotherapy in patients with metastatic breast cancer

Authors

Muss HB, Case LD, Richards F, *et al.* and the Piedmont Oncology Association

Reference

New England Journal of Medicine 1991; **325**:1342–1348

Summary

This trial registered 250 women with metastatic breast cancer to be treated with six courses of CAF (cyclophosphamide, doxorubicin, and 5-fluourouracil (5-FU)) given every 3 weeks. After completion of this induction period, women whose disease either regressed or remained stable were randomly assigned to receive either continued treatment with CMF (cyclophosphamide, methotrexate, and 5-FU) (maintenance therapy) or no further treatment (observation) followed by treatment with CMF when disease progression occurred. Of 250 women who entered the induction period, 145 were randomized. The median time to progression following randomization was 9.4 months for patients in the maintenance therapy group and 3.2 months for patients in the observation group ($p < 0.001$). After re-induction therapy, the median time to progression was 3.5 months. Thus, the median time without progression was 9.4 months versus 6.7 months in favour of the maintenance therapy group. The median length of survival from the time of initial therapy was 21.1 months for the maintenance therapy group and 19.6 months for the observation group ($p = 0.67$). Multivariate analysis showed that maintenance therapy was the most important determinant of time to progression, but was not significantly associated with prolonged survival. Performance status changes were similar in both groups, but nausea, vomiting, and mucositis were more frequent with maintenance therapy.

Related reference   **(1)**   Coates A, Gebski V, Bishop JF, *et al.* Improving the quality of life during chemotherapy for advanced breast cancer: a comparison of intermittent and continuous treatment strategies. *New England Journal of Medicine* 1987; **317**:1490–1495.

Key message

In women with metastatic breast cancer who received induction chemotherapy for 6 months, subsequent continuous chemotherapy was associated with a significant prolongation of the time to progression. Overall survival was not significantly different, however, and there were more nausea, vomiting, and mucositis in the continuous chemotherapy group.

Why it's important

This study, although published later than the study by Coates *et al.* described in Paper 4, was carried out over roughly the same time period and tested a similar question. This trial tested the question of six cycles of chemotherapy with no maintenance versus continued chemotherapy – a question that perhaps bears more relevance to standard practice than that asked by Coates and colleagues. Together with the Coates study, this trial confirmed the superiority of continued versus intermittent chemotherapy in this group of women. Both studies together, however, showed that overall survival was not significantly prolonged by the continuous approach.

Strength

This trial randomized women to a control group that represented more standard practice than did the control group in the study by Coates *et al.*

Weakness

No quality-of-life data were collected.

Relevance

This paper showed that continued chemotherapy can improve progression-free survival in metastatic disease. This trial, together with that by Coates *et al.*, helps clinicians to this day to recommend continuing or stopping chemotherapy in women with metastatic disease, based on firm data about clinical endpoints and quality of life.

Paper 7

Double-blind randomized trial of very-low-dose warfarin for prevention of thromboembolism in stage IV breast cancer

Authors

Levine MN, Hirsch J, Gent M, *et al.*

Reference

Lancet 1994; **343**:886–889

Summary

Women receiving chemotherapy for metastatic breast cancer are at high risk for thromboembolic disease, but long-term oral anticoagulation increases the risk of haemorrhagic complications. In this trial, 311 women receiving chemotherapy for metastatic breast cancer were randomly assigned to either low-dose warfarin (1 mg/daily for 6 weeks, adjusted upwards as required to maintain an international normalized ratio (INR) of 1.3–1.9) or placebo. Study treatment continued until 1 week after the end of chemotherapy. There were seven thromboembolic events (six deep-vein thromboses and one pulmonary embolism) in the placebo group and one (pulmonary embolism) in the warfarin group (a relative risk reduction of about 85%; $p = 0.031$). Major bleeding occurred in two placebo recipients and one warfarin-treated patient. There was no detectable difference in survival between the treatment groups.

Related reference   **(1)**   Pritchard KI, Paterson AHG, Paul NA, Zee B, Fine S, Pater J, and the National Cancer Institute of Canada Clinical Trials Group Breast Cancer Site Group. *Journal of Clinical Oncology* 1996; **14**:2731–2737.

Key message

The risk of thromboembolism was reduced by about 85% by the use of low-dose warfarin titrated to keep the INR at 1.3–1.9 in this group of women receiving chemotherapy for metastatic breast cancer. Haemorrhagic events were not increased with the use of this therapy.

Why it's important

Women with metastatic breast cancer have many complications related to their disease and to the therapy. Neutropenic sepsis, pathologic fractures, anaemia, and other problems reduce their quality of life. Deep vein thrombosis and pulmonary embolism are quite common. In this trial, they occurred in about 5% of women receiving chemotherapy, but in less than 1% of those treated with low-dose warfarin. Warfarin in these doses was not toxic and resulted in no increase in major haemorrhagic events.

Strengths

1. Although thromboembolism is known to be a complication in this setting, such an approach had never been previously tested.
2. This randomized trial clearly showed the benefit of low-dose warfarin.

Weakness

Other approaches to the treatment of thromboembolic disease, such as low-molecular-weight heparin, are now available. These approaches involve subcutaneous injections, however.

Relevance

For whatever reason, the results of this paper have not been widely applied in practice. On rereading this paper, one must think that there is strong benefit and little detriment to the use of low-dose warfarin in women receiving chemotherapy for metastatic breast cancer.

Papers 8 and 9

8: *Efficacy of pamidronate in reducing skeletal complications in patients with breast cancer and lytic bone metastases*

9: *Pamidronate reduces skeletal morbidity in women with advanced breast cancer and lytic bone lesions: A randomized, placebo-controlled trial*

Authors

8: Hortobagyi GN, Theriault RL, Porter L, *et al.* for the Protocol 19 Aredia Breast Cancer Study Group
9: Theriault RL, Lipton A, Hortobagyi GN, *et al.* for the Protocol 18 Aredia Breast Cancer Study Group

References

8: *New England Journal of Medicine* 1996; **335**:1785–1791
9: *Journal of Clinical Oncology* 1999; **17**:846–854

Summary

In these two trials, women with stage IV breast cancer who were receiving either cytotoxic chemotherapy (382 randomized patients) or hormonal therapy (372 randomized patients) were randomized to receive either placebo or pamidronate 90 mg as a 2-hour intravenous infusion for 12 cycles (with chemotherapy) or 24 cycles (with hormonal therapy). In both cases, the median time to the occurrence of first skeletal complications was greater in the pamidronate group than in the placebo group: 13.1 months versus 7 months ($p = 0.005$) for patients receiving chemotherapy and 10.4 months versus 6.9 months ($p = 0.049$) for patients receiving hormonal therapy. The proportion of patients in whom any skeletal complication occurred was also lower: 43% versus 56% ($p = 0.008$) with chemotherapy and 56% versus 67% ($p = 0.024$) with hormonal therapy. There was also significantly less increase in bone pain ($p = 0.046$ with chemotherapy and $p = 0.002$ with hormonal therapy) and less deterioration of performance status ($p = 0.027$ with chemotherapy) in the pamidronate group. In no instance was survival improved.

Related reference   (1)   Patterson AH, Powles TJ, Kanis JA, McCloskey E, Hanson J, Ashley S. Double-blind controlled trial of oral clodronate in patients with bone metastases from breast cancer. *Journal of Clinical Oncology* 1993; **11**:59–65.

Key message

These papers describe two large randomized studies of similar design, examining the role of pamidronate versus placebo in patients receiving either chemotherapy (Paper 8) or hormonal therapy (Paper 9). In both instances, skeletal complications were fewer and took longer to occur, bone pain was less, and deterioration of performance status was less in women receiving pamidronate.

Why they're important

Of women who develop recurrent breast cancer, 60% present with bone metastases and 80% will ultimately develop bone metastases. In the last months of life, many women with breast cancer develop serious complications related to bone metastases, including pathologic fractures and hypercalcaemia. The introduction of the bisphosphonates, by delaying or preventing these events, has truly changed the quality of life for many women with metastatic breast cancer.

Strength

These large randomized studies showed distinct differences between the pamidronate- and placebo-treated groups.

Weakness

Statistical analyses of these studies, because of the inter-related nature of the endpoints, have been problematic. Some statistical analyses were weighted by multiple endpoints in few patients rather than multiple endpoints in multiple patients. This has been considered misleading by some readers.

Relevance

The use of the bisphosphonates in metastatic disease has greatly improved quality of life for many women. The bisphosphonates are now being tested and/or used in the adjuvant setting, and may prevent or reduce metastases in bone and elsewhere.

Paper 10

Anastrozole versus megestrol acetate in the treatment of postmenopausal women with advanced breast cancer. Results of a survival update based on a combined analysis of data from two mature phase III trials

Authors

Buzdar AU, Jonat W, Howell A

Reference

Cancer 1998; **83**:1142–1152

Summary

This important paper reports on the results of a survival update based on combined data from two studies that compare the efficacy and tolerability of anastrozole 1 mg or 10 mg once daily and megestrol acetate 40 mg four times daily in the treatment of postmenopausal women with metastatic breast cancer whose disease had progressed after treatment with tamoxifen. Two randomized parallel group multicentre trials were conducted involving a total of 764 women. An overview analysis was carried out, with a median follow-up duration of 31 months.

Anastrozole 1 mg daily demonstrated a statistically significant survival advantage over megestrol acetate, with a hazard ratio of 0.78 ($p < 0.025$; 97.5% confidence interval 0.60–1.0). The 1 mg anastrozole group also had a longer median time to death (26.7 months, versus 22.5 months for the megestrol acetate group). This paper added to prior publications describing this trial in which no significant difference had been shown between overall response rate, time to progression, and percentage of patients gaining clinical benefit.

Related references **(1)** Kaufmann M, Bajetta E, Dirix LY, *et al.* Exemestane is superior to megestrol acetate after tamoxifen failure in postmenopausal women with advanced breast cancer: results of a phase III randomized double-blind trial. The Exemestane Study Group. *Journal of Clinical Oncology* 2000; **18**:1399–1411.

(2) Dombernowsky P, Smith I, Falkson G, *et al.* Letrozole, a new oral aromatase inhibitor for advanced breast cancer: double-blind randomized trial showing a dose effect and improved efficacy and tolerability compared with megestrol acetate. *Journal of Clinical Oncology* 1998: **16**:453–461.

Key message

This paper was the first to suggest that all endocrine agents for the treatment of metastatic breast cancer were not the same. It (together with related references 1 and 2) showed that aromatase inhibitors were not only less toxic but also somewhat more efficacious in the treatment of metastatic breast cancer.

Why it's important

Up to this time, all endocrine approaches to the treatment of breast cancer were believed to be roughly equivalent in terms of efficacy. Tamoxifen, for example, had replaced oestrogen as treatment for metastatic breast cancer in postmenopausal women, because it was equally effective but much less toxic. These papers were the first to suggest that different endocrine approaches – in this case aromatase inhibitors – were actually superior in terms of efficacy in the metastatic setting. This work opened the door to the concept that other endocrine approaches might be even more efficacious.

Strength

This was a large randomized study with detailed reporting of efficacy endpoints and toxicity. All endpoints were externally reviewed for consistency.

Weakness

This study included a number of patients whose oestrogen receptor (ER) and progesterone receptor (PgR) status was not known. It has become increasingly clear that all patients entered on studies of endocrine manoeuvres must have accurate ER and PgR determinations in order to most accurately explore the efficacy of these hormonal therapies.

Relevance

This study led to the examination of aromatase inhibitors versus tamoxifen in the metastatic and then the adjuvant setting. Early data from the large adjuvant ATAC (Arimidex, Tamoxifen, Alone or in Combination) trial has now shown that the aromatase inhibitor anastrozole (Arimidex) is superior to tamoxifen as adjuvant therapy in terms of disease-free survival at about 4 years of follow-up. Additional large studies comparing the other two major aromatase inhibitors (letrozole and exemestane) with tamoxifen in the adjuvant setting are underway. While more data from these studies and additional follow-up from the ATAC trial are required, the aromatase inhibitor anastrozole is now clearly established as a legitimate alternative for the treatment of postmenopausal women with endocrine-responsive disease in the adjuvant setting.

Paper 11

Multinational study of the efficacy and safety of humanized anti-HER2 monoclonal antibody in women who have HER2-overexpressing metastatic breast cancer that has progressed after chemotherapy for metastatic disease

Authors

Cobleigh MA, Vogel CL, Tripathy D, *et al.*

Reference

Journal of Clinical Oncology 1999; **17**:2639–2648

Summary

In this trial, 220 women with metastatic breast cancer that had progressed after one or two chemotherapy regimens and whose tumours overexpressed the HER2/*neu* (c-*erb*B-2) oncogene were treated with trastuzumab (Herceptin), with an objective response rate of 15% in the intent-to-treat population (95% confidence interval 11–21%). The median duration of response was 9.1 months and the median duration of survival 13 months. Side-effects included infusion-associated fever or chills, occurring usually only during the first infusion and of mild to moderate severity. Cardiac dysfunction occurred in 4.7% of patients.

Related reference   **(1)**   Slamon DJ, Leyland-Jones B, Shak S, *et al.* Use of chemotherapy plus a monoclonal antibody against HER2 for metastatic breast cancer that overexpresses HER2. *New England Journal of Medicine* 2001; **344**:783–792.

Key message

This trial showed that the recombinant humanized anti-HER2/*neu* monoclonal antibody trastuzumab administered as a single agent produced durable objective responses and was well tolerated by women with HER2-overexpressing metastatic breast cancer that had progressed after chemotherapy for metastatic disease. The common side-effects of chemotherapy such as alopecia, mucositis, and neutropenia were rarely seen.

Why it's important

This study was the first demonstration that immunotherapy of any type is effective in breast cancer. Trastuzumab, a recombinant monoclonal antibody designed to target the protein product of the HER2/*neu* oncogene, was shown to produce clearly measurable response rates in 15% of women whose tumours overexpressed the oncogene. Trastuzumab is not only the first immunotherapy to be effective in breast cancer, but also the first new type of targeted therapy for breast cancer since the development of hormonal therapy in 1896.

Strength

This well-conducted multicentre trial showed clinical efficacy of a targeted therapy developed from bedside to bench.

Weakness

The antibody that was used to measure the HER2/*neu* oncogene in this study, namely the clinical trials assay (CTA), was a polyclonal antibody that is no longer available, so the exact measurement of HER2/*neu* made in this study cannot now be duplicated. Subsequent analyses of these data have shown that better methods of measuring HER2/*neu* can select patients with closer to a 30% response rate to trastuzumab.

Relevance

Trastuzumab can be used to treat women whose tumours overexpress the HER2/*neu* oncogene in the metastatic setting. Because it has so few side-effects, trastuzumab may be the treatment of choice for some women whose tumours are HER2/*neu*-overexpressing. The combination of trastuzumab with paclitaxel also produces higher response rates than paclitaxel alone (see related reference 1). Trastuzumab is now being tested in several large randomized trials in the adjuvant setting for women whose tumours overexpress HER2/*neu*, and may prove useful there as well. The availability of this low-toxicity targeted therapy represents a step forward in the treatment of breast cancer.

Paper 12*

Conventional dose chemotherapy compared with high-dose chemotherapy plus autologous hematopoietic stem-cell transplantation for metastatic breast cancer

Authors

Stadtmauer EA, O'Neill A, Goldstein LJ, *et al.* for the Philadelphia Bone Marrow Transplant Group

Reference

New England Journal of Medicine 2000; **342**:1069–1076

Summary

This randomized trial comparing high-dose chemotherapy plus haematopoietic stem cell rescue with a prolonged course of monthly conventional-dose chemotherapy in women with metastatic breast cancer enrolled 553 patients, of whom 310 had complete or partial responses to induction chemotherapy. Of these 310 patients, 110 were randomized to high-dose therapy plus haematopoietic stem cells and 89 to conventional-dose chemotherapy. There was no difference in overall survival rate at 3 years between the two treatment groups (32% in the transplantation group and 38% in the conventional chemotherapy group). Nor was there any significant difference between the two treatments in median time to progression (9.6 months for high-dose chemotherapy plus haematopoietic stem cells and 9 months for conventional-dose chemotherapy).

Related references **(1)** Peters WP, Shpall EJ, Jones RB, *et al.* High-dose combination alkylating agents with bone marrow support as initial treatment for metastatic breast cancer. *Journal of Clinical Oncology* 1988; **6**:1368–1376.

(2) Crump M, Gluck S, Stewart D, *et al.* for the National Cancer Institute of Canada Clinical Trials Group. *Proceedings of the American Society of Clinical Oncology* 2001; **20**:21s (Abst 82).

Key message

This trial showed that high-dose chemotherapy plus autologous stem cell transplantation soon after the induction of a complete or partial remission with conventional-dose chemotherapy did not improve survival in women with metastatic breast cancer as compared with maintenance chemotherapy in conventional doses.

---

* See also Paper 15 in Chapter 14

Why it's important

Phase II trials performed in the late 1980s reported promising results for high-dose chemotherapy with autologous haematopoietic stem cell transplantation in patients with chemotherapy-responsive metastatic breast cancer. These results were perceived to be an improvement compared with historical controls. As a result, high-dose chemotherapy with autologous stem cell transplantation became widely used in the USA and in some other countries. Breast cancer became the most common indication for such transplantation in North America, despite the lack of randomized studies comparing stem cell transplantation with conventional-dose chemotherapy. This trial was one of the first (see related references 1 and 2) to show that such aggressive therapy does not improve survival in women with metastatic breast cancer, and indeed results in increased toxicity, including severe leukopenia, thrombocytopenia, anaemia, infection, diarrhoea, and vomiting, as well as one death from veno-occlusive disease of the liver.

Strength

This trial was one of the first randomized controlled trials to compare high-dose chemotherapy with autologous stem cell support versus conventional chemotherapy.

Weakness

No quality-of-life analysis was carried out.

Relevance

Following the publication of the results of this trial and the presentation of several other trials (see related references 1 and 2) showing a lack of benefit for this therapy, high-dose therapy with autologous stem cell transplantation was virtually dropped from use in the USA. Until some modification of this type of therapy is developed that can demonstrate improved progression-free and overall survival in a randomized trial and/or can be given with many fewer toxic side-effects, this therapy will not be used in women with metastatic breast cancer. This trial shows that although dosing is important in women with metastatic breast cancer, as shown by Tannock and colleagues (Paper 5), high-dose chemotherapy with stem cell support is not additionally beneficial. Thus, there must be a threshold beyond which increasing doses of chemotherapy are not additionally beneficial in this setting.

Index